This book is dedicated to Dr Dion Bell, author
and later editor of the first four editions of this
book, a gifted teacher of tropical medicine,
and an inspiration to generations of doctors
working in the tropics.

Lecture Notes
Tropical Medicine

EDITED BY

Geoff Gill
Professor of International Medicine
Liverpool School of Tropical Medicine
Liverpool, UK

Nick Beeching
Senior Lecturer in Infectious Disease
Liverpool School of Tropical Medicine
Liverpool, UK

Sixth Edition

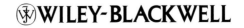
A John Wiley & Sons, Ltd., Publication

Blackwell Publishing was acquired by John Wiley & Sons in February 2007. Blackwell's publishing program has been merged with Wiley's global Scientific, Technical and Medical business to form Wiley-Blackwell.

Registered office: John Wiley & Sons Ltd, The Atrium, Southern Gate, Chichester, West Sussex, PO19 8SQ, UK

Editorial offices: 9600 Garsington Road, Oxford, OX4 2DQ, UK
              The Atrium, Southern Gate, Chichester, West Sussex, PO19 8SQ, UK
              111 River Street, Hoboken, NJ 07030-5774, USA

For details of our global editorial offices, for customer services and for information about how to apply for permission to reuse the copyright material in this book please see our website at www.wiley.com/wiley-blackwell

Library of Congress Cataloging-in-Publication Data   **1005731208**

Lecture notes. Tropical medicine. — 6th ed. / [edited by] Geoff Gill, Nick Beeching.
    p. ; cm.
    Rev. ed. of: Lecture notes on tropical medicine. 5th ed. 2004.
    Includes bibliographical references and index.
    ISBN 978-1-4051-8048-1
    1. Tropical medicine. I. Gill, Geoffrey V. II. Beeching, N. III. Lecture notes on tropical medicine.
IV. Title: Tropical medicine.
    [DNLM: 1. Tropical Medicine. WC 680 L471 2009]
RC961.L42 2009
616.9'883—dc22   2008042562

ISBN: 978-1-4051-8048-1

A catalogue record for this book is available from the British Library.

Set in 8/12 pt Stone Serif by Charon Tec Ltd (A Macmillan Company), Chennai, India
Printed in Singapore by Ho Printing Singapore Pte Ltd

1 2009

Contents

Contributors, vii
Preface, ix
List of Abbreviations, x
New Drug Names, xiii

Part 1: A General Approach to Syndromes/Symptom Complexes

1 Gastrointestinal presentations 3
2 Respiratory presentations 11
3 Neurological presentations 17
4 Febrile presentations 26
5 Dermatological presentations 32
6 The patient with anaemia 36
7 A syndromic approach to sexually transmitted infections 40
8 Splenomegaly in the tropics 49

Part 2: Major Tropical Infections

9   Malaria 55
10 Visceral leishmaniasis 73
11 Cutaneous leishmaniasis 80
12 Tuberculosis 85
13 HIV infection and disease in the tropics 101
14 Onchocerciasis, filariasis and loiasis 133
15 African trypanosomiasis 148
16 South American trypanosomiasis—Chagas' disease 155
17 Schistosomiasis 158
18 Leprosy 171

Part 3: Other Tropical Diseases

Gastrointestinal

19 Amoebiasis 185
20 Bacillary dysentery 192
21 Cholera 195
22 Giardiasis and other intestinal protozoal infections 199
23 Intestinal cestode infections (tapeworms) including cysticercosis 204
24 Soil-transmitted helminths 208
25 Viral hepatitis 215
26 Liver and intestinal flukes 226
27 Hydatid disease 229

Respiratory

28 Pneumonia 233
29 Lung flukes 241
30 Tropical pulmonary eosinophilia 244

Neurological

31 Pyogenic meningitis 246
32 Cryptococcal meningitis 254
33 Encephalitis 256
34 Acute flaccid paralysis 261
35 Spastic paralysis 264
36 Rabies 267
37 Tetanus 272

Fever

38 Brucellosis 275
39 Typhoid and paratyphoid fevers 280
40 Arboviruses 287
41 Viral haemorrhagic fevers 289
42 Dengue and yellow fever 296
43 Relapsing fevers 301
44 Rickettsial infections 304
45 Leptospirosis 306
46 Melioidosis 309

Miscellaneous

47 Tropical ulcer 311
48 Buruli ulcer 313
49 Myiasis 316
50 Cutaneous larva migrans 318
51 Scabies and lice 320
52 Strongyloidiasis 322

Contents

53 Guinea worm infection (dracunculiasis) 326

54 Histoplasmosis 328

55 Other fungal infections 330

56 Haemoglobinopathies and red cell enzymopathies 333

57 Haematinic deficiencies 338

58 Bites and stings 342

59 Non-communicable diseases 347

60 Refugee health 365

61 Syndromes of malnutrition 373

Index 380

Contributors

Imelda Bates Senior Lecturer, Liverpool School of Tropical Medicine, Pembroke Place, Liverpool L3 5QA
Chapters 6, 8, 56, 57

Nick Beeching Senior Lecturer, Liverpool School of Tropical Medicine, Pembroke Place, Liverpool L3 5QA; Clinical Lead, Tropical & Infectious Disease Unit, Royal Liverpool University Hospital, Liverpool L7 8XP
Chapters 1, 5, 18, 25, 29, 31, 38, 53

Tom Blanchard Honorary Senior Lecturer in Infection & Immunity, University of Liverpool; Honorary Fellow, Liverpool School of Tropical Medicine; Consultant in Infectious Diseases & Tropical Medicine, North Manchester General Hospital, Delaunays Rd, Manchester M8 5RB
Chapter 4

Martin Dedicoat Chief Specialist Physician, Polokwane Mankweng Hospital Complex, Polokwane, Limpopo 0700, South Africa
Chapter 13

Tom Doherty Senior Lecturer, London School of Hygiene & Tropical Medicine, London WC1E 7HT; Consultant Physician, Hospital for Tropical Diseases, Mortimer Market Centre, Capper Street, London WC1E 6AU
Chapter 61

Neil French Director, Karonga Prevention Study, Box 46, Chilumba, Malawi; Reader in Infectious Disease Epidemiology, London School of Hygiene & Tropical Medicine, London WC1E 7HT
Chapters 2, 28, 30

Geoff Gill Professor, Liverpool School of Tropical Medicine, Pembroke Place, Liverpool L3 5QA; and Honorary Consultant Physician, Aintree University Hospital, Liverpool L9 1AE
Chapters 44, 47, 49–52, 54, 59

Stephen Gordon Senior Lecturer, Liverpool School of Tropical Medicine, Pembroke Place, Liverpool L3 5QA
Chapters 2, 28, 30

Rachel Kneen Consultant Paediatric Neurologist, Alder Hey Children's NHS Foundation Trust, Alder Hey, Liverpool L12 2AP
Chapters 3, 33, 34

David Lalloo Clinical Director and Reader, Liverpool School of Tropical Medicine, Pembroke Place, Liverpool L3 5QA
Chapters 15, 16, 32, 37, 46, 55, 58

Diana Lockwood Professor, London School of Hygiene & Tropical Medicine, London WC1E 7HT; Consultant Physician and Leprologist, Hospital for Tropical Diseases, Mortimer Market Centre, Capper Street, London WC1E 6AU
Chapter 18

Alastair Miller Honorary Fellow, Liverpool School of Tropical Medicine; Consultant Physician, Tropical & Infectious Disease Unit, Royal Liverpool University Hospital, Liverpool L7 8XP
Chapter 45

Malcolm Molyneux Professor, Liverpool School of Tropical Medicine, Pembroke Place, Liverpool L3 5QA
Chapter 9

Contributors

Tim O'Dempsey Senior Lecturer, Liverpool
School of Tropical Medicine, Pembroke Place,
Liverpool L3 5QA
*Chapters 10, 11, 14, 19, 20, 22–24, 26, 27,
43, 48, 60*

Chris Parry Senior Lecturer, Department of
Medical Microbiology and Genitourinary
Medicine, University of Liverpool, Duncan
Building, Liverpool L69 3GA
Chapter 39

Paul Shears Consultant Microbiologist, Sheffield
Teaching Hospitals NHS Foundation Trust,
Sheffield S10 2JF
Chapter 21

Rebecca Sinfield Clinical Lecturer, Child and
Reproductive Health, Liverpool School of
Tropical Medicine, Pembroke Place, Liverpool
L3 5QA
Chapter 61

Tom Solomon Professor, Division of Neurological
Science, University of Liverpool, Liverpool L9 7LJ
Chapters 3, 33–36, 40–42

Bertie Squire Reader, Liverpool School of
Tropical Medicine, Pembroke Place, Liverpool
L3 5QA
Chapters 12, 17

Miriam Taegtmeyer Senior Lecturer, Liverpool
School of Tropical Medicine, Pembroke Place,
Liverpool L3 5QA
Chapters 7, 13

Maureen Wilkinson Consultant Psychiatrist,
Cheshire and Wirral Partnership NHS
Foundation Trust, Countess of Chester Health
Park, Chester CH2 1BQ
Chapter 59

Preface

The first edition of *Lecture Notes in Tropical Medicine* was published in 1981, conceived and entirely written by Dr Dion Bell of the Liverpool School of Tropical Medicine. It rapidly became a highly successful 'classic' due to its practical, authoritative and entertaining style. The next two editions continued as single author books, but by the time of the fourth edition in 1994, the spectrum of tropical disease had considerably expanded—HIV/AIDS in particular had become a major health problem. In view of this, other authors from the Liverpool School became involved to cover specific topics.

Dion Bell was one of the greatest tropical physicians and teachers of his time, and it has been a privilege for us to take over editorship of this book following his retirement and sadly his subsequent death. In the fifth edition, we continued the process of multi-authorship, though all contributors were either staff of the Liverpool School of Tropical Medicine or teachers on the Liverpool DTM&H course. We also introduced syndromic chapters on fever, splenomegaly, skin problems, etc., as well as new chapters on the emerging problems of non-communicable diseases and refugee health.

In this, the sixth edition, all chapters have been updated, and a new chapter on nutritional syndromes has been added, and a section on mental health has been included in the chapter on non-communicable diseases. We continue to use bullet points, tables and boxes, and lists of recommended reading, including websites. We say goodbye in this edition to three valued retiring authors Professor Charlie Gilks, Dr Fred Nye, and Dr George Wyatt and welcome to our team Dr Tom Doherty, Dr Rebecca Sinfield and Dr Maureen Wilkinson.

As well as continuing the style and philosophy of *Lecture Notes in Tropical Medicine* begun by Dr Dion Bell 28 years ago, we have also continued the same financial arrangements with the publishers. No author or editor of the book has ever accepted payment and all royalties are paid to the Liverpool School and used to award medical student bursaries for elective periods in the tropics.

We hope that this new edition is useful to both students and practitioners of tropical medicine. As always, we welcome any comments and criticisms.

Geoff Gill
Nick Beeching
Liverpool, UK

List of Abbreviations

AAFB acid- and alcohol-fast bacilli
Ab antibody
ABC abacavir
ACE angiotensin-converting enzyme
ACR adequate clinical response
ADLA acute dermatolymphangioadenitis
AFB acid-fast bacilli
AFL acute filarial lymphangitis
Ag antigen
AgB antigen B
AIDP acute inflammatory demyelinating polyneuropathy
AIDS acquired immune deficiency syndrome
ALA amoebic liver abscess
ALB albendazole
AMAN acute motor axonal neuropathy
APOC African Programme for Onchocerciasis Control
ARC AIDS-related complex
ARI annual risk of infection
ART antiretroviral therapy
ARV antiretroviral drug
AZT zidovudine
BB borderline leprosy
BCG bacille Calmette–Guérin
b.d. twice daily
BI bacterial index
BL borderline lepromatous leprosy
BMI body mass index
BP blood pressure
b.p.m. beats per minute
BT borderline tuberculoid leprosy
cAMP cyclic adenosine monophosphate
CATT card agglutination test for trypanosomes
CBT cognitive behaviour therapy
CCHF Crimean–Congo haemorrhagic fever
ComDT Community directed treatment with ivermectin

CFT complement fixation test
CHE complex humanitarian emergency
CHK chikungunya virus
CIATT card indirect agglutination test for trypanosomes
CL cutaneous leishmaniasis
CM cryptococcal meningitis
CMI cell-mediated immunity
CMR crude mortality rate
CMV cytomegalovirus
CNS central nervous system
COPD chronic obstructive pulmonary disease
CRP C-reactive protein
CSF cerebrospinal fluid
CT computerized tomography
CTC community based therapeutic care
CTF Colorado tick fever
CVP central venous pressure
CXR chest x-ray
DAT direct agglutination test
d4T stavudine
DCL diffuse cutaneous leishmaniasis
ddi didanosine
DD5 double diffusion test for arc 5
DEN dengue virus
DDS 4,4-diaminodiphenylsulphone
DDT dichlorodiphenyl-trichloroethane
DEC diethylcarbamazine citrate
DF dengue fever
DHF dengue haemorrhagic fever
DHFR dihydrofolate reductase
DHPS dihydropteroate synthetase
DIC disseminated intravascular coagulation
DKA diabetic ketoacidosis
DOT directly observed therapy
DOTS directly observed short course therapy
DSS dengue shock syndrome
DTH delayed-type hypersensitivity

DTM&H diploma in tropical medicine and hygiene
DTP diptheria, tetanus and pertussis
EBV Epstein–Barr virus
ECG electrocardiogram
EEE eastern equine encephalitis
EEG electroencephalography
EFV efavirenz
EIA enzyme immunoassay
EITB enzyme-linked immunoelectrotransfer blot
ELISA enzyme-linked immunoabsorbent assay
EMF endomyocardial fibrosis
ENL erythema nodosum leprosum
EPI extended programme of immunization
ERCP endoscopic retrograde cholangiopancreatography
ESR erythrocyte sedimentation rate
ETF early treatment failure
FAR fever–arthralgia–rash
FBC full blood count
FCPD fibrocalculous pancreatic diabetes
FES fasciola excretory–secretory
FEV$_1$ forced expiratory volume in 1 second
FGM female genital mutilation
FGT formol gel test
FTC emtricitabine
FUO fever of unknown origin
FVC forced vital capacity
G6PD glucose-6-phosphate dehydrogenase
GABA γ-aminobutyric acid
GAELF Global Alliance for the Elimination of Lymphatic Filariasis
GAVI Global Alliance for Vaccines and Immunization
GBS Guillain-Barré syndrome
GCS Glasgow coma score
GDP gross domestic product
GTT glucose tolerance test
HAART highly active antiretroviral therapy
HAV hepatitis A virus
HbA adult haemoglobin
HbF fetal haemoglobin
HbS sickle haemoglobin
HBeAg hepatitis B 'e' antigen
HBIg hepatitis B immunoglobulin
HBsAg hepatitis B surface antigen
HBV hepatitis B virus

HCC hepatocellular carcinoma
HCV hepatitis C virus
HDCV human diploid cell vaccine
HDV hepatitis D virus
HEV hepatitis E virus
HFRS haemorrhagic fever with renal syndrome
Hib *Haemophilus influenzae* type b
HIV human immunodeficiency virus
HLA human leucocyte antigen
HNK hyperosmolar non-ketotic coma
HPV human papilloma virus
HTLV-1 human T lymphotrophic virus type 1
HUS haemolytic uraemic syndrome
ICT immunochromatographic card test
IDP internally displaced person
IFAT indirect fluorescent antibody test
IFN interferon
Ig immunoglobulin
IGRA interferon gamma release assays
IL interleukin
i.m. intramuscular
IMAI Integrated Management of Adult Illness strategy
IMCI Integrated Management of Childhood Illness strategy
INR international normalized ratio
IPT intermittent presumptive therapy
IRD immune reconstitution disease
IRIS immune reconstitution inflammatory syndrome
i.v. intravenous
IVDU intravenous drug use
IVM ivermectin
JEV Japanese encephalitis virus
KS Kaposi's sarcoma
LACV La Crosse virus
LBRF louse-borne relapsing fever
LED light emitting diode
LF lymphatic filariasis
LL lepromatous leprosy
LP lumbar puncture
LR leishmaniasis recidivans
LRTI lower respiratory tract infection
LTF late treatment failure
MAEC minianion exchange column technique
MAT microscopic agglutination test

MCH mean corpuscular haemoglobin
MCHC mean corpuscular haemoglobin concentration
MCL mucocutaneous leishmaniasis
MCV mean corpuscular volume
MDR multidrug resistant
MDT multidrug therapy
Mf/mL microfilariae per millilitre
MHCT microhaematocrit
ML mucosal leishmaniasis
MMDM malnutrition-modulated diabetes mellitus
MOTT mycobacteria other than tuberculosis
MRDM malnutrition-related diabetes mellitus
MRI magnetic resonance imaging
MSF Médecins sans frontières
MTB *Mycobacterium tuberculosis*
MTCT mother to child transmission
MUAC mid-upper arm circumference
MVE Murray Valley encephalitis
NCD non-communicable disease
NGO non-governmental organizations
NK natural killer
NNN Novy, MacNeal and Nicolle's medium
NNRTI non nucleoside reverse transcriptase inhibitor
NRTI nucleoside reverse transcriptase inhibitor
NSAID non-steroidal anti-inflammatory drug
NTS non-typhi *Salmonella*
NVP nevirapine
OCP Onchocerciasis Control Programme
OEPA Onchocerciasis Elimination Program for the Americas
OLM ocular larva migrans
ONN o'nyong nyong virus
ORS oral rehydration solution
ORT oral rehydration therapy
OTF outpatient treatment facility
OTP outpatient therapeutic programme
PAS periodic acid–Schiff
PCECV purified primary chick embryo cell vaccine
PCP *Pneumocystis jirovecii* (formerly *P carinii*) pneumonia
PCR polymerase chain reaction
PCV packed cell volume
PDEV purified duck embryo vaccine
PE pre-erythrocytic

PEG pegylated
PI protease inhibitors
PID pelvic inflammatory disease
PF peak flow
PGL persistent generalized lymphadenopathy
PHC primary health clinic
PKDL post-kala-azar dermal leishmaniasis
PML progressive multifocal leucoencephalopathy
PMTCT prevention of mother to child transmission
PPD purified protein derivatives
PTSD post traumatic stress disorder
PUO pyrexia of unknown origin
PVCV purified vero cell vaccine
PVRV purified Vero cell vaccine
QBC quantitative buffy coat
q.d.s. four times a day
QTc corrected QT interval (electrocardiographic)
RAPLOA rapid assessment procedures for loiasis
RDT rapid diagnostic test
RIG rabies immune globulin
r.p.m. revolutions per minute
RR respiratory rate
RRV Ross River virus
RUTF ready to use therapeutic food
RVF Rift Valley fever
SACD subacute combined degeneration of the spinal cord
SAM severe acute malnutrition
SAT standard agglutination test
SFP selective feeding programme
SLE systemic lupus erythematosus
SLE St Louis encephalitis
SMB suckling mouse brain
SP sulfadoxine–pyrimethamine
STD sexually transmitted disease
STI sexually transmitted infection
TB tuberculosis
TBE tick-borne encephalitis
TBRF tick-borne relapsing fever
TCBS thiosulphate citrate bile salt sucrose
TDF tenofovir
t.d.s. three times daily
TFC therapeutic feeding centre
TIF thiomersal, iodine and formol
TNF tumour necrosis factor
TPE tropical pulmonary eosinophilia

TT tuberculoid leprosy
U&E urea and electrolytes
UFM under-fives mortality
UN United Nations
UNICEF United Nations Children's Fund
UTI urinary tract infection
VCT voluntary counselling and testing
VEE Venezuelan equine encephalitis
VHF viral haemorrhagic fever
VIMTO vascular, infectious, metabolic, tumours
    trauma and toxins, other

VL visceral leishmaniasis
VLM visceral larva migrans
W/H weight-for-height index
WBC white blood cell count
WBCT20 20-min whole blood clotting test
WHO World Health Organization
WNV West Nile virus
XDR extremely drug resistant
YF yellow fever

New Drug Names

New	Old
aciclovir	acyclovir
amoxicillin	amoxycillin
anthelmintic	antihelminthic
beclometasone	beclomethasone
chlorphenamine	chlorphenyramine
hydroxycarbamide	hydroxyurea
lidocaine	lignocaine
nonoxinol '9'	non-oxynol 9
phenobarbital	phenobarbitone
sulfamethoxazole	sulphamethoxazole
tiabendazole	thiabendazole
thioacetazone	thiacetazone

Part 1

A General Approach to Syndromes/Symptom Complexes

Chapter 1

Gastrointestinal presentations

The most important gastrointestinal presentation in the tropics is diarrhoea, and the majority of this chapter is devoted to this problem. However, other presentations of gastrointestinal disease are discussed first.

Dysphagia

Significant recent-onset dysphagia should always raise the possibility of oesophageal carcinoma. This malignancy is particularly common in certain parts of the tropics, for example, some areas of Central and East Africa. Oesophageal candidiasis (AIDS-related) is also a common cause of tropical dysphagia. In South America, the mega-oesophagus of Chagas' disease should be considered. Finally, peptic strictures, corrosive chemical ingestion and foreign bodies (fish bones especially in some areas) may also be important causes of impaired swallowing.

Haematemesis

In all areas of the world, an upper gastrointestinal haemorrhage can be caused by peptic ulceration, gastritis, oesophagitis and gastric or oesophageal carcinoma. Gastritis, gastric erosions and gastric

Lecture Notes: Tropical Medicine, 6th edition.
By G.V. Gill and N.J. Beeching. Published 2009 by
Blackwell Publishing, ISBN: 978-1-4051-8048-1.

ulcers may be drug related, for example, corticosteroids and non-steroidal anti-inflammatory drugs (NSAIDs). *Helicobacter pylori* is recognized globally as a major cause of gastric and duodenal inflammation and/or ulceration. Oesophageal varices may be a particularly common cause of haematemesis in many tropical areas—at least 25% of all cases in some series. The underlying liver disease can be the late result of chronic viral hepatitis or schistosomal hepatic fibrosis.

Abdominal pain

In 'western' populations, severe abdominal pain can result from appendicitis, mesenteric adenitis, perforated peptic ulcers, biliary colic, cholecystitis and intestinal obstruction (commonly because of adhesions or malignancy). This list is far from exhaustive, but serves to demonstrate that the spectrum of causes in the tropics is much wider. The following 'exotic' causes of acute severe abdominal pain may need to be considered.
- Abdominal tuberculosis (TB)
- Typhoid (including typhoid perforation)
- Hydatid cyst rupture
- Amoebic colitis (including perforation)
- Amoebic liver abscess (which may rupture)
- Intestinal obstruction caused by *Ascaris lumbricoides*
- Ectopic ascariasis (e.g. biliary and/or pancreatic obstruction)

3

- Sickle cell crisis
- Splenic rupture
- Hyperinfection syndrome of strongyloidiasis.

Malabsorption

Malabsorption can be a feature of infection with *Giardia lamblia*, *Strongyloides stercoralis*, intestinal TB, as well as AIDS. Perhaps the most common cause, however, is the temporary lactase-deficient situation that may occur after any significant acute infective diarrhoeal illness. Milk and milk products may need to be avoided, although yoghurt is usually tolerated, because of its high bacterial lactase content.

Tropical sprue

A particularly well-described form of tropical malabsorption is 'tropical sprue'. This occurs predominantly in India and South East Asia, as well as in the Caribbean and Central America. Patients develop non-bloody diarrhoea (sometimes steatorrhoea) often with abdominal bloating and significant weight loss. There may be a history of initial acute diarrhoeal illness, which is thought to be the precipitant (although the exact mechanism is unknown). Duodenal biopsy, as well as biochemical features of malabsorption, typically shows partial villous atrophy. The illness can be prolonged and debilitating. Traditional treatment with tetracycline (for associated bacterial small bowel overgrowth) and folic acid is often highly effective.

Diarrhoea

Diarrhoeal illness is one of the most important causes of morbidity and mortality in the tropics, causing over six million deaths per year, and is clearly linked with poor hygiene and contamination of water and food. A wide variety of viral, bacterial and parasitic pathogens have been implicated in the pathogenesis of diarrhoea, but it is impossible and unnecessary to test for all these in individual cases. Systematic review of epidemiological, clinical and host factors usually enables a sensible working aetiological diagnosis to be established. The working diagnosis can be used to decide whether specific investigation should be performed, or to direct empirical antimicrobial therapy in the minority of cases in which it is required. The mainstay of management of diarrhoeal illness is the assessment and maintenance of adequate hydration and electrolyte balance, irrespective of the aetiology, as well as the introduction of control measures in an epidemic setting to prevent further cases.

History

It is essential to establish that both the doctor and the patient are talking about the same thing, especially if interpreters are being used to take the clinical history. A useful working definition of diarrhoea is the passage of three or more loose or watery bowel motions in 24h. The distinction between soft and loose diarrhoea is more difficult, but bowel motions can be described as diarrhoeal, when they assume the shape of the collecting container. This definition works with acute diarrhoeal illness but is less satisfactory with chronic diarrhoeal illness related to malabsorption in which bulky, sticky soft bowel motions are abnormal but may not be fluid enough to move around in the container. Key features in the history are the presence or absence of visible blood in the stool (dysentery), the presence and degree of abdominal pain, the presence of tenesmus and the presence of fever. The duration of illness is important—chronic diarrhoea can usefully be defined as diarrhoea lasting more than 14 days, although a more precise definition (especially in the context of an immunocompromised host) is the passage of three or more loose or watery stools a day for 28 days or more.

In the historical assessment of fluid balance, the volume and frequency of faecal loss should be estimated together with the frequency and approximate volume of any vomiting. The amount of fluid intake should be checked, as should the frequency of urinary output during the last 24h.

The epidemiological setting is important. Illness in close family contacts should be ascertained, and enquiry should be made about whether the patient has attended any functions or eaten unusual foods in the preceding 48–72h. If so, have any other guests had similar illness? Point source outbreaks can be caused by toxin-mediated food poisoning in which case vomiting is often a predominant feature and incubation periods are usually shorter than 24 h. This may be difficult to distinguish from outbreaks of norovirus infection in which vomiting is a predominant feature and contacts are readily infected. Unusual systemic pathogens (e.g. anthrax of the gut) or non-infectious poisoning caused by adulterated or contaminated food products must always be considered. Bacterial pathogens causing small or large bowel diarrhoea usually have intermediate incubation periods of 12–72 h. More detailed food histories are not otherwise very helpful, except in the case of expatriates who have unwisely overindulged in very spicy foods ('tasting the chilli twice') or who have recently arrived in the tropics (traveller's diarrhoea). Diarrhoea developing in patients who are already hospitalized suggests a nosocomial or antibiotic-associated cause, while outbreaks of diarrhoeal illness in a refugee or camp setting imply specific infections such as shigellosis or cholera (see later) (Fig. 1.1).

Other illness

Diarrhoea can be a prominent feature of many systemic illnesses, including malaria, pneumonia and enteric fever, especially in children, and evaluation of the patient should exclude these as potential causes. Surgical and other intra-abdominal conditions may mimic gastroenteritis, as can inflammatory bowel disease. In older or immobile patients,

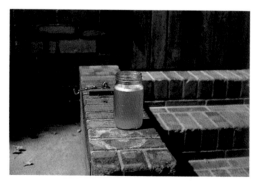

Figure 1.1 Though it looks like urine, this is the 'ricewater' stool from a patient with cholera.

constipation with overflow diarrhoea must be excluded. Alcohol and drugs frequently cause diarrhoea with or without nausea and vomiting.

Host factors

Conditions that cause hypochlorhydria (e.g. gastric surgery, H_2 antagonists and proton pump inhibitors) reduce the gastric acid barrier to many bacterial pathogens, so a smaller infective dose is required. Patients with established cardiovascular or renal disease are less likely to tolerate dehydration, as are those on diuretics and patients with poorly controlled diabetes. Pre-existing large bowel problems such as inflammatory bowel disease predispose to complications of dysenteric infections such as toxic megacolon, signs of which may be partly masked by concurrent steroid therapy. Bowel tumours can produce diarrhoea with or without blood or weight loss. Small bowel problems, including lymphoma, can cause prolonged diarrhoea. Immunosuppression of the patient, particularly by HIV, predisposes to increased invasiveness (local and systemic) of bacterial pathogens such as non-typhoidal *Salmonella*, increased recurrence of such pathogens and chronic diarrhoea caused by a variety of protozoa.

Examination

General examination must include assessment of the state of hydration. This is more difficult to quantify clinically in adults than in children, but key features are summarized in Table 1.1. Measurement of any postural drop in blood pressure (BP) is particularly useful. Rectal examination should be performed, except in obvious cases of cholera, and is particularly important in older patients who are more likely to have non-infectious bowel problems. Systemic causes of diarrhoea and signs of immunosuppression (e.g. zoster scars and oral candidiasis) should be sought out.

Clinical syndromes of diarrhoea

Apart from acute toxin-mediated food poisoning, diarrhoeal illness can be broadly classified into small bowel secretory diarrhoea, small

Table 1.1 Clinical classification of severity of dehydration in adults

	Mild	Moderate	Severe
Subjective			
General state	Alert, active, up and about	Weak, lethargic, able to sit and walk	Dull, inactive, unable to sit or walk
Ability to perform daily activities	Able to perform daily activities without difficulty	Able to perform daily activities with some difficulty, for example, stays away from work and needs support	Unable to perform daily activities, stays in bed or needs hospitalization
Thirst	Not increased	Increased thirst	Feels very thirsty
Objective			
Pulse	Normal	Tachycardia	Tachycardia
Blood pressure	Normal	Normal or decrease, 10–20 mmHg systolic	Decrease >20 mm Hg systolic
Postural hypotension	No	Yes or no	Yes
Jugular venous pressure	Normal	Normal or slightly flat	Flat
Dry mucosa (mouth, tongue)	No	Slight	Severe
Skin turgor	Good	Fair	Poor
Sunken eye balls	No	Minimal	Sunken
Body weight loss	<5%	5–10%	>10%

Table 1.2 Clinical features of inflammatory and non-inflammatory diarrhoea

Non-inflammatory	Inflammatory
Symptoms	
Nausea, vomiting; abdominal pain and fever not major features	Abdominal pain, tenesmus, fever
Stool	
Voluminous, watery	Frequent, small volume; blood-stained, pus cells present, mucus
Site	
Proximal small intestine	Distal ileum, colon
Mechanism	
Osmotic or secretory	Invasion of enterocytes leading to mucosal cell death and inflammatory response

bowel malabsorption and large bowel inflammatory diarrhoea. Each of these groups may be acute or chronic, and there is considerable overlap (Table 1.2).

Small bowel secretory diarrhoea is exemplified by cholera and non-invasive *Escherichia coli* infections in which toxins specifically promote secretion of water and electrolytes into the bowel lumen and inhibit their reabsorption. Such secretion can be competitively overcome by a steady intake of balanced electrolyte solutions containing adequate amounts of glucose but not too much to produce an osmotic diarrhoea. This is the scientific basis for the success of oral rehydration therapy in which the correct quantities of salts and glucose are added to sterile water for rehydration.

Table 1.3 Pathogens in inflammatory and non-inflammatory diarrhoea

Inflammatory	Non-inflammatory
Viruses	
Nil	Rotavirus
	Adenovirus 40/41
	Astrovirus
	Norovirus (Norwalk agent)
	Calicivirus
	Small round structureless virus
	Coronavirus
	Torovirus
	Bredavirus
	Picobirnavirus
Bacteria	
Enteroinvasive *Escherichia coli* (EIEC)	Enterotoxigenic *E. coli* (ETEC)
Enterohaemorrhagic *E. coli* (EHEC), for example, 0157	Enteropathogenic *E. coli* (EPEC)
Enteroaggregative *E. coli* (EAggEC)	*Vibrio cholerae*
Aeromonas hydrophila	*Vibrio parahaemolyticus*
Campylobacter spp.	*Campylobacter* spp.
Salmonella spp.	*Salmonella* spp.
Shigella spp.	*Plesiomonas shigelloides*
Yersinia enterocolitica	*Bacillus cereus*
Clostridium difficile	*Clostridium perfringens*
Protozoa	
Entamoeba histolytica	*Cryptosporidium* spp.
Balantidium coli	*Giardia intestinalis*
	Cyclospora cayetanensis
	Isospora belli
	Microsporidia (e.g. *Enterocytozoon bieneusi*)
Helminths	
Schistosoma spp.	*Strongyloides stercoralis*

Malabsorption is a common complication of infectious diarrhoea in the tropics, as many races have relatively low disaccharidase activity in the small bowel enterocytes. Disruption of 'normal' bowel activity readily leads to failure to break down sugars and a moderately prolonged lactose intolerance. This is particularly common after infections that cause flattening of the small bowel mucosa (such as giardiasis and cryptosporidiosis). Large bowel diarrhoea is usually caused by direct invasion of the bowel by pathogens such as *Entamoeba histolytica*, bacteria such as *Campylobacter* species or *Clostridium difficile* after antibiotic therapy. Other parasites such as *Schistosoma mansoni* can also cause prolonged large bowel diarrhoea. In heavy *Trichuris trichiura* infections, oedema of the rectal mucosa together with continued efforts to defaecate resulting from tenesmus can lead to rectal prolapse. A summary of the major pathogens in inflammatory and non-inflammatory diarrhoea is shown in Table 1.3.

Investigations

A useful algorithmic approach to individual patient diagnosis and management is shown in Figure 1.2. In most tropical settings, microbiological investigation proves impossible or very

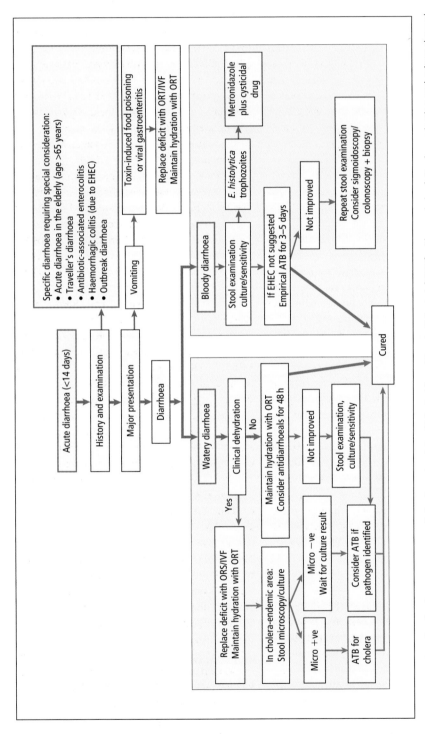

Figure 1.2 Algorithm for the management of diarrhoea in adults. (Adapted from Manatsathit et al. [2002] with permission.) Stool examination and culture depend on local availability, affordability and practice. In suspected cholera, dark field microscopy is ideal (or, if not available, a search for 'shooting star' bacteria on light microscopy will do). In epidemic situations, a clinical diagnosis is sufficient. When antibiotics are used, the choice depends either on culture and sensitivity results or on local experience. If available, ciprofloxacin is a good choice except in Asia where resistant campylobacter responds better to azithromycin. ATB, antibiotic; EHEC, enterohaemorrhagic *Escherichia coli*; IVF, intravenous fluids; ORT, oral rehydration therapy.

limited. Microscopic inspection of faeces for leuco-cytes, suggestive of invasive pathogens in the large bowel, is commonly advocated but is of question-able time-effectiveness compared with macro-scopic inspection of faeces for blood (and smell) when resources are limited. However, cholera vibrios may be observed with their characteristic 'shooting star' motility even without dark ground facilities, and this is very useful when culture is not available. Investigations for faecal parasites should be limited to specific settings (e.g. chronic diarrhoea complicating HIV) and are almost never indicated in nosocomial diarrhoea. Fresh stool microscopy for active trophozoites should only be requested when amoebic dysentery is truly sus-pected. Blanket requests for faecal microscopy for 'ova, cysts and parasites' on all patients are a waste of time in most settings. Such requesting patterns overload laboratories, demoralize their staff and lead to reports of questionable quality with little effect on clinical management decisions.

In an outbreak setting, full microbiological identification of the pathogen and assessment of the antimicrobial resistance patterns are very helpful, and it should be pursued even if outside assistance is required. In sporadic cases, detailed microbiological tests may be inappropriate, but clinicians need to be aware of the local antibi-otic sensitivities of organisms such as *Shigella*, *Salmonella* and *Campylobacter* if they are to use empirical antimicrobial therapy in a responsible and effective manner. Other investigations, such as serum electrolytes, peripheral white cell count and blood cultures, are performed in a hospital setting but again may not be available routinely.

Management

Detailed management of individual pathogens is beyond the scope of this chapter. The key is the correction of fluid and electrolyte imbalance. Severely dehydrated patients need rapid intrave-nous replacement of fluid loss, preferably using a physiologically balanced electrolyte solution such as Ringer's solution (see Chapter 21, p. 197). Large volumes of dextrose solution can be dan-gerous. Intravenous fluid can be supplemented

and rapidly replaced by oral rehydration, which is more successful if small volumes of fluid are taken steadily rather than large volumes at a time. Specific World Health Organization (WHO) oral rehydration solution (ORS) is ideal, but the water in which it is dissolved must be clean and safe to drink—preferably by prior boiling and cooling. Alternative oral rehydration therapy mixtures can also be used for adults, and food, including milk products, is usually reintroduced as early as possi-ble after initial resuscitation of children. Fluid bal-ance should be carefully monitored, and a cholera bed is useful for less mobile patients with profuse diarrhoea. The fluid faeces can then be collected through a hole in the middle of the bed directly into a measuring bucket. If a large-bore disposable Foley's urinary catheter is available, this can be inserted into the rectum when diarrhoea is pro-fuse and watery (e.g. in cholera), removing the need for frequent evacuation, and allowing accu-rate measurement of faecal losses by volume.

Antidiarrhoeal agents such as codeine or lop-eramide should be avoided in patients with acute invasive or large bowel disease and should not be used in young children. Antiemetics should be used sparingly and again avoided in young children. Zinc supplementation is beneficial for children, but the roles of probiotics and use of lactose-free feeds are less clear. Empirical or spe-cific antimicrobial treatment should be reserved for specific situations such as proven amoebiasis, prolonged severe infection in a vulnerable host or in outbreak settings—for example cholera or shigellosis. Chronic diarrhoea presents a different challenge and patients with HIV-related diarrhoea often progress through successive therapeutic trials of co-trimoxazole, metronidazole, fluo-roquinolones, albendazole or nitazoxanide. Such patients may need 'hospital at home' support including provision of adequate antidiarrhoeal medications.

In a refugee camp outbreak setting, logisti-cal support must be requested at an early stage for detailed epidemiological investigation, triage and treatment facilities, as well as provision of an adequate water supply, rehydration solutions and latrines (Chapter 60).

Further reading

Al-Abri SA, Beeching NJ, Nye FJ. Traveller's diarrhoea. *Lancet Infect Dis* 2005; 5: 349–360. [Overview of aetiology, epidemiology, management and prevention of this common problem for travellers.]

Elliott EJ. Acute gastroenteritis in children. *BMJ* 2007; 334: 35–40. [Concise evidence based review, very practical and useful.]

Hart CA. Introduction to acute infective diarrhoea. In: Cook GC, Zumla A, eds. *Manson's Tropical Diseases*, 21st edn. London: Elsevier Science, 2003: 907–913. [Good overview with references of both adult and paediatric diarrhoea causes and effects.]

Manatsathit S, DuPont H, Farthing M *et al.* Guideline for the management of acute diarrhoea in adults. *J Gastroenterol Hepatol* 2002; 17 (Suppl): S54–S71. [Superb working party report produced by acknowledged experts from Thailand, India and Africa as well as 'western' authorities. Detailed definitions, practical approaches and many references.]

Thomas PD *et al.* Guidelines for the investigation of chronic diarrhoea, 2nd edition. *Gut* 2003; 52: 1–15. [British guidelines for assessment of both infectious and non-infectious causes of chronic diarrhoea.]

WHO. *Handbook IMCI Integrated Management of Childhood Illness*. WHO 2005. Chapter 8 Diarrhoea—assessment and management of diarrhoea in children in tropical settings pages 25–31. [Summary of WHO guidelines for use at clinic level. Full manual and other IMCI and nutrition-related resources freely downloadable from WHO child and adolescent health development website http://www.who.int/child_adolescent_health/topics/en/]

WHO. *Implementing the New Recommendations on the Clinical Management of Diarrhoea. Guidelines for Policy Makers and Programme Managers.* WHO 2006. [Summary of new recommendations for use of the 2003 low osmolarity ORS mixture and zinc supplementation, plus programme guidance.]

WHO. *The Treatment of Diarrhoea. A Manual for Physicians and Other Senior Health Workers*, 4th edn. WHO 2005. [Comprehensive review with algorithms for assessment and management of children and adolescents in particular, appropriate for resource poor settings.]

Chapter 2

Respiratory presentations

Disorders of the respiratory tract are the most important cause of ill health in human populations around the world. The normal physiological functioning of the respiratory tract exposes it to prolonged and intimate contact with the external environment, leading to a steady exposure to airborne pollutants and pathogens with disease-causing potential.

Infectious diseases dominate acute respiratory illness in the tropics in all age groups; acute viral and bacterial infections in childhood, and tuberculosis and bacterial pneumonia in adults. The enormous global burden of respiratory impairment due to chronic obstructive pulmonary disease (COPD) has recently been described and shown to be worst in South Africa and China, where the disease is mainly caused by the exposure to tobacco smoke in men and by indoor air pollution from cooking with biomass fuel in women. Global concern regarding the health effects of tobacco smoke has now resulted in important international treaties to limit tobacco products.

Assessment

History

The predominant symptoms of respiratory illness are breathlessness, cough and chest pain. Symptom

Lecture Notes: Tropical Medicine, 6th edition.
By G.V. Gill and N.J. Beeching. Published 2009 by Blackwell Publishing, ISBN: 978-1-4051-8048-1.

duration and the concurrence of fever are useful discriminators—common presentations in adults and children are summarized in Table 2.1.

Breathlessness

Shortness of breath should be characterized by duration, progression and whether it is constant or intermittent. Orthopnoea (breathlessness when lying flat) suggests a cardiac cause or a structural abnormality of the thoracic cage. Nocturnal dyspnoea is a feature of asthma and obstructive airways disease.

The effort required to precipitate breathlessness provides a good gauge of the level of respiratory impairment. Breathlessness at rest or inability of a young child to feed indicates severe restriction. Shortness of breath in an adult should be quantified in terms of tasks completed or failed, or distance walked.

Cough

Cough is a reflex from any part of the vagal supply and a conscious act. Therefore, discriminating between causes of cough can be difficult. Cough may be productive or non-productive, but a 'productive' cough is often evidence of pulmonary infection.

The quantity of sputum produced may provide diagnostic information about COPD or bronchiectasis. The expectoration of mucopurulent

Table 2.1 Shortness of breath in adults and children

Sudden (hours)	Acute (days)	Chronic (weeks, months)
Adults		
Pneumothorax	Pneumonia	Tuberculosis
Pulmonary embolus	Bronchitis	COPD
Asthma	Lung abscess	Kaposi's sarcoma
	Acute left ventricular failure	Lung cancer
	Allergic alveolitis	Heart failure
	Pulmonary eosinophilia	Silicosis/asbestosis
Children		
Pneumothorax	Pneumonia	Tuberculosis
Inhaled foreign body	Bronchitis	Heart failure
Asthma		

material is an indicator of neutrophil activity and infection.

Haemoptysis is often an indicator of serious underlying pathology, but it is important to establish that blood is being coughed and not coming from the upper airway or enteric tract. Tuberculosis, bronchiectasis and neoplasia are primary concerns.

Extreme paroxysms of coughing in a child, particularly in association with the characteristic whoop, indicates a diagnosis of whooping cough. A 'barking' cough with inspiratory stridor is the hallmark of laryngotracheobronchitis—croup.

Chest pain

Complaints of chest pain should be assessed for their association with breathing and coughing. Pain derived from the pleura will be noticeable on breathing and is lateralized. Tracheal pain has a tearing or burning quality and is felt retrosternally, particularly on coughing.

Respiratory history

In addition to the presenting symptoms, it is important to enquire about
- *tobacco smoking* (quantify in pack years);
- *occupation*—identify occupationally related symptoms and exposures including asbestos, inhaled proteins and fumes;

- risk factors for *HIV* infection and contact with *tuberculosis* cases, particularly in children failing to thrive.

Non-respiratory illness

Non-respiratory illness may present with predominantly respiratory symptoms. Breathlessness is a feature of metabolic acidosis which may be caused by diabetic ketoacidosis, poisoning, severe sepsis or renal failure. Chronic breathing difficulties are a feature of anaemia and thyroid disease. Alteration of breathing pattern and breathlessness can occur with neurological injury, during the early stages of tetanus and botulism and following envenomation.

Examination in respiratory cases

A respiratory examination is used to test hypotheses generated by the history. The signs elicited are rarely diagnostic in isolation.

The general condition of an individual provides clues to a diagnosis. In particular, cachexia, or failure to thrive in a young child, will indicate malnutrition or chronic underlying illness. Oral thrush, skin rashes and old herpes zoster scars are highly suspicious of HIV infection, heightening the possibility of pneumococcal pneumonia or tuberculosis.

Tachypnoea (rapid breathing) can be a feature of any respiratory illness. In the context of an acute presentation, rates in adults above 30/min suggest severe disease particularly in association with systolic blood pressure below 90 mmHg and/or a tachycardia in excess of 120 beats per minute. The criteria for tachypnoea in childhood are very different from adults. It is diagnosed only if the respiratory rate is over 60/min before the age of 2 months, over 50/min from 2 to 12 months, over 40/min from 1 to 5 years and over 30/min (as for adults) over the age of 5 years.

Cyanosis should be looked for in the oral mucosa but is a difficult sign in pigmented people. When present it indicates at least 10% desaturation of haemoglobin and the need for supplemental oxygen. Pulse oximetry is becoming increasingly widespread and provides more reliable information.

Altered consciousness and confusion usually indicate severe acute disease and can necessitate specific management to protect the airway. Meningism can be found with severe pneumonia, with or without pneumococcal meningitis.

Percussion of the chest will identify a large pleural effusion (dull note). Lobar consolidation is common in pneumonia or tuberculosis and can be diagnosed on the basis of bronchial breathing. Many patients present with non-specific signs or scanty chest signs. In these cases, a suggestive history should lead to further investigation as a normal chest examination does not exclude significant pathology.

Investigation of respiratory disease

Chest X-ray

Limited resources must be carefully rationed in order to optimally investigate respiratory patients in the tropics. In particular, a chest X-ray should be used to extend the examination in difficult cases and not simply to confirm diagnosis made confidently on auscultation. Patients with severe acute respiratory illness or those who fail to respond to therapy including smear-negative cases of chronic cough are the ones most frequently requiring a chest X-ray.

Sputum/respiratory secretions

Sputum examination is essential in the management of suspected TB (see Chapter 12) and is of less value in other cases. Ziehl–Neelsen staining for mycobacteria and Gram staining for bacteria are the most common investigations. Occasionally, an unstained wet preparation of sputum examined under low power may be useful for identifying *Strongyloides*, paragonimiasis or fungal elements. Cytology for malignant cells can also be performed on sputum but requires a skilled pathologist. Other sputum tests include direct immunofluorescence for viruses and *Pneumocystis jirovecii*, antigen detection for pneumococci and molecular techniques for several organisms including tuberculosis, but these methods are not resource-efficient in developing countries.

Sputum must be from the lower respiratory tract and a macroscopic mucopurulent appearance makes this probable. Microscopic sputum quality assessment is described in Chapter 28. Sputum samples are best collected in the open air (outside) to limit the hazard of cross-infection. When sputum cannot be produced, placing the patient in a head down position or simple chest physiotherapy (drumming) for 2–3 min will help. Lung aspiration increases the diagnostic yield in young children with lung consolidation. A needle and syringe primed with 1 mL normal saline or sterile water is passed into the consolidated tissue through the thoracic wall and aspirated. The aspirated material can be smeared onto slides for examination and injected into liquid culture media. In young children when sputum is difficult to collect, gastric washings may be considered for the investigation of possible tuberculosis (mycobacteria are gastric acid resistant).

Blood cultures

Blood cultures are a valuable investigation in all febrile patients. Recovery of a pathogen allows confident treatment and is frequently the investigation by which an unusual cause of pneumonia is established, for example, *Salmonella typhi*,

Cryptococcus spp, *Burkholderia pseudomallei* (melioidosis), *Rhodococcus equi*.

Pleural fluid

Sampling of pleural fluid is simple to perform and should be considered for most effusions, as the management of simple effusion and empyema is different. Fluid is aspirated by using a needle and syringe, avoiding the neurovascular bundle at the inferior margin of each rib. Occasionally, this fails because pleural fluid is loculated and has formed a thick empyema or the chest findings result from chronic pleural scarring. Protein measurements may be helpful in confirming an effusion to be a transudate—a protein level below 30 g/dL and an absence of inflammatory cells.

Lung function testing

Although lung function can now be measured using hand-held technology and stored on a laptop computer, this is not yet widely used. Now that asthma prevalence is increasing and COPD is recognized as a significant burden of chronic disease in Africa, this may change.

Common presentations

In general, respiratory presentations in the general medical clinic tend to fall into a small number of syndromes.

Acute breathlessness and fever in a small child

Lower respiratory tract infection (LRTI) is a leading killer of children. Consequently, the early assessment and management of this syndrome is a core component of the Integrated Management of Childhood Illness (IMCI) strategy promoted by the WHO. Vaccination against pneumococcal and *Haemophilus* infection are also global priorities.

Simple assessment at the primary care level using features of rapid breathing and subcostal recession (chest indrawing) of a child with fever and cough is used to distinguish children with an LRTI who require antibiotics and possible hospital admission, from those with an upper respiratory tract infection (see Figure 28.1). Early initiation of therapy is essential for a good outcome.

Although many LRTIs are initiated by viral infections, amongst which respiratory syncytial virus, parainfluenza, adenovirus and measles are important, super-added bacterial infections are frequent. *Streptococcus pneumoniae* and *Haemophilus influenzae* type b are common. The presentation of tuberculosis in infants is often occult.

Acute breathlessness, cough and fever in adults

Acute bacterial pneumonia is the principal diagnostic consideration, and the diagnosis and management of this is covered in Chapter 28. Non-infectious causes become more prevalent in older adults.

Chronic cough and malaise

Most chronic respiratory problems present in this way. It is important to exclude or confirm tuberculosis which represents a serious public health threat but is readily treatable (Chapter 12). A small number of conditions are specific to the tropics and may need to be considered under the right epidemiological circumstances: paragonimiasis in South East Asia and restricted areas of West Africa (Chapter 29); endemic mycoses in South and Central America (Chapter 54); and pulmonary complications of schistosomiasis in endemic regions (Chapter 17). The incidence of tobacco smoking associated lung cancer is increasing in developing countries.

Breathlessness and wheeze

Asthma is an increasingly important problem in the tropics, particularly in urban centres. The expiratory wheeze or whistling associated with lower airways obstruction must be differentiated from inspiratory phase stridor, which indicates upper airway obstruction. The presence of paroxysmal or diurnal cough, breathlessness and wheeze preferably supported by variation in peak flow measurements reliably indicates airways obstruction. An important differential diagnosis of asthma is tropical pulmonary eosinophilia (Chapter 30). Although the symptoms are identical, a high peripheral eosinophil count above 1×10^9/L, demonstration of microfilaria in blood and clinical response to filaricides support the diagnosis.

Pleural effusion

Symptoms associated with pleural effusions can be of short or long duration depending on the nature of the underlying problems, but large effusions are straightforward to find on examination.

Pleural fluid should be sampled as described earlier. In HIV endemic regions, TB is the most common cause of pleural effusion. Parapneumonic effusions, empyema or tuberculous effusions should be suggested by the history. Malignant effusions must be considered when an infective aetiology is not readily apparent. Effusions may indicate extrapulmonary or systemic problems (Table 2.2).

Respiratory disease in the HIV-infected adults

Respiratory problems head the list of conditions leading to hospital admission of HIV-infected adults (Table 2.3). Bacterial (particularly pneumococcal) pneumonia is strongly associated with HIV infection. It has a similar predictive value for HIV infection in adults to herpes zoster—around 90% in eastern and southern Africa. HIV infection

Table 2.2 Causes of pleural effusion

Common	Infrequent	Rare
• Tuberculosis	• Neoplasia	• Thoracic duct damage
• Parapneumonic	– Lung carcinoma	• Pancreatitis
• Empyema	– Kaposis's sarcoma	• Haemorrhagic fever
• Heart failure	– Burkitt's lymphoma	• Filariasis
	– Mesothelioma	• Hypothyroidism
	• Constrictive pericarditis	

Table 2.3 Respiratory problems complicating HIV infection

Common	Infrequent
• Bacterial pneumonia	• *Pneumocystis jirovecii* pneumonia[a]
• Tuberculosis	• *Rhodococcus equi* infection
• Acute bronchitis	• Nocardiasis
• Sinusitis	• Lymphoid interstitial pneumonitis[b]
• Bronchiectasis	• Lymphoma
• Pulmonary cryptococcosis	• Pulmonary hypertension
• Pulmonary Kaposi's sarcoma	• Penicillinosis[c]
	• Melioidosis[c]
	• Invasive mycoses[d]

[a]Common in children under 1 year old.
[b]Common in children.
[c]South East Asia.
[d]South and Central America.

is the principal factor driving the tuberculosis epidemic in Africa. Thus, HIV coinfection varies between 50% and 70%. HIV testing should be considered in all cases of pneumonia and tuberculosis.

Cough is a frequently reported symptom in individuals with advanced immunosuppression. Although tuberculosis always requires exclusion, hypostatic pneumonia, bronchial mucus hypersecretion, pharyngeal thrush, acute bronchitis and postnasal drip from sinus disease all contribute to the causes of cough. Management is especially difficult; the patient appears ill and multiple courses of antibiotics are often prescribed. Therapeutic trials of antituberculosis therapy are frequently required, but are often disappointing.

Chronically ill AIDS patients frequently present with intractable breathlessness. These cases are difficult to manage as pulmonary Kaposi's sarcoma, sputum-negative TB, bacterial pneumonia, pulmonary cryptococcosis and fungal pneumonia can all potentially be present at one time—each of these diagnoses is hard to make and treatment unlikely to be successful. Careful consideration must be made of when symptom-directed palliative care is the most appropriate strategy.

Further reading

Ait-Khaled N, Odhiambo J, Pearce N *et al.* Prevalence of symptoms of asthma, rhinitis and eczema in 13- to 14-year-old children in Africa: the International Study of Asthma and Allergies in Childhood Phase III. *Allergy* 2007; 62: 247–258.

Buist AS, McBurnie MA, Vollmer WM *et al.* International variation in the prevalence of COPD (the BOLD Study): a population-based prevalence study. *Lancet* 2007; 370: 741–750.

http://www.fctc.org. The website of the Framework Convention Alliance, an NGO supporting the actions of the Framework Convention for Tobacco Control (last accessed 4/12/07).

Chapter 3

Neurological presentations

Neurological presentations are more common in the tropics than in the developed industrial world. Infectious diseases make a major contribution, but non-infectious causes are also important (Table 3.1). A complex mixture of socio-economic and environmental factors contribute to the increased incidence.

Reasons for increased incidence of neurological disorders in the tropics

• Non-infectious neurological disorders—trauma is more common in the tropics, especially road-traffic accidents. Patterns of vascular disease are catching up with those in the developed world, but the usage of drugs to control those lag behind.
• Infectious neurological diseases—the climate supports transmission of insect-borne pathogens (malaria, trypanosomiasis, arthropod-borne viruses). Environmental factors include the close proximity of homes to zoonotic infections. Vaccine-preventable diseases are more common (e.g. measles, tetanus, diphtheria, polio). There is also unregulated use of over-the-counter antibiotics leading to the partial pretreatment of central nervous system (CNS) infections, which hampers

diagnosis and therapy, and promotes the development of antibiotic resistance.
• Poverty, overcrowding, poor sanitation and lack of education about disease, risk factors and prevention are important. These may lead, for example, to cysticercosis and typhoid.
• Immunosuppression, particularly as a result of HIV, allows many other infections such as cryptococcal and tuberculous meningitis. Many patients with HIV have no access to highly active antiretroviral therapy (HAART).

Neurological syndromes

Neurological diseases—particularly infections—can present with a range of syndromes.
• *Encephalopathy*—a reduced level of consciousness from any cause (infectious, metabolic, vascular, traumatic).
• *Meningism*—clinical signs of meningeal irritation (headache, neck stiffness, Kernig's sign; discussed later).
• *Paralysis*—weakness of one or more limb, respiratory or bulbar muscles, which may be a result of damaged upper motor neurones, lower motor neurones, peripheral nerves or muscles.
• *Chronic neurological presentations*—insidious presentation over weeks or months, often with changes in personality, behaviour or other psychiatric illness. Fever may not be prominent, even with an infectious cause (Table 3.2).

Lecture Notes: Tropical Medicine, 6th edition.
By G.V. Gill and N.J. Beeching. Published 2009 by Blackwell Publishing, ISBN: 978-1-4051-8048-1.

Table 3.1 Causes of neurological disease—VIMTO.

Vascular
Ischaemia/infarct
Subarachnoid/subdural/extradural/intracerebral
  haemorrhage
Hypertension/hypotension
 	
Infectious
Direct effect on CNS
Bacteria
  Meningococcus, streptococci, *Haemophilus*
  influenzae, tuberculosis, leprosy, *Mycoplasma*
  pneumoniae, *Listeria spp*, *E. coli* (neonates),
  Mycobacterium tuberculosis
Viruses
  Arboviruses, herpes viruses, enteroviruses,
  rabies, paramyxoviruses (measles, mumps),
  influenza and parainfluenza viruses, adenoviruses,
  Nipah virus
Parasites
  Protozoans
    malaria (*Plasmodium falciparum*)
    African trypanosomiasis (*Trypanosoma gambiense*
    and *T. rhodesiense*)
    toxoplasmosis (*Toxoplasma gondii*)
    amoebiasis (*Naegleria fowleri, Balamuthia*
    mandrillaris)
  Trematodes (flukes)
    paragonimiasis
    schistosomiasis (especially *Schistosoma japonicum*)
  Cestodes (tapeworms)
    cysticercosis (*Taenia solium*)
    hydatidosis (*Echinococcus granulosus*)
  Nematodes (roundworms)
    ascariasis (*Ascaris lumbricoides*)
    parastrongyliasis (*Parastrongylus cantonensis*)
    gnathostomiasis (*Gnathostoma spinigerum*)
    trichinosis (*Trichinella spiralis*)
Spirochetes
  Neurosyphilis (*Treponema pallidum*)
  Lyme disease (*Borrelia burgdorferi*)
  Leptospirosis (*Leptospira* species)
  Louse-borne/epidemic relapsing fever (*B. recurrentis*)
  Tick-borne/endemic relapsing fever (*B. duttonii*)
Rickettsiae
  Epidemic/louse-borne typhus (*Rickettsia prowazekii*)
  Endemic/murine/flea-borne typhus (*R. typhi/R.*
  mooseri)
	Scrub typhus (*Orientia tsutsugamushi*)
	  Rocky Mountain spotted fever (*R. rickettsii*)
	Fungi
	  Cryptococcosis
	  Histoplasmosis
	  Aspergillosis
	  Coccidioidomycosis
	  Candidiasis
	  Paracoccidiomycosis
	  Blastomycosis
	  Nocardiasis[a]
	Prion
	Creutzfeldt–Jakob disease (sporadic, new-variant,
	  iatrogenic)
	
	Indirect effect of infection
	Toxin-mediated infectious diseases (tetanus, diphtheria,
	  shigellosis)
	Immune-mediated postinfectious inflammatory (GBS,
	  acute disseminated encephalomyelitis, transverse
	  myelitis)
	
	Metabolic
	Hypoglycaemia
	Diabetic ketoacidosis
	Hepatic encephalopathy
	Uraemia
	Hyponatraemia
	Hypothyroidism/hyperthyroidism
	Mitochondrial encephalopathies (e.g. Leigh Syndrome)
	Addison's disease
	
	Tumours/trauma/toxins
	Alcohol
	Drugs (medical, recreational, traditional)
	Pesticides
	Poisons
	
	Other
	Hydrocephalus
	Hypertensive encephalopathy
	Epilepsy (non-convulsive status epilepticus)
	Psychiatric disease (hysteria)
	Inflammatory
	Vasculitis
	Nutritional
	Degenerative

Abbreviations: CNS, central nervous system; GBS, Guillain–Barré syndrome.

[a]*Nocardia* are actinomycete bacteria which are grouped with fungi because of their morphology and behaviour.

Table 3.2 Causes of chronic neurological presentations in the tropics

Infectious	Other
Sleeping sickness (especially *Trypanosoma rhodesiense*, *T. gambiense*)	Tumours
	Chronic subdural haemorrhages
Tuberculous meningitis	Lead, other heavy metal poisoning
HIV encephalopathy	
Toxoplasma gondii and other parasitic space-occupying lesions	Dementia
	Vitamin deficiencies
Bacterial abscesses	Drugs
Partially treated bacterial meningitis	Toxins
Neurosyphilis	
Cryptococcal meningitis and other fungi	
Subacute sclerosing panencephalitis	

Table 3.3 Causes of CNS space-occupying lesions in the tropics

> Tumours and metastases
> Haemorrhage
> Bacterial abscesses
> Tuberculomas
> Parasites
>   Protozoa (toxoplasmosis, amoebiasis)
>   Trematodes (paragonimiasis, schistosomiasis)
>   Cestodes (cysticercosis, hydatidosis)
>   Nematodes (ascariasis)
> Fungi
>   Aspergillosis, blastomycosis, nocardiasis
> HIV related —toxoplasmosis, primary CNS lymphoma, tuberculomas

• *Headache*—may be the only symptom (e.g. in cryptococcal meningitis).
• *Other focal neurological signs*—including hemispheric signs, brainstem signs, seizures, and movement disorders.

Pathological processes

These neurological syndromes are explained by a range of pathological processes.
• *Encephalitis*—inflammation of the brain substance, not only in response to viral infection, but also in response to other pathogens.
• *Meningitis*—inflammation of the meningeal membranes covering the brain, in response to bacterial, viral or fungal infection.
• *Myelitis*—inflammation of the spinal cord. This may occur across the whole cord (causing transverse myelitis, which is often postinfectious) or be confined to the anterior horn cells).
• *Neuropathy*—damage to peripheral nerves (e.g. Guillain–Barré syndrome, diphtheria, leprosy, rabies, vitamin deficiencies, unwanted effects of antiretroviral therapy (ART)).

• *Mononeuritis multiplex*—damage to at least two individual nerves. Can be caused by HIV, leprosy, Lyme disease, hepatitis A.
• *Polyradiculopathy*—inflammation of the nerve roots, often presents as a cauda equina syndrome. May occur in HIV infection caused by cytomegalovirus (CMV), syphilis and HSV2.
• *Space-occupying lesions* (Table 3.3)—these cause pathology in the brain or spinal cord directly (by interrupting neuronal pathways), and indirectly (by causing localized swelling, raised intracranial pressure and brainstem herniation syndromes). Typically, they present with focal signs or a chronic insidious deterioration.

Rapid assessment of patient with coma in the tropics

1 *Stabilize the patient*, and treat any immediately life-threatening conditions.
• Airways.
• Breathing—give oxygen; intubate if breathing is inadequate or gag reflex impaired.
• Circulation—establish venous access.
  – Obtain blood for immediate bedside blood glucose test (hypoglycaemia?).
  – Malaria film (look for parasites and pigment of partially treated malaria).
  – Full blood count, serum biochemistry, blood cultures, arterial blood gases.

19

- Disability.
  - Give intravenous (i.v.) glucose (e.g. 10% glucose 50 mL in adults, 5 mL/kg in children), irrespective of blood glucose.
  - Give adults 100 mg thiamine i.v., especially if alcohol abuse is suspected.
  - Immobilize cervical spinal cord if neck trauma is suspected.
- Rapidly assess AVPU scale (Alert, responds to Voice, to Pain or Unresponsive).
  - If patient responds to pain or is unresponsive, examine the pupils, eye movements, respiratory pattern, tone and posture for signs of cerebral herniation (discussed later).
  - If herniation is suspected start treatment as stated below.
- If purpuric rash is present, give penicillin or chloramphenicol (or third generation cephalosporin) for presumed meningococcal meningitis, after taking blood cultures.
- Look for and treat generalized seizures, focal seizures and subtle motor seizures (mouth or finger twitching, or tonic eye deviation).

2 *Take a history*, while preliminary assessment and resuscitation proceeds. This is the single most useful tool in determining the cause of coma, in particular.
- Duration of onset of coma.
  - Rapid onset (minutes–hours) suggests a vascular cause, especially brainstem cerebrovascular accidents or subarachnoid haemorrhage. If preceded by hemispheric signs, then consider intracerebral haemorrhage. Coma caused by some infections (e.g. malaria, encephalitis) can also develop rapidly, especially when precipitated by convulsions.
  - Intermediate onset (hours–days) suggests diffuse encephalopathy (metabolic or, if febrile, infectious).
  - Prolonged onset (days–weeks) suggests tumours, abscess or chronic subdural haematoma (see Table 3.2).
- Any drugs?
- Any trauma?
- Important past medical history (e.g. hypertension)?
- Family history (e.g. tuberculosis)?

- Known epidemic area (e.g. viral encephalitis)?

3 *Perform a rapid general medical examination*, and in particular:
- Check pockets for drugs.
- Note temperature (febrile or hypothermia) and blood pressure (hypo- or hypertensive).
- Examine for signs of trauma (check ears and nose for blood or cerebrospinal fluid [CSF] leak).
- Smell the breath for alcohol or ketones (diabetes?).
- Examine the skin for:
  - rash (meningococcal rash, dengue or other haemorrhagic fever, typhus, relapsing fever);
  - needle marks of drug abuse;
  - recent tick bite or eschar (tick-borne encephalitis, tick paralysis, tick-borne typhus or relapsing fever);
  - chancre, with or without circinate rash (trypanosomiasis, especially *Trypanosoma rhodesiense*);
  - healed dog bite (rabies); or
  - snake bite.
- Examine for lymphadenopathy (e.g. Winterbottom's sign of posterior cervical lymphadenopathy in African trypanosomiasis).
- Examine the fundi for papilloedema (long-standing raised intracranial pressure) or signs of hypertension.

4 *Determine the coma score* to allow subsequent changes to be accurately monitored. The scale in Box 3.1 is for adults and children over 5 years of age and in Box 3.2 for young children.

5 *Neurological examination.* A detailed description of the neurological examination is beyond the scope of this chapter. For most practical purposes the ability to recognize the following four clinical patterns (and combinations of them) will allow appropriate classification and subsequent investigation and treatment.
- *Meningism*—with or without encephalopathy.
- *Diffuse encephalopathies*—usually metabolic or infectious.
- *Supratentorial focal damage* (above the cerebellar tentorium)—usually manifests as hemispheric signs.

Box 3.1 Modified Glasgow coma scale for adults and children over 5 years

Best motor response

6	Obeys command
5	Localizes supraorbital pain
4	Withdraws from pain on nail bed
3	Abnormal flexion response
2	Abnormal extension response
1	None

Best verbal response

5	Oriented
4	Confused
3	Inappropriate words
2	Incomprehensible sounds
1	None

Eye opening

4	Spontaneous
3	To voice
2	Pain
1	None

Total score is the sum of best score in each of the three categories (maximum score 15). 'Unrousable coma' reflects a score <9

Box 3.2 Blantyre coma scale for young children.

Best motor response

2	Localizes painful stimulus
1	Withdraws limb from pain
0	Non-specific or absent response

Best verbal response

2	Appropriate cry
1	Moan or inappropriate cry
0	None

Eye movements

1	Directed (e.g. follows mother's face)
0	Not directed

Total score is the sum of best score in each of the three categories (maximum score 5). 'Unrousable coma' reflects score <2

• *Damage in the diencephalon or brainstem* (midbrain, pons or medulla)—may indicate a syndrome of cerebral herniation through the tentorial hiatus or the foramen magnum

(Figure 3.1). The importance of these syndromes is being increasingly recognized in non-traumatic coma, particularly that caused by infections. Although the level of brainstem damage is given in brackets below (and in Figure 3.1), recognizing the presence or absence of brainstem signs, and in particular early signs of reversible damage, is usually more important than determining their exact localization.

Assessment of the following five points allows most patients to be classified.

1 *Check for neck stiffness* (if no trauma) *and Kernig's sign* (extension of knee when hip is already flexed causes pain).

2 *Examine pupil reaction to light* (Figure 3.1). A normal reaction (constriction) is seen in a diffuse encephalopathy. A unilateral large pupil is seen in herniation of the uncus of the temporal lobe. The pupils are reactive (small or mid-sized) in the diencephalic syndrome. Unreactive pupils occur in brainstem lesions (mid-sized in midbrain or pontine lesions; large in medullary lesions). Pinpoint pupils occur following opiate or organophosphate overdose, or in isolated pontine lesion. Other drugs can cause large unreactive pupils.

3 *Assess eye movements* (holding eyelids open if necessary).

• *Spontaneous eye movements*—eyes spontaneously roving or eyes following indicates the brainstem is intact (a diencephalic syndrome or a diffuse encephalopathy).

• *Oculocephalic (doll's eye) reflex*—when rotating the head, the eyes normally deviate away from the direction of rotation. A normal response indicates that the brainstem is intact (diffuse encephalopathy). Reduced or absent responses occur in uncal herniation, brainstem damage or, rarely, deep metabolic coma.

• *Oculovestibular reflex*—caloric response to water should be tested if the result of the oculocephalic reflex is unclear. Check that the eardrum is not perforated, then irrigate by injecting 20 mL ice-cold water. Nystagmus is the normal response and indicates 'psychogenic coma'. Both eyes deviate towards the irrigated ear in coma with the brainstem intact.

A reduced or absent response indicates an uncal syndrome or a damaged brainstem.

4 *Assess breathing pattern* A normal pattern occurs in diffuse encephalopathy. Cheyne–Stokes breathing and hyperventilation occur in reversible herniation syndromes. Shallow, ataxic or apnoeic respiration occurs in more severe syndromes (Figure 3.1). Hyperventilation also occurs in acidosis or may be caused by aspiration pneumonia, which is common in coma.

5 *Assess response to pain* by applying painful stimulus to the supraorbital ridge and nail bed of each limb.

- *Hemiparesis*—most often indicates supratentorial hemispheric focal pathology (other signs include asymmetry of tone and focal seizures), but also occurs in uncal herniation.
- *'Decorticate posturing'*—flexion of arms with extension of legs, indicating damage in the diencephalon, and *'decerebrate posturing'*

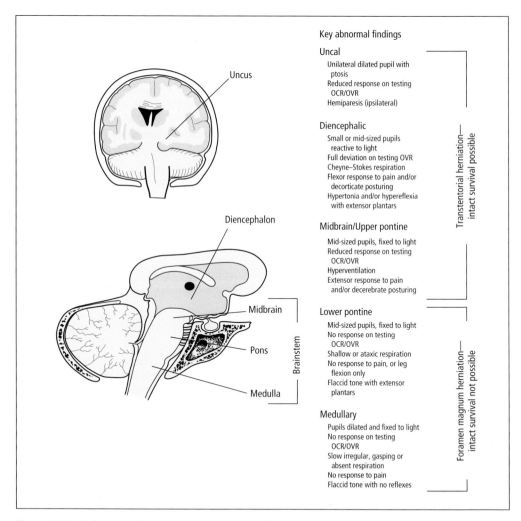

Figure 3.1 Sagittal section of brain showing anatomy and key abnormal findings of midline herniation syndromes, and (above) coronal section showing herniation of the uncus of the temporal lobe—this compresses the ipsilateral third nerve (to cause a palsy of CN III), and the contralateral cerebral peduncle (to cause an ipsilateral hemiparesis).

(extension of arms and legs caused by mid-brain/upper pontine damage) may both be reversible. No response, or leg flexion only, are more severe.

Symmetrical posturing (decorticate or decerebrate) and hemiparetic focal signs are also occasionally seen in metabolic encephalopathies (e.g. hypoglycaemia; hepatic, uraemic or hypoxic coma; sedative drugs), cerebral malaria, and intra- or postictally. Other pointers to metabolic disease include asterixis, tremor and myoclonus preceding the onset of coma.

Classification and further investigation of patients with coma

At this stage, if the history, general examination and preliminary investigation have not made one diagnosis extremely likely, most comatose patients will fall into one of three categories, based on the presence or absence of meningism, supratentorial and brainstem signs.

1 *Coma only* (no hemispheric signs, brainstem signs or meningism—'sleeping beauties').
  • If patient is febrile (or has a history of fever), suspect CNS infection (especially cerebral malaria) or metabolic coma plus secondary aspiration pneumonia.
  • If afebrile, coma is likely to be metabolic (hypoglycaemia, drugs, alcohol, diabetic ketoacidosis, toxins), psychogenic (test caloric response to water—causes nystagmus), or, occasionally, resulting from subarachnoid haemorrhage or other cerebrovascular accident.
2 *Coma with meningism*, but no focal signs.
  • If febrile, CNS infection (especially bacterial meningitis) is likely.
  • If afebrile, subarachnoid haemorrhage is likely.
3 *Coma with focal signs* (with or without meningism). Decide if the signs are 'hemispheric signs', 'brainstem signs', or both.
  • *Hemispheric signs only*. If febrile, consider CNS infection (especially encephalitis, bacterial meningitis, abscess, etc.). If afebrile, consider space-occupying lesion (Table 3.3), cerebrovascular accident or trauma.

  • *Brainstem signs only* may be caused by either focal pathology within the brainstem (e.g. encephalitis) especially if markedly asymmetrical signs or by herniation of the brainstem through the foramen magnum, secondary to a diffuse process (e.g. diabetic ketoacidosis or late bacterial meningitis) causing raised intracranial pressure.
  • *Hemispheric and brainstem signs* may be a result of either a supratentorial lesion causing hemispheric signs and sufficient swelling to precipitate brainstem herniation (e.g. cerebral bleed, abscess) or patchy focal pathology in the hemispheres and brainstem (e.g. toxoplasmosis, viral encephalitis).

Indications and contraindications for lumbar puncture in suspected CNS infections (Table 3.4)

For many years lumbar puncture was performed in all patients with suspected CNS infections, in both the tropics and western industrialized nations. It has gone out of fashion in the latter, following concerns that it was being performed

Table 3.4 Guidelines for lumbar puncture in patients with suspected CNS infections

All patients with suspected CNS infection should have a lumbar puncture, except those with the following contraindications:
• Obtunded state with poor peripheral perfusion or hypotension
• Deteriorating level of consciousness, or deep coma (responsive only to pain, GCS <8)
• Focal neurological signs present:
  – Unequal, dilated or poorly responsive pupils
  – Hemiparesis/monoparesis (in patients with coma)
  – Decerebrate or decorticate posturing
  – Absent 'doll's eye' movements
  – Papilloedema
• Hypertension and relative bradycardia
• Within 30 min of a short convulsive seizure
• Following a prolonged convulsive seizure or tonic seizure

Abbreviation: CNS, central nervous system; GCS, Glasgow coma score.

on patients with contraindications, and may have precipitated herniation.

In patients with a contraindication, treatment should be started and then a lumbar puncture reconsidered later. In many tropical settings in Africa and Asia, where CNS infections are very common, lumbar puncture is still considered an essential investigation. Here the benefits of accurate diagnosis and appropriate treatment may outweigh the theoretical risk of herniation, and even patients with relative contraindications often receive lumbar punctures with no apparent harm.

Cerebrospinal fluid findings in CNS infections

Although most patients with CNS infections will have findings that are straightforward to interpret, there may be considerable overlap (Table 3.5). Ideally, the decision about starting antibiotics should await the result of the lumbar puncture (if it is available quickly). However, antibiotics should be started immediately for patients with a typical meningococcal rash, because of the speed with which meningococcal septicaemia can become fatal. In such patients if it is certain that

Table 3.5 CSF findings in central nervous system infections

	Acute bacterial meningitis	Viral meningo-encephalitis	Tuberculous meningitis	Fungal	Normal
Opening pressure	Increased	Normal/increased	Increased	Increased	10–20 cm
Colour	Cloudy	'Gin' clear	Cloudy/yellow	Clear/cloudy	Clear
Cells/mm³	High–very high 1000–50 000	Normal–high 0–1000	Slightly increased 25–500	Normal–high 0–1000	<5
Differential	Neutrophils	Lymphocytes	Lymphocytes	Lymphocytes	Lymphocytes
CSF:plasma glucose ratio	Low	Normal	Low–very low (e.g. <30%)	Normal–low	66%
Protein (g/L)	High >1	Normal–high 0.5–1	High–very high 1–5	Normal–high 0.2–5.0	<0.5

Normal values

Normal CSF opening pressure is <20 cm water for adults, <10 cm for children below age 8.

A normal CSF glucose is usually quoted to be 66% that of the plasma glucose, but in many tropical settings a cut-off of 40% is found to be more useful.

A bloody tap will falsely elevate the CSF white cell count and protein. To correct for a bloody tap, subtract 1 white cell for every 700 red blood cells/mm³ in the CSF, and 0.1 g/dL of protein for every 1000 red blood cells.

Some important exceptions

In patients with acute bacterial meningitis that has been partially pretreated with antibiotics (or patients <1 year old) the CSF cell count may not be very high and may be mostly lymphocytes.

In viral CNS infections, an early lumbar puncture may show predominantly neutrophils, or there may be no cells in early or late lumbar punctures.

Tuberculous meningitis may have predominantly CSF polymorphs early on.

Listeriosis can give a similar CSF picture to tuberculous meningitis, but the history is shorter.

CSF findings in bacterial abscesses range from near normal to purulent, depending on location of the abscess and whether there is associated meningitis or rupture.

An Indian ink test, and if negative a cryptococcal antigen test, should be performed on the CSF of all patients in whom cryptococcosis is possible.

the rash is meningococcal, it has been argued that the lumbar puncture is not necessary because the diagnosis is already made, though others advocate always doing a lumbar puncture.

Further reading

Kirkham FJ. Non-traumatic coma in children. *Arch Dis Child* 2001; 85: 303–312. [An excellent review of pathophysiology and management.]

Kneen R, Solomon T, Appleton RA. The role of lumbar punctures in CNS infections. *Arch Dis Child* 2001; 87: 181–183. [Detailed discussion of the use of lumbar puncture.]

Chapter 4

Febrile presentations

Pathogenesis and symptomatic treatment of fever

Fever is a physiological response to infection, but there are other non-infective causes of inflammation and fever to be considered. The principal cytokines initiating fever are interleukin 1 and interleukin 6; these alter thermoregulation in the hypothalamus mediated by prostaglandins. Antipyretics in common use act by inhibition of pyrogenic prostaglandin production: these are either non-steroidal anti-inflammatory drugs or paracetamol (acetaminophen). Although antipyretics are widely used and have beneficial properties in terms of analgesic effects and reducing discomfort, they have never been proved to improve the outcome of infection or to reduce the complications of pyrexia. Paracetamol is the antipyretic of choice because it is free of side effects at normal dosage and, unlike aspirin, it is not associated with Reye's syndrome in children.

Clinical approach to the patient with fever

History

Patients often complain of symptoms, such as generalized myalgia and arthralgia, that suggest

Lecture Notes: Tropical Medicine, 6th edition.
By G.V. Gill and N.J. Beeching. Published 2009 by
Blackwell Publishing, ISBN: 978-1-4051-8048-1.

the presence of fever, but are actually afebrile (temperature <37.5°C). Such patients rarely have significant underlying pathology and are best managed conservatively. A history of rigors or night sweats is much more suggestive of fever and, even if initially afebrile, they are best managed as if a fever were present. Similarly, significant weight loss is also indicative of underlying organic disease. Localizing symptoms should be sought, but these carry far more weight if they are volunteered at the outset. Important symptoms are headache, photophobia, cough, sputum, pleurisy, localized pain, diarrhoea (especially if bloody) and urinary symptoms. Coryza and upper respiratory symptoms generally suggest a viral illness. Prior treatment with antibiotics may make diagnosis difficult. Freshwater exposure suggests schistosomiasis (Katayama fever). Recent travel (within 3 weeks) to high risk countries should always raise the possibility of viral haemorrhagic fever so that appropriate precautions are taken. The pattern of fever is rarely helpful in making a diagnosis in practice, but duration of fever is useful. Older children will give a history in the same way as adults. For infants and babies, enquiry should be made about feeding, weight gain (often charted), general activity and the health of the parents.

Examination

A temperature >37.5°C is clinically significant. If there is a convincing history of fever but no significant pyrexia on presentation, and if the patient is not sick enough to be admitted, a self-recorded temperature chart usually resolves the matter. A pulse rate >125 or systolic blood pressure <100 mmHg in an adult suggests the patient is seriously ill and in need of empirical treatment. Spontaneous haemorrhage suggests a viral haemorrhagic fever. The eyes should be inspected for anaemia, jaundice, conjunctival injection (measles and leptospirosis) and the fundi examined if lumbar puncture is likely to be needed or bacterial endocarditis is possible. The mouth should be examined for candidiasis (HIV infection), Koplick's spots (measles) and pharyngitis. The tympanic membranes of all young children should be inspected, but only in adults if there are relevant symptoms. Cervical and axillary lymphadenopathy should be sought (pharyngitis, HIV, CMV, Epstein–Barr virus [EBV], tuberculosis, lymphoma, toxoplasmosis, syphilis) and also occipital lymphadenopathy (rubella, trypanosomiasis). The skin should be carefully inspected for rash (viral exanthems, non-blanching meningococcal petechiae), an eschar (tick-borne rickettsial infection) or anaesthetic patches with pigmentary change (leprosy). Skin sepsis and cellulitis are common causes of fever (streptococcal or staphylococcal). Conscious level, orientation and neck stiffness need to be assessed. Psychosis may be a manifestation of typhoid.

A more detailed neurological examination is not required unless the history suggests a neurological problem, a lumbar puncture is likely to be needed or leprosy is possible. The chest and heart require examination for signs of consolidation (pneumonia often fails to give respiratory symptoms), pleural or pericardial effusion (tuberculosis, HIV, empyema) and heart murmurs (bacterial endocarditis, rheumatic heart disease). In infants and babies a raised respiratory rate may be the only evidence of pneumonia. Abdominal tenderness and peritonism should be sought (appendicitis, peritonitis, pelvic inflammatory disease). Localized right lower intercostal tenderness suggests amoebic liver abscess. Hepatomegaly (malaria, tuberculosis, hepatitis, schistosomiasis, hepatoma, amoebic liver abscess) and splenomegaly (malaria, typhoid,

leishmaniasis, HIV, infectious mononucleosis, lymphoma and leukaemia, portal hypertension, brucellosis, disseminated tuberculosis) are important signs. Demonstrable ascites requires a diagnostic tap. Any detectable joint effusion should also be tapped. Urinalysis should, of course, be part of the examination.

Initial investigation

Laboratory tests that are useful to discriminate those who require further investigation and treatment from those who require symptomatic management only are malaria films and full blood count. A malaria film should always be performed if there has been a visit to a malarious area and there is fever or symptoms suggestive of fever, irrespective of the patient's presentation. It is useful triage to arrange a malaria film as soon as a febrile patient presents, even before seeing a doctor. Where facilities are available, measurement of urea and electrolytes (renal failure in septicaemic shock, severe malaria, leptospirosis, haemolytic uraemic syndrome; hyponatraemia in tuberculosis), liver function tests (viral hepatitis) and C-reactive protein (CRP) are helpful. If the CRP is <10 mg/L, significant underlying pathology is unlikely, unless the erythrocyte sedimentation rate (ESR) is raised: this may suggest a rare case of systemic lupus erythematosus (SLE). The ESR is simple to perform and may be helpful as a non-specific marker of inflammation (bearing in mind that the ESR may be raised in the elderly and in the general population in the tropics). It is good practice to save a specimen of acute serum, if you have facilities to analyse acute and convalescent viral titres, to make a retrospective diagnosis. A chest X-ray should be performed if no obvious cause of fever is present. Appropriate bacterial cultures are important and, where available, should always be performed prior to starting antibiotic treatment. These include blood cultures, especially if typhoid or paratyphoid is possible; urine culture, where symptoms or urinalysis suggest urinary tract infection; and stool microscopy and culture, if bloody diarrhoea is present. At least two sets (aerobic and anaerobic on each occasion) of blood cultures should be taken: these do not have to coincide with spikes of fever, but should be taken from different sites and as little as 10–20 min apart if antibiotic treatment is urgent. If bacterial endocarditis is suspected then at least three sets of blood cultures should be taken, preferably spaced over several hours. Sputum culture is generally not helpful, except for tuberculosis, and is often unavailable in resource-poor settings. Sputum microscopy for acid-fast bacilli should be available in most settings and is important if pulmonary tuberculosis is suspected (chronic cough, weight loss, night sweats). Lumbar puncture is necessary if symptoms and signs suggest meningitis. In well-resourced settings, there is massive overuse of CT scanning prior to lumbar puncture: CT scan is only indicated if there are recent onset seizures, focal neurology, significantly depressed Glasgow coma score (<13), papilloedema, or immunosuppression (e.g. by HIV) is likely. Unnecessary CT scans are a waste of money, impair bacteriological diagnosis and cause significant delays in lumbar puncture and appropriate treatment. In a western or low HIV prevalence setting, high-dose corticosteroids should be given prior to or with the first dose of antibiotics if pneumococcal meningitis is possible, in order to improve survival and prevent neurological handicap. In practice, dexamethasone (0.15 mg/kg qds for 4 days, maximum 10 mg qds) should usually be given first if antibiotics are deemed necessary for suspected meningitis, but then stopped promptly unless CSF findings confirm neutrophil leucocytosis or the presence of pneumococci on Gram's stain, latex agglutination or culture. It is inappropriate to use corticosteroids in suspected meningococcal septicaemia or during outbreaks of meningococcal meningitis, or in areas of high prevalence of HIV, such as sub Saharan Africa (see Chapter 31, p. 251). Infants and babies may show no specific clues of meningitis, so lumbar puncture should be performed if they are significantly unwell with no other identifiable cause of fever and a negative malaria film. An adult patient who has severe headache but no meningism, and in whom HIV is known or suspected, requires lumbar puncture in order to exclude cryptococcal

> **Box 4.1 Acute fevers with a negative malarial blood film**
>
> *Polymorphonuclear leucocytosis?*
>
> | Yes | No |
> | --- | --- |
> | Pyogenic infection | Viral infections |
> | Leptospiral infection | Rickettsial infections |
> | Relapsing fevers | Typhoid |
> | Amoebic liver abscess | Brucellosis |
> | Gout | Q fever |

meningitis. Usually, evidence of raised intracranial pressure is a contraindication to lumbar puncture, but it has a therapeutic role in cryptococcal meningitis provided that space occupying lesions such as cerebral toxoplasmosis have been excluded. Genital swabs for microscopy and culture should be taken if sexually transmitted infection is suspected; syphilis serology is also relevant, especially with a rash extending to the palms and soles. Viral tests are usually restricted to serology, generally for HIV and hepatitis B, in resource-poor settings.

Acute fevers with a negative malarial blood film

The white blood cell count (WBC) divides this group into two, as shown in Box 4.1.

Treatment of common causes of fever lasting <2 weeks

It is important to remember that in general in at least 50% of adults and older children with genuine fever, no cause will be identified and the fever will resolve spontaneously in a few days. These patients come to no harm from their presumed infection, and the important thing is to keep diagnostic procedures and therapeutic intervention to a minimum. In young children and babies many infections are viral, and if the cause is not immediately apparent, it may become so in a few days. Such infections require symptomatic treatment only, with the exception of suspected measles (requiring high-dose vitamin

A supplements). In adults, even when there is likely to be an underlying cause for infection, it is preferable to delay anti-infective treatment until the diagnosis is established, and certainly cultures should always be taken first where possible. In children with neutrophilia who appear unwell there may be a case for giving antibiotics. There are instances where empirical treatment should be started immediately, but treatment has to be guided by the diagnostic and therapeutic options available. For example, it is bad practice to blindly give treatment for malaria unless there are no diagnostic facilities whatsoever. Semi-immune people in endemic areas may have a few detectable malaria parasites circulating harmlessly, with their fever caused by something entirely different. Malaria does not cause a raised neutrophil count, but thrombocytopenia is very common and requires no intervention unless very low with spontaneous bleeding. Empirical treatment should be started immediately for meningitis if the patient is ill (with appropriate symptoms and signs) or if there is going to be a delay in obtaining the results of lumbar puncture. In practice, this usually means treatment with chloramphenicol or a third generation cephalosporin. Similarly, a shocked septicaemic patient will require empirical antibiotics immediately after blood cultures have been taken. Supportive care of such a patient is critical, and in a well-equipped hospital the best evidence favours implementation of the Rivers early goal-directed therapy protocol for sepsis. Rickettsial infection is often a clinical diagnosis; the patient should be treated with tetracycline once investigations have been performed to exclude malaria and typhoid. Dengue fever should be suspected if there is general body pain and severe retro-orbital headache with generalized blanching erythema and a negative malaria film. Treatment is supportive only, and the diagnosis is only established retrospectively when serology is available. The fever should not last longer than 2 weeks and classically has a saddleback pattern. Treatment for pneumonia should be started on clinical grounds, although chest X-ray is certainly helpful. A low threshold for treating severe pharyngitis with penicillin V is reasonable in the tropics, partly because post-streptococcal complications are seen much more frequently, and because the rare but severe Lemierre's syndrome has increased in frequency as antibiotic treatment for sore throat has become unfashionable.

Common causes of fever lasting >2 weeks

The following list contains the most common causes of prolonged fever, simply subdivided according to the most usual WBC picture.

1 Chronic fever with neutrophilia:
- deep sepsis
- amoebic liver abscess
- erythema nodosum leprosum
- cholangitis
- relapsing fever

2 Chronic fever with eosinophilia:
- invasive (toxaemic) *Schistosoma mansoni* and *S. japonicum* infections
- invasive *Fasciola hepatica* infection
- acute lymphangitic exacerbations of *Brugia malayi* and *Wuchereria bancrofti* infections
- gross visceral larva migrans caused by *Toxocara canis*

3 Chronic fever with neutropenia:
- malaria
- disseminated tuberculosis
- visceral leishmaniasis
- brucellosis

4 Chronic fever with normal WBC:
- HIV related (discussed later)
- localized tuberculosis
- brucellosis
- secondary syphilis
- trypanosomiasis
- toxoplasmosis
- bacterial endocarditis
- SLE
- chronic meningococcal septicaemia

5 Chronic fever with a variable WBC picture:
- tumours
- lymphomas
- drug reactions.

Omitted from the list are those conditions where the localizing signs are so obvious that they could not be overlooked, such as pyogenic arthritis.

Fever in HIV-infected patients

The likely cause of fever in HIV infection changes according to the CD4 count, but this piece of information and even HIV serostatus may be unavailable. HIV and/or AIDS in infants and young children presents with a different spectrum of febrile infections compared with adults; often they are simply common childhood infections (e.g. acute respiratory infection, measles, respiratory syncytial virus, chickenpox) but with greater severity and duration. In a recent study in Malawi, it was found that the mortality of perinatally acquired HIV infection reached 89% by 3 years of age in the absence of antiretroviral treatment. Symptoms suggestive of HIV infection in a child are cough, ear discharge, oropharyngeal ulcers, fever and skin rash (when present for >2 weeks). Signs suggestive of HIV infection are malnutrition (wasting and stunting), oral thrush, oropharyngeal ulcers, lymphadenopathy and evidence of pulmonary infection. As in adults, tuberculosis is more common, especially extrapulmonary forms.

Symptoms and signs suggestive of HIV infection in adults are chronic diarrhoea and weight loss, dysphagia (especially when associated with oral thrush), symptomatic sexually transmitted infection, chronic cough and night sweats, herpes zoster (vesicles or scars in dermatomal distribution), oropharyngeal candidiasis, generalized lymphadenopathy and skin lesions suggestive of Kaposi's sarcoma or persistent herpes simplex. Symptomatic HIV seroconversion (a febrile illness reminiscent of infectious mononucleosis, sometimes accompanied by aseptic meningitis) is rarely identified in sub-Saharan Africa. Apart from this initial illness, HIV does not directly cause fever. Fever in early HIV infection may signify underlying pneumococcal pneumonia, tuberculosis (often extrapulmonary), staphylococcal pyomyositis or the onset of herpes zoster, although these infections can still occur in late-stage HIV disease. Once the CD4 count drops below 200×10^6/L,

fever may signify opportunistic infections such as cryptococcosis and toxoplasmosis. Non-typhoid *Salmonella* septicaemia is particularly common. In South East Asia, *Penicillium marneffei* septicaemia may be found on blood culture (pulmonary infiltrates and skin lesions). Histoplasmosis resembles *Penicillium* infection clinically but has a more global distribution. Tuberculosis is a very common finding at postmortem in HIV positive African patients. Disseminated leishmaniasis (chronic fever, splenomegaly, pancytopenia, amastigotes in bone marrow and/or splenic aspirates) is a feature of late-stage HIV infection, being found in Mediterranean patients as well as Africans. *Mycobacterium avium*-complex, *Pneumocystis jirovecii* pneumonia and active CMV infection can all cause fever in African patients in a developed world setting but are less common in sub-Saharan Africa, perhaps because mortality occurs before these manifestations of advanced immunosuppression can become apparent, and diagnostic facilities are lacking. Although the majority of HIV-related fevers are infective, other causes include lymphomas (usually non-Hodgkin's), drug fevers (often accompanied by rash) and immune reconstitution inflammatory syndrome (IRIS). Malaria is statistically associated with a higher parasitaemia and fever in HIV infection (see Chapter 13).

Common clinical problems with febrile patients

Managing a febrile patient with no localizing symptoms or signs and little or no laboratory or radiological back-up is a realistic problem. If the patient is unwell, empirical treatment has to be given. In a malarious area, the first line should be antimalarials, and a significant fall in fever would be expected after 3–4 days. If there is no response, then the next pathogen of importance is typhoid. Empirical treatment with chloramphenicol is appropriate in Africa, but elsewhere resistance is widespread and alternatives such as a fluoroquinolone or a third generation cephalosporin is preferred (Chapter 39). Typhoid fever should respond to appropriate treatment in 4–5 days, but it can take longer if there is low-grade ciprofloxacin resistance or if third gen-eration cephalosporins are used. If there is still no response, empirical antituberculous therapy may be indicated, although regimens containing rifampicin will treat other infections as well as tuberculosis.

Another difficult scenario is a fever (>38.3°C on at least two occasions) which has lasted >4 weeks and has not resolved after at least 3 days of inpatient investigation; that is, pyrexia/fever of unknown origin (PUO or FUO). Such patients should be clinically assessed at regular intervals in case new signs or symptoms come to light. There is very little information regarding underly-ing causes of PUO in the tropics. When PUO in the developed world is investigated, then infec-tion accounts for about one-third of cases (mainly intra-abdominal abscess, tuberculosis, infective endocarditis and complications of HIV infection), neoplasia for 20% (especially lymphoma and occasionally renal cell carcinoma), autoimmune disorders for 10% (e.g. adult Still's disease, tempo-ral arteritis, Wegener's granulomatosis, systemic lupus erythematosus and polyarteritis nodosa), miscellaneous causes for 15% (e.g. drug fever, non-infective granulomatous disorders, haemato-mas, e.g. subdural), and the cause is unknown in 25%. Travel and exposure history, symptoms and signs should guide investigation and laboratory tests. If available, an ultrasound is non-invasive and helpful for demonstrating hepatic disease (e.g. tumour, abscess, schistosomiasis, fascioliasis), splenomegaly, ascites and renal tract disorders. A CT scan of the thorax, abdomen and pelvis is relatively non-invasive and has a high diagnos-tic yield for abscesses, tumours and lymphaden-opathy but is not widely available in the tropics. Other potentially useful investigations include lymph node biopsy (if enlarged), bone marrow aspirate, trephine and culture, and liver biopsy. In the tropics, tuberculosis, osteomyelitis, dental sep-sis, hepatoma and SLE appear more common than in adults with PUO in Europe. There is very little written about PUO affecting babies and children in the tropics, but it is safe to say that infections secondary to HIV-induced immunosuppression

are increasing in importance, and neoplasia is less common than in adults.

PUO in HIV-infected adults in the tropics presents a different spectrum of disease, and is usu-ally associated with a CD4 count <200 × 10⁶/L (Chapter 13). PUO has become less common since the advent of HAART, but the causes of PUO remain essentially unchanged. A series of patients investigated in Brazil found (in descending order): tuberculosis; *Pneumocystis jirovecii*; *Mycobacterium avium* complex; non-Hodgkin's lymphoma; cryp-tococcal meningitis; sinusitis; salmonellosis; his-toplasmosis; neurosyphilis and isosporiasis. A similar investigation in Thailand found tuberculo-sis, *Cryptococcus neoformans*, *Pneumocystis jirovecii*, *Toxoplasma gondii* and salmonella bacteraemia. It is important to note that up to 25% of HIV-infected patients with PUO will have two or more oppor-tunistic infections simultaneously. PUO is associ-ated with a high mortality in HIV infection, so it is unwise to wait the statutory 4 weeks before investi-gating thoroughly. Traditionally, infectious disease physicians have waited to obtain a clear response to treatment of opportunistic infection before ini-tiating ART, because of the complexity of interac-tions and interpreting the side-effects of all the drugs involved with the added difficulty of recog-nizing IRIS. Evidence now suggests that better out-comes are obtained if ART is started earlier rather than later in such patients.

Finally, there are many exotic and uncommon infective causes of fever. Some, like trypanosomia-sis, *Borrelia recurrentis* and babesiosis, will show up unexpectedly on examination of the blood film. Others have to be thought of and deliberately sought, such as bartonellosis, *Borrelia burgdorferi* and Q fever.

Further reading

Rivers EP, Ahrens T. Improving outcomes for severe sepsis and septic shock: tools for early detection of at-risk patients and treatment pro-tocol implementation. *Crit Care Clin* 2008; 24: S1–47.

Chapter 5

Dermatological presentations

Skin disease is ubiquitous among the poor of underdeveloped countries. Bacterial infections often secondary to insect bites or scabies are particularly likely in childhood, and superficial fungal infections, especially pityriasis versicolor, are present in many adults. Several of the major tropical diseases also have skin manifestations and it is essential that the clinician should not miss the diagnosis of leprosy.

Whenever possible take a systematic history that includes details of any travel, contact with insects or sensitizing agents, use of drugs or skin applications, similar rashes in family or contacts, and the evolution of the skin problem. Examine the entire skin surface together with the scalp and mucous membranes in a good light, and note the character and distribution of all skin lesions, distinguishing the original lesions from modifications caused by scratching or secondary infection.

Skin ulcers

Trauma and insect bites account for many acute skin ulcers but these usually heal quickly. All the causes of chronic ulceration seen in temperate climates (including diabetic ulcers, venous and arterial ulcers) are seen but their frequency is much

Lecture Notes: Tropical Medicine, 6th edition.
By G.V. Gill and N.J. Beeching. Published 2009 by Blackwell Publishing, ISBN: 978-1-4051-8048-1.

less in most young tropical populations. Some of the more important causes of chronic ulcers are given in Table 5.1.

Skin itching

A very wide range of dermatological conditions and health problems may cause itching but in the tropics the most common causes include the following:
• Scabies—typical distribution but burrows often masked by secondary infection
• Insect bites—papular urticaria on exposed surfaces
• Superficial fungal infection—examine scrapings for hyphae after clearing in 10% potassium hydroxide
• Eczema—often a personal or family history of allergy, or recent exposure to drugs or topical sensitizer
• Onchocerciasis—geographical distribution, examine for nodules and take skin snips.

Creeping eruptions

• Larva migrans from dog hookworms form a slowly extending, persistent, itching track most often on the foot or lower leg. Multiple infections cause severe itching
• Track-like lesions from the larvae of some species of *Paragonimus*, *Gnathostoma spinigerum* or from some fly larvae are less common.

Table 5.1 Chronic ulcers

Type of ulcer	Main characteristics	How diagnosis is established
Tropical ulcer	Painful; rapid onset, usually lower leg	Heals on non-specific regimen
Buruli ulcer	Extensive; mainly painless; very deep undermined edges	Finding acid-fast bacilli in edge of ulcer
Cutaneous leishmaniasis	Single or multiple; often with infiltrated edges; not undermined	Amastigotes in edges of lesions. Culture or PCR
Desert sore, veld sore (cutaneous diphtheria)	Usually single, painful onset with vesicle; adherent slough, undermined, paralysis from toxin	Culture, as well as the clinical combination of ulcer with neurological deficit
Tertiary syphilis (gumma)	Chronic, usually painless ulcers on extremity	Serological tests for syphilis. Spirochaetes cannot be found
Tuberculous ulcer	Frank ulcers often follow subcutaneous TB; there may be adjacent cold abscess or evidence of TB elsewhere	Microscopy for AAFB. Culture
Sickle cell disease in adults	Rare in Africa where few adults with the disease survive. Ulcers often symmetrical on lower legs	Patient obviously anaemic and sickling test positive
Dracunculiasis (guinea worm)	The pearly prolapsed uterus is seen early	By identifying the worm or larvae expelled after exposure to water
Trophic ulcer of leprosy	Painless; may be deeply penetrating on the sole	Associated evidence of nerve damage: thick nerves, loss of sensation
Diabetic ulcer	In the tropics usually neuropathic. On soles of feet over bony prominences. Usually painless.	Evidence of neuropathy. Known or newly diagnosed diabetes
Malignant ulcer	Squamous cell carcinoma usually	Biopsy and histology
Mycoses (subcutaneous or deep)	Usually ulcerates within a preformed granulomatous nodule	Biopsy, culture and histology. Microscopy for hyphae and spores

Abbreviations: AAFB, acid- and alcohol-fast bacilli; PCR, polymerase chain reaction; TB, tuberculosis.

• Larva currens is the name given to rapidly moving tracks caused by migrating *Strongyloides stercoralis* larvae. These urticaria-like tracks are found between the neck and the knees, and last for hours, or a day or two only.

Papules

• Milia
• Onchocerciasis
• HIV related
• Scabies
• Insect bites
• Acne

• Cercarial dermatitis
• Tungiasis

Skin nodules

• Furuncle
• Furuncular myiasis
• Leprosy—The nodules are frequently over the ears, eyebrows and face. The diagnosis is readily confirmed by slit skin smears for acid-fast bacilli
• Erythema nodosum resulting from leprosy is sometimes widespread on the body. Tuberculosis, streptococcal infection and sarcoidosis are other causes

• Leishmaniasis—Single or multiple nodules may take months to ulcerate; they are predominant on exposed surfaces but spread along lymphatics also occurs. Diffuse cutaneous leishmaniasis and nodular post-kala-azar dermal leishmaniasis can resemble nodular leprosy

• Kaposi's sarcoma—Chiefly affecting limbs of older persons in endemic areas, but any skin surface and mucosae often with lymph node enlargement in AIDS

• Fungal infections including chromoblasto-mycosis, sporotrichosis, *Histoplasma capsulatum* and *H. duboisii, Paracoccidioides brasiliensis, Penicillium marneffei*. Some are particularly common as secondary infections in the immunosuppressed

• Subcutaneous nodules are a feature of onchocerciasis

• Cysticercosis

• Juxta-articular nodules are found in late yaws

Remember also 'non-tropical' causes such as rheumatoid nodules, gouty tophi and neurofibromata.

Changes in pigmentation

Hypopigmented macules

• Postinflammation and scarring

• Pityriasis versicolor—'Raindrop' patches over trunk with slight scaling

• Leprosy—Loss of sensation; enlarged nerves

• Onchocerciasis—Patches chiefly over shins; nodules and positive skin snips

• Yaws—Mainly affects palms and soles; positive syphilis serology

• Vitiligo—Usually white sometimes hyperpigmented borders; symmetrical; association with autoimmune disease

• Post-kala-azar dermal leishmaniasis

Hyperpigmentation

• Pellagra—Affects sun-exposed skin

• Pregnancy

• Chronic arsenic poisoning—Slaty-grey colour of trunk with small areas of normal skin; hyperkeratosis of palms and soles

• Addison's disease—Look for pigment in oral mucosa

• Hypertrophic lichen planus—Warty patches typically involving calves, forearms and lower back

• Kaposi's sarcoma

Urticaria

Acute urticaria may follow jellyfish stings or other envenomation, contact with plants, arthropods or drugs such as penicillin. The diagnosis of the cause of chronic urticaria can be very difficult because such a wide variety of both internal and external causes may be responsible. Some common causes acquired in the tropics are as follows:

• Papular urticaria from insect bites

• Katayama syndrome in schistosomiasis—Follows freshwater exposure by days to months and associated with cough, wheeze and marked eosinophilia

• Intestinal helminths including roundworms and hookworms, and migrating larvae of *Strongyloides stercoralis*

• Filarial infection

• Drugs

• Food additives

Bullae

Large fluid-filled blisters may result from a variety of causes; some of the more common ones in the tropics include the following:

• Bullous impetigo

• Insect bites

• Sunburn

• Burns and scalds

• Drug eruptions

• Snake bite and other causes of envenoming

• Larva migrans

• Pemphigus including Brazilian pemphigus foliaceous

• Porphyria associated with sun exposure

Petechial rashes

• Meningococcal septicaemia

• Chikungunya infection

- Dengue and dengue haemorrhagic fever
- Viral haemorrhagic fevers including Lassa, Ebola and Crimean-Congo
- Vasculitis including Henoch-Schönlein purpura
- Disseminated intravascular coagulation
- Infective endocarditis

Further reading

Caumes E, Carriere J, Guermonprez G *et al.* Dermatoses associated with travel to tropical countries: a prospective study of the diagnosis and management of 269 patients presenting to a tropical disease unit. *Clin Infect Dis* 1995; 20: 542–548. [A description of travellers with dermatological conditions acquired abroad.]

Hay R, Bendeck SE, Chen C *et al.* Skin diseases. In: Jamison DT, Breman JG, Measham AR *et al*, eds. *Disease Control Priorities in Developing Countries*, 2nd edn. OUP, Oxford 2006: 707–721. [Useful review of prevalence and economic importance of key skin disorders and their treatments. Available free from http://www.dcp2.org/pubs/dcp.]

Naafs B. The skin. In: Parry EPO, Godfrey R, Mabey D, Gill, GV, eds. *Principles of Medicine in Africa*, 3rd edn. Cambridge University Press, Cambridge 2004: 1264–1305.

Saw S-M, Koh D, Adjani MR *et al.* A population-based survey of skin diseases in adolescents and adults in rural Sumatra, Indonesia, 1999. *Trans R Soc Trop Med Hyg* 2001; 95: 384–388. [Gives comparative prevalence data for skin disease in various developing countries.]

Chapter 6

The patient with anaemia

Anaemia is the most common medical condition worldwide, but it is not a diagnosis in itself. Whenever possible the underlying cause should be determined and alleviated to prevent recurrence. It is important to have knowledge of the local causes of ill health as this can help to prioritize investigations and treatment, especially when diagnostic resources are limited. Where schistosomiasis is common this may be a frequent local cause of anaemia, whereas amongst rural farming communities it may be chronic hookworm infestation. In poorer countries the aetiology of anaemia is often multifactorial and exacerbated by poor nutrition and high levels of infections and infestations.

Clinical diagnosis of anaemia

Examination of the degree of pallor of tongue, nails and conjunctiva can provide a reasonable indication of anaemia when it is severe but is not helpful for detecting mild/moderate anaemia. Clinical examination alone is 66% sensitive and 68% specific for haemoglobin levels of 5–8 g/100 mL in Malawian children, and 82% sensitive and 65% specific for haemoglobin levels

of <7 g/100 mL in pregnant women in Kenya. A laboratory test to estimate haemoglobin levels is therefore necessary to detect and guide treatment of mild/moderate anaemia and to prevent the development of severe anaemia. A good clinical history and examination are essential in determining the cause of anaemia (Box 6.1).

> **Box 6.1 History and examination of the anaemic patient**
>
> **Enquire about:**
> - Symptoms of hypotension/heart failure/anaemia
> - Diet (specifically iron and folate content)
> - Blood loss (from gastrointestinal, urogenital or gynaecological systems)
> - Childhood or family history of haemoglobinopathy
> - Chronic diseases
> - Tendency to bleed or excessive infections (suggesting bone marrow dysfunction)
>
> **Examine for:**
> - Heart failure/postural hypotension
> - Pallor
> - Jaundice
> - Fever
> - Spoon-shaped nails
> - Skeletal abnormalities (suggesting haemoglobinopathy)
> - Splenomegaly
> - Tuberculosis and other chronic disorders
> - Petechiae, lymphadenopathy, gum infiltration (suggesting leukaemia)

Lecture Notes: Tropical Medicine, 6th edition.
By G.V. Gill and N.J. Beeching. Published 2009 by Blackwell Publishing, ISBN: 978-1-4051-8048-1.

Laboratory investigations

At smaller hospitals, the laboratory may provide tests such as haemoglobin, blood film examination and malaria slide microscopy. It may also offer a transfusion service. Accurate haemoglobin estimation and a good blood film examination will enable the diagnosis and cause of anaemia to be established in the majority of cases. Features on the blood film can indicate the presence of iron or folate deficiency, haemoglobinopathies, enzymopathies and malignant or proliferative haematological disorders. Well-resourced hospitals may be able to estimate ferritin, folate and vitamin B_{12} levels, perform haemoglobin electrophoresis, examine bone marrow samples and carry out a range of other tests including endoscopy to determine the cause of anaemia.

Measurement of haemoglobin

Although haemoglobin estimation is the most commonly performed laboratory test and is used to guide blood transfusions, it is also one of the least accurate. The reference method for haemoglobin, the haemoglobin cyanide method, requires a spectrophotometer and well-supervised and qualified technicians, and the cyanide buffer is increasingly difficult to source. Any method that depends on manual dilution of the sample (e.g. Sahli, Lovibond) requires careful pipette technique to maintain accuracy. The HemoCue Hb 301 system has been designed specifically for tropical countries and provides rapid, accurate results directly from a finger-prick sample. The haemoglobin colour scale also uses finger-prick blood, is rapid and cheap and is probably better than clinical diagnosis for detecting mild/moderate anaemia. It is essential that clinicians satisfy themselves that their laboratory's results are reliable before using haemoglobin measurements to guide patient management. Test performance can be improved through participation in an external quality monitoring scheme, which may simply comprise exchanging samples between neighbouring laboratories. Other ways of maintaining the quality of results include the following:
• Repeat testing of the same sample with each batch of tests.

• Compare packed cell volume (PCV) with haemoglobin results (PCV should be approximately three times the haemoglobin value).
• Plot weekly cumulative averages of haemoglobin results to determine any 'drifting' of results.
• Ensure that reagents are within their shelf life, technical staff are qualified and regularly supervised, and the method in use is appropriate for the level of health care and local infrastructure.

Examination of peripheral blood film

If the cause of anaemia remains elusive after basic investigations, determining whether the anaemia is microcytic, macrocytic or normocytic (using the mean corpuscular volume [MCV] from a haematology analyzer) will narrow down the possibilities.

Microcytic anaemia

The most common cause of microcytic anaemia is iron deficiency (Figure 6.1). Questions should be asked about blood loss and dietary insufficiency; stool examination for parasites and occult blood, and endoscopic examination of the gastrointestinal tract to exclude occult malignancy, may be required. The thalassaemias also cause microcytosis, but the clinical setting and further investigations such as haemoglobin electrophoresis demonstrating raised HbA_2 and HbF may help to confirm the diagnosis. Thalassaemia trait may be particularly difficult to diagnose and referral to a specialist centre may be necessary. If the patient presents with mixed microcytic and macrocytic anaemia, nutritional deficiency of both iron and folate is likely.

Macrocytic anaemia

A high mean cell volume with oval macrocytes and hypersegmented neutrophils (Figure 6.2) is highly suggestive of folate or vitamin B_{12} deficiency (Chapter 57). A high MCV may also indicate the presence of early red cells. These may be produced in response to blood loss or destruction, or in response to haematinics, and can be detected

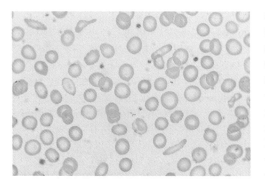

Figure 6.1 Iron-deficient red cells. The cells are paler and more irregular in shape than normal red cells. From Bain B. *Blood Cells: A Practical Guide*, 3rd edn. Oxford: Blackwell Publishing, 2002.

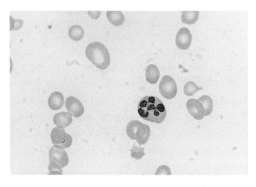

Figure 6.2 Oval macrocytes and hypersegmented neutrophils in folate deficiency. (From Bain B. *Blood Cells: A Practical Guide*, 3rd edn. Blackwell Publishing, Oxford, 2002.)

non-haematological disease. Investigations should include screening for renal disease, infections, autoimmune diseases and neoplasia. In the presence of anaemia, a lack of polychromasia and reticulocytes suggests failure of erythropoiesis due to true or functional lack of haematinics, or bone marrow suppression. A combination of fever, anaemia and thrombocytopenia may indicate acute leukaemia and a blood film should be examined urgently for the presence of blasts. Examination of the bone marrow may be helpful to detect aplastic anaemia, infiltrations, infections (e.g. tuberculosis) or myelodysplastic syndrome. Bone marrow examination is not always necessary for the diagnosis of leukaemia as immunophenotyping can be performed on the abnormal peripheral blood.

Management of anaemia in the absence of a laboratory

At health centres without laboratory facilities, the management of anaemia will be guided by knowledge of the locally prevalent diseases. Good clinical skills are essential to elicit relevant information and to detect possible causes. Mild anaemia is likely to be missed if haemoglobin cannot be measured (for management of anaemia see Box 6.2).

In children under 5 years in malaria-endemic regions, local policy may recommend treating all fevers as malaria. The majority of these children

as polychromatic cells on a peripheral blood film. A specific stain can be used to confirm that these cells are reticulocytes. A high MCV can also be associated with alcohol excess and liver disease, or drugs such as hydroxycarbamide, stavudine or zidovudine. A combination of red cell fragments, thrombocytopenia and polychromasia on the blood film indicates microangiopathic haemolytic anaemia and the need for further tests such as coagulation studies, assessment of renal function and a search for infection or neoplastic disease.

Normocytic anaemia

Normochromic normocytic anaemia is usually caused by inflammation or an underlying chronic

---

Box 6.2 Suggested management of anaemia if no laboratory tests are available

• Give iron, folate and antihelmintics and monitor response (clinically detectable improvement should occur within 4 weeks and the haemoglobin should rise at the rate of 0.5–1.0 g/100 mL each week).

• Continue iron for at least 3 months after normal haemoglobin is achieved.

• If acute life-threatening haemolysis is suspected (anaemia with jaundice and dark urine) and there is no obvious cause or underlying infection, a trial of folate and prednisolone 0.5–1 mg/kg (1–2 weeks) may be worthwhile until transfer to a higher level facility can be arranged.

• If still no response, refer to specialist centre.

are also anaemic and their consultation at the health centre should be used as an opportunity to detect and treat anaemia and any underlying conditions and also to provide relevant education for the child's carer.

Blood transfusion in developing countries

Blood transfusions should only be given for specific clinical indications and in accordance with local or international guidelines (Box 6.3). Transfusions carry serious risks of transmitting infections such as HIV and hepatitis B and C, and can also be responsible for acute and delayed immune reactions. These risks are increased in laboratories without rigorous quality-checking processes. Although international guidelines stipulate that blood for transfusion should be donated by

---

Box 6.3 Prescribing blood: a checklist for clinicians

Always ask yourself the following questions before prescribing blood or blood products for a patient.
1 What improvement in the patient's clinical condition am I aiming to achieve?
2 Can I minimize blood loss to reduce this patient's need for transfusion?
3 Are there any other treatments I should give before making the decision to transfuse, such as intravenous replacement fluids or oxygen?
4 What are the specific clinical or laboratory indications for transfusion in this patient?
5 What are the risks of transmitting HIV, hepatitis, syphilis or other infectious agents through the blood products that are available for this patient?
6 Do the benefits of transfusion outweigh the risks for this particular patient?
7 What other options are there if no blood is available in time?
8 Will a trained person monitor this patient and respond immediately if any acute transfusion reactions occur?
9 Have I recorded my decision and reasons for transfusion on the patient's chart and the blood request form?
Finally, if in doubt, ask yourself the following question.
 If this blood was for myself or my child, would I accept the transfusion in these circumstances?

---

voluntary donors, many blood transfusions in developing countries are donated by family members and hospitals that have no, or very little, blood stocks for emergency use. The problem has been worsened by the increasing prevalence of HIV infection amongst potential blood donors. Patients with severe anaemia, usually children with malaria or obstetric emergencies, need blood transfusion rapidly as an emergency life-saving measure. Before prescribing blood transfusions, clinicians need to carefully balance the risks and benefits. They should satisfy themselves that all other options, such as intravenous fluids and haematinics, have been excluded. Transfusions should only be used as a last resort.

Further reading

Cheesbrough M. *District Laboratory Practice in Tropical Countries*. Volume 2, 2nd edn. Cambridge, UK: Tropical Health Technology, 2006. [Widely recognized as a leading standard laboratory manual for developing countries. Clearly written and well illustrated with basic explanations of rationale and principles of tests.]

Critchley J, Bates I. Haemoglobin colour scale for anaemia diagnosis where there is no laboratory: a systematic review. *Int J Epidemiol* 2005; 34: 1425–1434. [Review of techniques used for anaemia diagnosis where there is no laboratory with focus on haemoglobin colour scale.]

World Health Organization. Methods Recommended for Essential Clinical Chemistry and Haematological Tests for Intermediate Hospital Laboratories. WHO/LAB/86.3, 1986. [Provides information about recommended validated methods and standards for tests used in diagnosis and management of common conditions including anaemia.]

World Health Organization. The Clinical Use of Blood. WHO/BTS/99.2, 1999. [Provides prescribers of blood with information to assist them to make appropriate decisions about the use of blood and to avoid unnecessary transfusions. A pocket handbook is available to accompany this publication.]

Chapter 7

A syndromic approach to sexually transmitted infections

The global prevalence of chronic viral sexually transmitted infections (STIs) is likely to be over a billion. In some populations, almost every adult has either active or latent infection with viruses such as genital herpes virus, genital human papilloma virus (HPV), hepatitis B or HIV. In addition, in 2005 the WHO estimated that the incidence of curable bacterial STIs such as gonorrhoea, chlamydia and syphilis was 340 million annually. In view of this, it is hardly surprising that the management of individuals with STIs and the consequences thereof constitutes the bulk of the outpatient workload in high-prevalence settings.

The need for a public health approach

The rapid spread of the HIV epidemic has renewed interest in the early detection and treatment of curable STIs. From early on in the HIV epidemic, it was clear that STIs have a role in the spread of HIV. Individuals with recurrent presentations of genital ulcer or discharge were shown to be at a higher risk of acquiring HIV. In addition, HIV-infected individuals with an ulcer or discharge were found to have higher rates of viral

shedding of HIV and therefore to be more infectious to partners. Because rates of shedding revert to lower levels after treatment, the appropriate management of STIs reduces the risk of HIV transmission. It makes sense, therefore, to include STI management as an HIV prevention strategy. Currently, however, the public health benefits of this approach have not been realized on a large scale.

Syndromic management

In 1991, the WHO developed a system of syndromic management for STIs. The aim was effective management of STIs in resource-poor countries with high prevalence rates of STIs. The emphasis was on an integrated approach at primary healthcare centres with no requirement for specialist clinics, highly trained personnel or laboratory facilities. Syndromic management is based on the identification of consistent groups of symptoms and easily recognized signs (syndromes) (Table 7.1). A patient with an STI syndrome presents to a health facility for care and the practitioner has merely to tell the difference between a genital ulcer and a discharge. Once identified, a step-by-step flow chart guides the practitioner. A single course of treatment is provided at the first clinic visit, which deals with the majority of the organisms responsible for producing each syndrome in a given area.

Lecture Notes: Tropical Medicine, 6th edition.
By G.V. Gill and N.J. Beeching. Published 2009 by Blackwell Publishing, ISBN: 978-1-4051-8048-1.

Table 7.1 Some common syndromes and their aetiologies

Syndrome	Infectious causes	Aetiological agent[a]	Non-infectious causes
Urethral discharge	Gonococcal urethritis	***Neisseria gonorrhoeae***	Physiological
	Non-gonococcal (NSU)	No aetiology (25%)	Trauma
		Chlamydia trachomatis (most of the rest)	
		Ureaplasma urealyticum	
		Trichomonas vaginalis	
		Candida albicans	
	Intra-urethral ulcers or warts	Herpes simplex	
		HPV	
Vaginal discharge	Vaginal infections	*C. albicans*	Physiological, trauma,
		Gardnerella vaginalis	retained products,
		T. vaginalis	tampons
	Cervical infections	***C. trachomatis***	Carcinoma of cervix
		N. gonorrhoeae	(linked with HPV
		Herpes simplex	infection)
		HPV	
		Treponema pallidum	
Genital ulcer			
Multiple and painful	Herpetic	Herpes simplex	Behçet's disease
	Chancroid	*Haemophilus ducreyi*	Stevens–Johnson
	Scabies	*Sarcoptes scabiei*	syndrome
Single and painful	TB	*Mycobacterium tuberculosis*	Carcinoma
	Superinfection of painless ulcers	***Staphylococcus aureus***	
Multiple and painless	Secondary syphilis	*T. pallidum*	
Single and painless	Primary syphilis	*T. pallidum*	
	LGV	*C. trachomatis* (LGV strains)	
	Granuloma inguinale	*Calymmatobacterium granulomatis*	
Bubo			
Genital ulcer visible	Chancroid	*H. ducreyi*	
No genital ulcer visible	LGV	*C. trachomatis*	
Non-sexually transmitted infections	Plague		
	Filariasis		
	Infections of the lower limb		

Abbreviations: HPV, human papilloma virus; LGV, lymphogranuloma venereum; NSU, non-specific urethritis; TB, tuberculosis.
[a]Bold italic indicates infections targeted by syndromic management.

Local adaptations

Local data on aetiology and bacterial sensitivity patterns must be taken into consideration when designing a flow chart. For example, penicillin resistance amongst *Neisseria gonorrhoeae* is on the increase globally. In some countries, as many as 50% of gonorrhoea cases are resistant to penicillin. This represents a major threat to the cheap and effective treatment of urethral and cervical discharge syndromes. Moreover, as in the treatment of pneumococcal disease, penicillin resistance is associated with resistance to multiple antibiotics including macrolides. The inevitable consequence has been therapeutic failures and higher priced therapies such as ciprofloxacin being included in syndromic management.

The successful implementation of syndromic management programmes requires that the appropriate drugs be accessible, available and affordable. Unfortunately, many of the antibiotics used for the treatment of STIs in the West (such as quinolones) are too expensive for STI control programmes or individuals to afford in resource-poor countries. The choice of drugs in most countries is therefore often a compromise between what is affordable and what is therapeutically

required. Drugs are generally dispensed at health centre level where other more urgent conditions may put demands on supplies originally intended for STI treatment only. Ensuring that the supply of STI drugs is used for the treatment of STIs, and guarding it against drug theft are additional challenges for a strained system.

Each country, therefore, has a slightly different flow chart validated in its own setting according to local prevalence and incidence rates of STIs. This chapter contains simplified versions of the WHO flow charts in use that manage the following common clinical situations:
- urethral discharge syndrome in men (Figure 7.1);
- vaginal discharge (Figure 7.2);
- lower abdominal pain in women (Figure 7.3);
- genital ulcer disease (Figure 7.4).

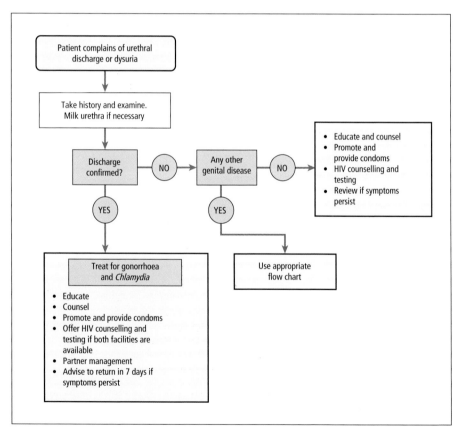

Figure 7.1 Urethral discharge in men.

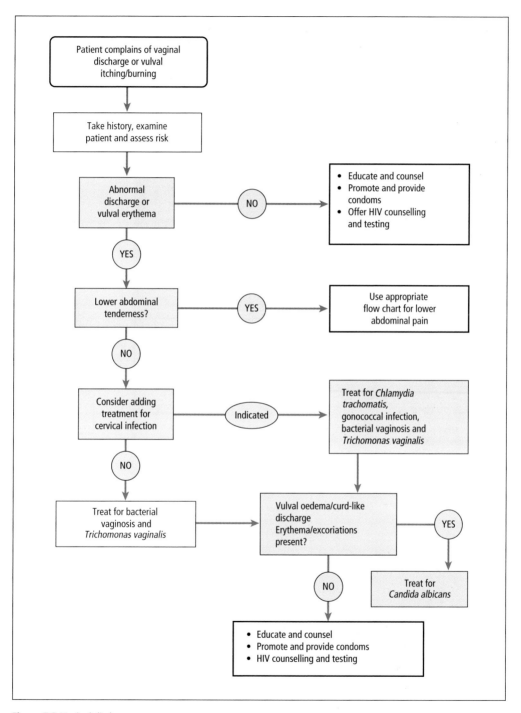

Figure 7.2 Vaginal discharge.

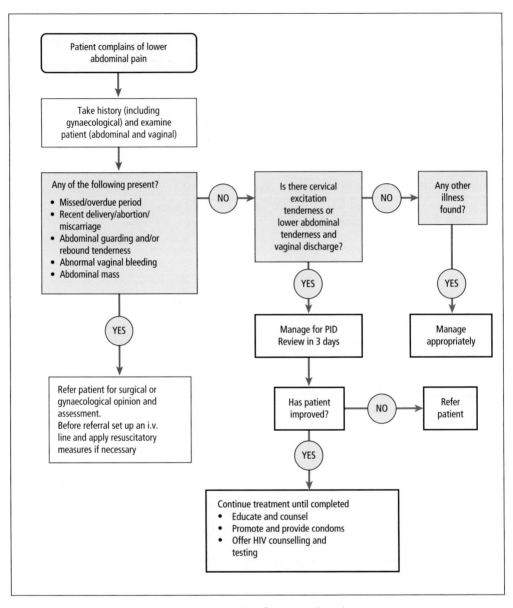

Figure 7.3 Lower abdominal pain in women. (PID = pelvic inflammatory disease)

How to use the flow charts

1 Symptoms determine which flow chart to select. Patients should be specifically asked about the onset of symptoms and whether the condition is associated with pain.

2 Signs indicate the likelihood of pathology. Patients must be examined for the presence of ulcers; in males the urethra milked for discharge, and in females a bimanual examination should be performed. Speculum examination of the cervix should be performed if available, as a cervix that bleeds easily when touched or a mucopurulent discharge from the cervix are indications for which treatment for cervical infection should be added.

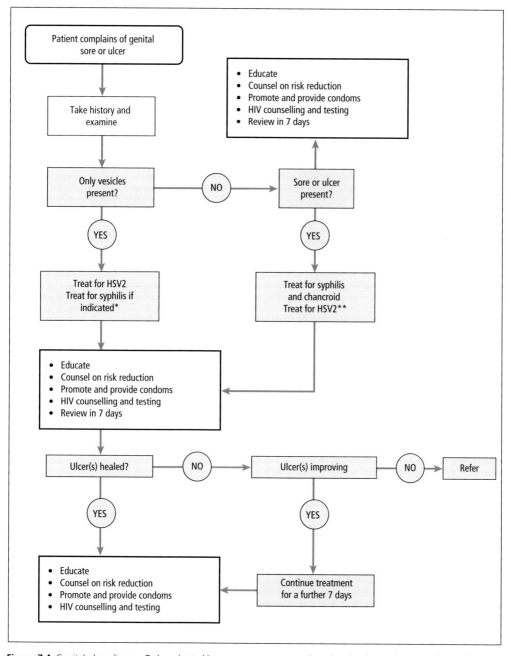

Figure 7.4 Genital ulcer disease. To be adapted by programme manager based on local prevalence. *Indication for syphilis treatment; RPR positive and no recent syphilis treatment. **Treat for HSV2 where prevalence is 30% or higher, or adapt to local conditions.

3 Investigations are limited in many settings. If a microscope is available, a Gram's stain provides a sensitive indicator of gonococcal infection in urethral discharge. A wet mount from the vaginal specimen will reveal *Candida albicans*, *Trichomonas vaginalis* and clue cells of bacterial vaginosis. However, investigation with microscopy does not improve the sensitivity and specificity of the flow charts for lower abdominal pain and vaginal discharge in women. To identify women at greater risk of cervical infection, questions have been added about partners' symptoms, sex work and whether the woman feels she has been exposed to an STI. Laboratory-assisted diagnosis is rarely helpful in genital ulcer disease as mixed infections are common.

4 Management should be guided by the local guidelines. Alternatives are recommended on the locally produced flow charts for patients with allergies. Special circumstances such as pregnancy are also covered. In general, quinolones are recommended to treat gonorrhoea and tetracyclines to cover chlamydial infection. Concurrent therapy for *Chlamydia* and gonorrhoea should be given to all patients with gonorrhoea, as dual infection is common. Although the treatment of choice for syphilis remains intramuscular benzylpenicillin, the penicillins and tetracyclines have no place in the treatment of chancroid due to widespread resistance in all geographical areas. To cover chancroid, a quinolone or macrolide must be added.

5 Some patients fail to respond to treatment. The likeliest causes are reinfection from partner, poor compliance or drug resistance. In the case of persistent urethral discharge, *T. vaginalis* should be considered before referral, as there are high-prevalence rates in some geographical settings. In the case of genital ulcer disease, if symptoms persist after adequate treatment of the index case and partner, the patient should be referred to rule out other causes, including chronic viral STIs, coinfection with HIV, carcinoma or a non-sexually transmitted disease. Where prevalence rates of HIV infection are high, a large number of genital ulcers are likely to be brought about by atypical herpes simplex virus infection.

The 'four Cs' of syndromic management

One of the greatest barriers to the successful implementation of syndromic management has been the attitude of healthcare workers. Training on the use of flow charts, therefore, always includes training on basic counselling skills. This is the first 'C'. Emphasis in training is also put on contact tracing, compliance and condoms.

Advantages of syndromic management

The syndromic approach to STI management is simple and problem orientated and can be integrated into existing health facilities without requiring specialist clinics, doctors or nurses. It allows for rapid diagnosis and treatment of the individual at the first visit, thus saving resources for the client and the provider, and improving surveillance. Flow charts developed for the treatment of urethral discharge in men are robust and well validated in numerous settings. Cases of genital ulcer disease resulting from chancroid and syphilis have dropped dramatically in Nairobi, Kenya as a result of intensive syndromic management in high-risk cohorts. Studies of a population-wide approach to syndromic management in Mwanza, Tanzania showed a 42% reduction in rural HIV incidence rates in those receiving access to syndromic management of STIs. However, reduction of HIV incidence was not demonstrated in a study conducted in neighbouring Rakai district in Uganda where a similar cohort was enrolled in a mass STI treatment campaign. A closer analysis of the two data sets reveals different baseline HIV and gonococcal prevalence rates as well as different risk behaviour levels. Syndromic management is therefore most likely to influence HIV incidence in areas with high levels of risk behaviour and low prevalence of HIV.

Disadvantages of syndromic management

The focus on syndromic management has public health limitations. The main disadvantage is that the uninfected are not targeted, and therefore asymptomatic infections are not detected and there is no provision for screening. In addition, there is insufficient emphasis on partner notification and a lost opportunity to promote condom use and provide information on STIs. The approach relies entirely on the self-presentation of those who perceive themselves to have symptoms. In the majority of settings, the flow charts have a low sensitivity and specificity for cervical gonococcal and chlamydial infections in symptomatic women. This frequently leads to overtreatment of the individual and possible increased rates of antibiotic resistance. A lack of consideration of the differential diagnoses is commonplace.

The design of STI control programmes in the tropics has been much enhanced by the widespread use of the syndromic management approach. However, programmes need to combine the simple management of syndromes with interventions that target the general population, promote condoms and educate on other prevention methods. Levels of appropriate health-seeking behaviour are low (Figure 7.5). Work in the community and with healthcare workers themselves is therefore needed to challenge stigma, gender roles and myths surrounding STIs. Partner notification and treatment are essential to interrupt the chain of transmission and prevent reinfection, and programmes should be accompanied by access to other services such as counselling and testing. Efforts to improve partner notification should be voluntary and ensure

the confidentiality of patients and their partners, as fear of rejection and domestic violence are very real concerns that underlie poor rates of partner notification recorded in many programmes. Good STI management challenges traditional views of medicine as clinicians work closely with public health specialists and all sectors of the community for it to be a success.

HIV testing in STI clinics

Coinfection with HIV should be excluded as part of routine practice in STI management. New guidance on provider-initiated HIV testing and counselling in many countries allows for rapid HIV testing to be conducted by trained personnel in STI clinics. This is of particular importance where the client is unaware of their status, and other forms of client-initiated testing (often called voluntary counselling and testing or [VCT]) are unavailable. Knowledge of HIV status allows appropriate referral to HIV treatment and care as well risk reduction counselling and behaviour change (see Chapter 13). To maximize uptake STI, clinics should operate an 'opt-out' policy on HIV testing.

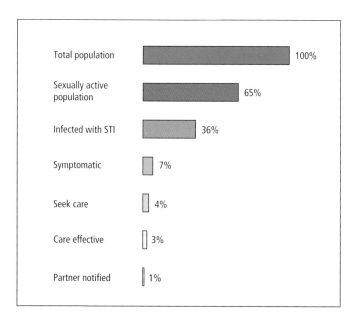

Figure 7.5 Operational model of treatment-seeking behaviour of STI patients.

Further reading

Dallabetta G, Laga M, Lamptey P *et al. Control of Sexually Transmitted Diseases: A Handbook for the Design and Management of Programmes.* Arlington: AIDSCAP/Family Health International, 2001. [This manual was developed primarily for programme managers in resource-poor settings.]

Grosskurth H, Mosha F, Todd J *et al.* Impact of improved treatment of sexually transmitted diseases on HIV infection in Tanzania: randomized, controlled trial. *Lancet* 1995; 346: 530–536. [Showed a 42% reduction in HIV incidence following effective syndromic management.]

Mayaud P, Ndowa F, Richens J, Mabey D. Sexually transmitted infections. In: Parry EPO, Godfrey R, Mabey D, Gill GV, eds. *Principles of Medicine in Africa*, 3rd edn. Cambridge: Cambridge University Press, 2004: 241–283. [A detailed and exhaustive chapter on the modern approach to tropical sexually transmitted diseases (STDs).]

Wawer M, Sewankambo N, Serwadda D *et al.* Control of sexually transmitted diseases for AIDS prevention in Uganda: a randomized community trial. *Lancet* 1999; 353: 525–535. [Showed a reduction in some STIs, but no significant reduction in HIV incidence despite mass treatment.]

Wisdom A. *A Colour Atlas of Sexually Transmitted Disease.* London: ELBS edition, 1992. [Available at low cost and still popular after all these years.]

www.who.int/Reproductive_health. [Useful source for the latest guidelines for the management of sexually transmitted infections with several flow charts that can be downloaded.]

Chapter 8

Splenomegaly in the tropics

Enlarged spleens are common in tropical practice. The disorders that cause splenomegaly in temperate regions are also present in the tropics but, in addition, there is a heavy burden of infections and parasitic infestations. The spleen responds to this by augmenting its major physiological functions of phagocytosis and antibody production. The subsequent splenic enlargement is particularly common in children living in areas of high malaria transmission, where the rates of splenomegaly are used as an indicator of transmission intensity in the population. Where transmission is intense, the 'spleen rate' may reach 100% in children and then decline to less than 10% in adults as they acquire clinical malarial immunity. In areas with stable endemic malaria, adults' spleens are about twice as large as those in non-malarious areas.

Reasons for enlarged spleens

Spleens can enlarge
- in response to a need for excess physiological activity (e.g. phagocytosis of abnormal red cells as in haemoglobinopathies; antibody production to combat infection); and
- because of a structural abnormality (e.g. portal hypertension; infiltration by malignant cells).

Lecture Notes: Tropical Medicine, 6th edition.
By G.V. Gill and N.J. Beeching. Published 2009 by Blackwell Publishing, ISBN: 978-1-4051-8048-1.

The degree to which the spleen enlarges depends on the underlying cause, but in most cases the spleen size rarely exceeds 10 cm when measured from the left costal margin to the spleen tip. Acutely enlarged spleens are often tender and soft on examination and are associated with a higher risk of rupture than chronically enlarged spleens which tend to be firmer and more fibrous. Conditions in which the spleen may be moderately (<10 cm) enlarged include chronic haemolysis (e.g. recurrent malaria, haemoglobinopathies, spherocytosis), portal hypertension and haematological malignancies such as chronic lymphocytic leukaemia, lymphomas, acute leukaemias and myeloproliferative disorders.

Massive tropical splenomegaly

The most common causes of massive splenomegaly in the tropics are hyper-reactive malarial splenomegaly (formerly called tropical splenomegaly syndrome), lymphomas, schistosomiasis, visceral leishmaniasis, haemoglobinopathies, chronic myeloid leukaemia, myelofibrosis and miscellaneous disorders such as splenic cysts, tumours and lipid storage diseases (Figure 8.1). Although massive splenomegaly has been reported to be common in many tropical African countries there are few data available on prevalence. Published rates in Africa vary from 1–2% in Nigeria to 0.4–1.2% in Gambia. The highest prevalence of massive

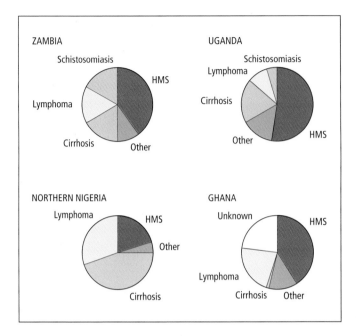

Figure 8.1 Causes of massive splenomegaly in various African countries.

splenomegaly is in Papua New Guinea where up to 80% of some ethnic groups are affected by hyper-reactive malarial splenomegaly. The diagnosis and management of most of the conditions associated with massive splenomegaly are discussed elsewhere in this book.

Hyper-reactive malarial splenomegaly

Hyper-reactive malarial splenomegaly is caused by an abnormal response to repeated malarial infections that results in overproduction of immunoglobulin M (IgM). The consequent immune complexes are removed by the spleen, which can enlarge to huge proportions (Figure 8.2). The disorder is more common in women and predominantly affects those aged between 20 and 40 years. Patients are surprisingly asymptomatic but eventually develop symptoms of anaemia, malaise and abdominal discomfort. Pregnant women with hyper-reactive malarial splenomegaly commonly experience sudden episodes of haemolysis which may be life-threatening. A mild

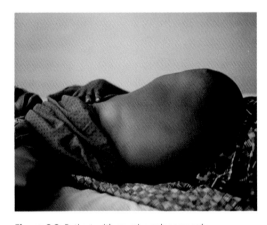

Figure 8.2 Patient with massive splenomegaly.

reduction in platelets and white cells secondary to hypersplenism is common in hyper-reactive malarial splenomegaly and almost all patients have anaemia and hepatomegaly.

Criteria for diagnosis include splenomegaly over 10 cm from the left costal margin and a sustained reduction in spleen size of at least 40% on anti-malarial treatment. Differentiation from splenic involvement by lymphoma may be difficult without sophisticated techniques, but a diagnosis of hyper-reactive malarial splenomegaly is more likely if the patient is under 40 years of age and has a peripheral blood lymphocyte count of less than 10×10^9/L. Lifelong treatment is necessary as hyper-reactive malarial splenomegaly may recur if treatment is stopped. Proguanil 100mg/day is the drug of choice as it is safe for continued use over many years. On this treatment the haemoglobin increases and the spleen slowly shrinks although it may never become impalpable.

Splenectomy in the tropics

The indications for splenectomy in tropical practice are similar to those in temperate regions but the balance between risk and benefit may be altered by the lack of blood products, intensive care and other support services in poorer countries. Elective splenectomy for patients with enlarged spleens in Uganda had an early postoperative mortality of 4.8%. Particular risks of splenectomy in tropical countries include the following:

• Larger spleens make the procedure technically difficult.

• Hypersplenism leads to reduced platelet counts with increased risk of peri-operative bleeding. The risk of morbidity from haemorrhage is exacerbated by the lack of emergency blood supplies and platelet transfusions.

• Increased susceptibility to bacterial infections, especially encapsulated organisms. Septicaemia with these organisms can be associated with disseminated intravascular coagulation, which has a mortality of 50–80% in established cases. Lifelong antibiotic prophylaxis and vaccination for *Haemophilus influenza* type b, *Neisseria meningitidis* and *Streptococcus pneumoniae* should be given if available.

• Very few data are available about the risk of malarial infection post-splenectomy. It is likely that the risk is less if the individual acquired malarial immunity at an early age and has been a long-term resident in a malarious area.

To reduce the risk of post-splenectomy infections, a partial rather than total splenectomy could be performed, leaving a portion of spleen with arterial structures *in situ*.

Further reading

Bedu Addo G, Bates I. Causes of massive tropical splenomegaly in Ghana. *Lancet* 2002; 360: 449–454. [Review of causes of massive splenomegaly in tropical, malaria-endemic country determined using current technology.]

Doherty T, Mabey D. The spleen. In: Parry EPO, Godfrey R, Mabey D, Gill GV, eds. *Principles of Medicine in Africa,* 3rd edn. Cambridge: Cambridge University Press, 2004: 1026–1029.

Part 2

Major Tropical Infections

Chapter 9

Malaria

Importance and distribution

Malaria is the most important of all tropical parasitic diseases, causing many deaths and much morbidity. It is widely distributed in the tropical and subtropical zones. There are four parasite species that commonly cause human malaria, all of which belong to the genus *Plasmodium*. In order of their prevalence worldwide, these are *Plasmodium falciparum* (the cause of nearly all of the deaths due to malaria), *P. vivax*, *P. malariae* and *P. ovale*. *P. knowlesi,* a primate parasite, is increasingly recognised as a fifth cause of human malaria in parts of South East Asia.

A malarial infection can occasionally be transferred directly from one person to another by blood transfusion, accidental inoculation or across the placenta. However, transmission usually depends on an insect vector, in which the parasite spends several weeks undergoing the sexual part of its life cycle.

Life cycle (Figure 9.1)

Malaria is usually transmitted by the bite of an infected female anopheline mosquito. The infecting agent is the sporozoite, a microscopic spindle-shaped cell which is in the mosquito's saliva.

Lecture Notes: Tropical Medicine, 6th edition.
By G.V. Gill and N.J. Beeching. Published 2009 by
Blackwell Publishing, ISBN: 978-1-4051-8048-1.

Thousands of sporozoites may be injected in a single bite. The sporozoites disappear from the blood within 8 h and the successful ones enter the liver cells. The process by which the malaria parasites multiply asexually is called schizogony—whether this takes place in a hepatocyte or in an erythrocyte.

Inside the liver cell, the sporozoite divides asexually by fission to form a cyst-like structure called a pre-erythrocytic (PE) schizont, which contains tens of thousands of merozoites. Each merozoite consists of a small mass of nuclear chromatin within a tiny sphere of cytoplasm. When the PE schizont is mature, it ruptures and liberates its contained merozoites. These merozoites now enter the bloodstream to penetrate red cells.

The time between the bite of the infecting mosquito and the appearance of parasites in the blood is the prepatent period. It is 7–30 days in *P. falciparum* (usually around 10 days) and longer in the other species. Only in the case of *P. vivax* and *P. ovale*, some hepatic-stage parasites may persist in a dormant form or *hypnozoite* which may then resume replication after a period of months or years to cause relapses of malaria.

Merozoites, released into the bloodstream from hepatic PE schizonts, attach themselves to red cells by means of surface receptors. The parasite then penetrates the red cell and resides in a vacuole with a lining derived from the red cell surface. Here the parasite grows, feeding on the haemoglobin of the

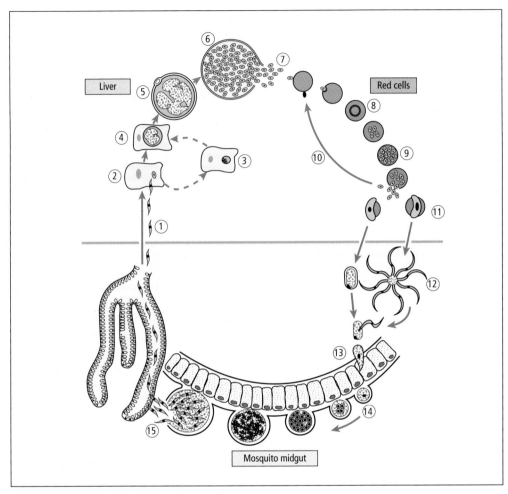

Figure 9.1 Malaria life cycle. 1, Sporozoites, injected through the skin by female anopheline mosquito; 2, sporozoites infect hepatocytes; 3, some sporozoites develop into 'hypnozoites' (*Plasmodium vivax* and *P. ovale* only); 4, liver-stage parasite develops; 5–6, tissue schizogony; 7, merozoites are released into the circulation; 8, ring-stage trophozoites in red cells; 9, erythrocytic schizogony; 10, merozoites invade other red cells; 11, some parasites develop into female (macro-) or male (micro-) gametocytes, taken up by mosquito; 12, mature macrogametocyte and exflagellating microgametes; 13, ookinete penetrates gut wall; 14, development of oocyst; 15, sporozoites penetrate salivary glands. (Reproduced with permission from Zaman V. *Atlas of Medical Parasitology*. Australia: ADIS Press, 1978.)

erythrocyte, and after about 24–36 h it begins a second episode of asexual division or 'blood schizogony', this time resulting in 12–24 merozoites per infected erythrocyte. Schizogony occurs in the circulating blood in the cases of *P. vivax*, *P. ovale* and *P. malariae*, so in all these infections schizonts are commonly seen in the peripheral blood films of infected patients. In *P. falciparum*,

schizogony occurs only in capillaries deep within the body. At the stage of the maturing trophozoite, parasite antigens are expressed on the surface of the red cell. Some of these antigens are capable of linking to receptors expressed on the endothelial cells lining capillaries in various organs and tissues of the body. The resulting cytoadherence of parasitized erythrocytes to endothelial surfaces leads to the gathering or sequestration of large numbers of mature parasites in deep tissues.

The periodicity of schizogony characteristically coincides with paroxysms of fever and this led to the traditional names of the different types of human malaria.

- *Tertian malaria*—fever every third day, if the first day is given the number 1: *P. vivax* and *P. ovale*.
- *Subtertian malaria*—fever slightly more often than every third day: *P. falciparum*.
- *Quartan malaria*—fever every fourth day if the first day is given the number 1: *P. malariae*.

P. falciparum malaria was sometimes called malignant tertian malaria because of its much greater lethal potential than the other tertian malarias. These antique names for malaria are best avoided, not only because they can be confusing, but because the periodicity they imply often fails to develop. Many patients have lost their lives from *P. falciparum* malaria because they never developed the periodic fever that their doctors wrongly believed to be invariable.

Some of the merozoites entering red cells do not develop into schizonts, but develop more slowly into solid-looking parasites called gametocytes. These may persist in the circulation for many weeks without destroying the red cells containing them and they are the forms infective to the mosquito. In each species of malaria, the gametocytes are differentiated into male and female. When the female mosquito swallows the male and female gametocytes in her blood meal, they develop further in her stomach. The male gametocytes rapidly develop to produce spermatozoon-like microgametes and the female gametocyte becomes the egg-like macrogamete.

Clinical features

There are no recognized symptoms associated with the liver stage of malarial infections or (as far as we know) with rupture of tissue schizonts. The development of a blood stage infection is necessary for malarial illness.

Infections with each of the different malaria species have many clinical features in common.

These result from the release, when red cell schizonts rupture, of 'malaria toxins' or pyrogens. The common features are as follows:

- *Fever*—This is often irregular. Fever is believed to be mediated by host cytokines, which are secreted by leucocytes and other cells in response to the released pyrogens. The pattern of regularly periodic fever often does not occur until the illness has continued for a week or more. It depends on synchronized schizogony. Why schizogony should ever become synchronized is unknown, but an intriguing explanation has been suggested. High temperatures slow the growth of mature, more than of young, parasites. Fever itself may therefore allow young parasites to 'catch up' with older ones, leading to increasing synchrony with successive cycles.
- *Anaemia*—This is caused by a combination of haemolysis and bone marrow suppression. Haemolysis is usually most severe in *P. falciparum* malaria because cells of all ages can be invaded in this infection.
- *Splenomegaly*—The spleen enlarges early in the acute attack in all types of malaria. When a patient has had many attacks, the spleen may be of enormous size and lead to secondary hypersplenism.
- *Jaundice*—A mild jaundice caused by haemolysis may occur in all types of malaria. Severe jaundice is unusual in malaria, only occurs in *P. falciparum* infection, and results from a combination of haemolysis and impaired liver function.

Classical stages of fever

In a paroxysm of malaria, the patient may notice the following stages:

1 *Cold stage*—The patient shivers or has a frank rigor; the temperature rises sharply.

2 *Hot stage*—The patient is flushed, has a rapid full pulse and a high temperature is sustained for a few hours.

3 *Sweating stage*—The patient sweats freely or is even drenched, and the temperature falls rapidly.

These stages are most often recognized in *P. vivax* infection. For the clinician or epidemiologist, the important point is that an individual with a symptomatic malarial infection or even with severe disease, may be afebrile at one particular time; a history of recent febrile symptoms and/or repeated measurements are important. In rare cases, a patient may be persistently afebrile in the presence of a very severe *P. falciparum* infection. Hyperpyrexia may complicate malaria, especially in attacks of *P. falciparum*.

Progress of the untreated attack

The natural history of untreated malaria differs with each species.

Following a single exposure to *P. falciparum* or *P. malariae* infection, the patient will either die in the acute attack (an outcome in a minority of infections, even with *P. falciparum)* or survive with the development of some immunity and residual anaemia. Attacks may recur over the course of the next year, but then die out spontaneously in the absence of reinfection. A recurrence of malaria illness is called a recrudescence if it is caused by the persistence of blood forms in small numbers between attacks or a reinfection if it is due to a new inoculation of sporozoites from a vector. If no treatment is given to clear the blood forms of the parasite, recrudescences may occur from time to time for more than 30 years. The severity of the attacks tends to diminish as time goes by, until bouts of fever last only a few days.

P. vivax and *P. ovale* malaria cause very similar illnesses with bouts of fever that relapse periodically but irregularly over a period of up to 5 years. These are true relapses and not simple recrudescences, because they may occur despite drug treatment that entirely eliminates the parasites from the blood. The relapses are caused by reinvasion of the blood by merozoites produced when hypnozoites awake from dormancy and develop into PE schizonts. Although causing much less severe disease and mortality than *P. falciparum,* *P. vivax* has been reported to cause altered consciousness, convulsions, severe thrombocytopenia and multiorgan failure in a minority of patients in whom concomitant *P. falciparum* infection has been ruled out by extensive molecular analysis of parasite DNA.

Peculiarities of infection

The important difference between *P. falciparum* and the other plasmodia that infect humans is the capacity of *P. falciparum* to cause severe (or complicated) disease. Nearly all of the million or more malaria deaths that occur each year result from *P. falciparum* infections. In endemic areas, most of the clinical impact of *P. falciparum* infection falls on young children. Nevertheless, the majority of infections cause only a self-limiting febrile illness or, as immunity increases, no illness at all. For reasons that are still not understood, some infections progress to severe disease and some of these are fatal. In areas with limited or unstable transmission, both adults and children with *P. falciparum* infection may develop severe or complicated disease, especially if diagnosis is neglected or delayed.

Complicated *P. falciparum* malaria, also known as 'severe' malaria, may take a number of clinical forms, which are listed in Table 9.1. In young children, in endemic areas, who suffer the greatest malaria mortality, five clinical syndromes predominate: prostration, severe anaemia, cerebral malaria, acidosis and hypoglycaemia. A child may suffer from just one of these complications or from any combination of them. Other complications seen in adults are unusual in children in endemic areas. Non-immune adults may develop any combination of these or of the other syndromes listed in Table 9.1.

Specific syndromes caused by *P. falciparum*

Altered consciousness and coma

In a patient with *P. falciparum* malaria and coma, several possible causes of altered consciousness must be considered.
• A metabolic explanation, such as *hypoglycaemia* (especially in a young child or pregnant woman) or *acidosis*. Correction of either of these may restore consciousness.
• The patient may be having a *seizure*. This is sometimes manifested by only very minor twitching movements or none at all, but an anticonvulsant drug may restore consciousness.

Table 9.1 Microcirculatory arrest in *P. falciparum* infection

Organs most affected	Main symptoms or signs	Typical misdiagnosis
Stomach and intestines	Vomiting and diarrhoea	Gastric flu; cholera (diarrhoea is not bloody)
Brain	Delirium Disorientation Stupor Coma Convulsions Focal neurological signs	Encephalitis, meningoencephalitis (there may be misleading CSF abnormalities)
Kidneys	Renal failure, with or without oliguria or haemoglobinuria	Nephritis
Liver	Jaundice and fever	Hepatitis
Lungs	Pulmonary oedema	Pneumonia, heart failure

- The patient may be *postictal* after a recent seizure, when recovery is likely within a few minutes or hours.
- *Very severe anaemia* may also impair consciousness.

If none of these complications accounts for the coma or if coma persists despite finding and correcting these, then the patient may have 'cerebral malaria'. When a diagnosis of cerebral malaria is made, it is important not to overlook other possible explanations of the illness (e.g. meningitis, encephalitis, severe pneumonia or head injury) in an individual who happens to be parasitaemic.

Cerebral malaria

This common complication is one of the important causes of malaria deaths. It is a diffuse disturbance of cerebral function, characterized by altered consciousness, commonly accompanied by convulsions. The onset may be gradual or sudden, usually within hours or days of the first febrile symptoms of malaria. It is not uncommon for a child to become comatose without any preceding fever or other symptoms. Coma may be accompanied by flaccidity of limbs or by any combination of hypertonicity, posturing and opisthotonos. Any repetitive muscular movement,

even of a minor degree, may reflect underlying seizure activity.

Recently, a characteristic retinopathy has been observed in children and adults with cerebral malaria. A short-acting mydriatic can be used to dilate the pupils, and the retinopathy can then be seen with a direct ophthalmoscope and with practice. The changes consist of areas of retinal whitening, best seen immediately around the fovea (but always sparing the fovea itself), and orange or white discoloration of retinal vessels and capillaries in scattered parts of the retina. These features are sufficiently distinctive to be diagnostically helpful. Most children with cerebral malaria also have white-centred retinal haemorrhages and about 10% have some degree of papilloedema, neither of these being distinctive of malaria (Figure 9.2).

For research purposes, a strict definition of cerebral malaria requires that the parasitaemic patient be unable to localize a painful stimulus (Glasgow coma score ≤8; Blantyre coma score ≤2), that coma persists despite correction of metabolic defects and seizures and that no other explanation for the coma can be found. If effective antimalarial drugs are given, together with supportive care, about 80% of patients with cerebral malaria recover. Coma usually persists for

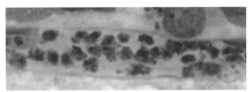

Figure 9.3 Brain smear in fatal malaria. A cerebral venule is packed with late-stage *P. falciparum* parasites (late trophozoites and schizonts). As a result of such sequestration in various deep tissues, these stages of *P. falciparum* are not usually seen in the peripheral blood. (Photo D Milner. Oil immersion, 1000×, reversed Field's stain.)

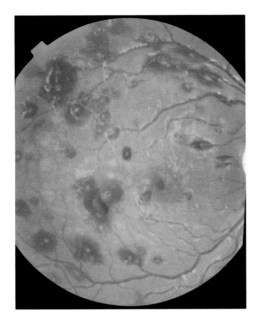

Figure 9.2 Fundus of a child with cerebral malaria showing malarial retinopathy. The edge of the optic disc is on the extreme right. In addition to many white–centred haemorrhages, there are multiple patches of retinal whitening which are most evident temporal to the macula (left-hand side of the photo). Retinal whitening is due to focal areas of retinal ischaemia. (Photo courtesy of Nick Beare.)

1–3 days after the start of treatment, on average somewhat longer in adults than in children. If recovery does occur, a minority of patients (5–25%) are left with a neurological deficit, such as hemiparesis, cerebellar ataxia, amnesia, diffuse spasticity or epilepsy. Clinically obvious sequelae may resolve over a period of months, but some are permanent. We do not know how many individuals may suffer more subtle impairment (e.g. of memory or intelligence) after cerebral malaria.

The pathogenesis of cerebral malaria remains unclear. The usual histopathological finding in fatal cases is the presence of large numbers of erythrocytes containing mature parasites in the capillaries and venules of many organs, including the brain. Because irreversible brain damage is unusual in those who recover, it seems unlikely that the microcirculation is totally obstructed by these sequestered cells. The highly active, developing and dividing parasites may consume essential nutrients such as glucose and release toxic products, including lactate, detrimental to surrounding tissues. As the schizont ruptures the red cell, substances that are known to stimulate the release of cytokines from host cells are released; in excessive local and systemic concentrations, these may contribute to coma and other complications of *P. falciparum* malaria (Figure 9.3).

Perivascular 'ring haemorrhages' are commonly found in the brain at autopsy. Their numbers correlate with the number of retinal haemorrhages visible by ophthalmoscopy during life, but their pathogenetic significance is not known. Raised intracranial pressure is usual in children with cerebral malaria, but there is no firm evidence that the raised pressure itself contributes to mortality. Factors contributing to raised intracranial pressure include cerebral oedema and, probably to a lesser extent, the mass of sequestered, parasitized erythrocytes.

Severe anaemia

This complication is most common in children between 6 and 24 months of age in areas of intense transmission of *P. falciparum*. There is direct red cell destruction when schizonts rupture, and further haemolysis, both of parasitized and unparasitized erythrocytes, occurs through autoimmune mechanisms.

Red cell destruction is not, however, the whole story. One would expect a brisk reticulocytosis in a haemolytic anaemia, but this is usually absent in acute malaria, reflecting impaired bone marrow function. Like fever, this bone marrow dysfunction is believed to be mediated by a host cytokine response to the infection. Marrow aspirates often show evidence of dyserythropoiesis, including phagocytosis of parasitized red cells by macrophages and of apparently uninfected red cells.

Severe anaemia may be found by chance when a patient attends for some unrelated problem or it may lead to breathlessness, weakness and, occasionally, impaired consciousness. Dyspnoea in a child with severe malarial anaemia is most commonly a manifestation of acidosis; occasionally, dyspnoea is a result of heart failure.

Acidosis

Tissue anoxia leads to anaerobic metabolism and the release of lactic and other acids. The resulting acidosis is initially compensated for by deep breathing, which eventually may be insufficient to prevent the arterial blood pH from falling. Factors contributing to tissue anoxia include: the sequestration of parasitized red cells, which may impair tissue perfusion; anaemia; hypovolaemia; and hypotension. Rapid fluid volume replacement, with whole blood if necessary, may be life-saving.

Hypoglycaemia

Hypoglycaemia is a common complication of untreated *P. falciparum* malaria in children, as it is of many other infections in children. Hypoglycaemia may also occur in adults with malaria, pregnant women being particularly susceptible. The principal mechanism of malarial hypoglycaemia is probably cytokine-induced impairment of hepatic gluconeogenesis, although the consumption of glucose by millions of parasites may also contribute. Hypoglycaemia sometimes develops as a complication of quinine or quinidine therapy, probably because these drugs stimulate the pancreas to secrete insulin; again, pregnant women are particularly susceptible.

'Blackwater fever'

This obsolete term used to be applied to the syndrome that sometimes occurs in *P. falciparum* malaria when severe intravascular haemolysis is associated with haemoglobinuria and renal failure. The syndrome still occurs, especially in non-immune adults with severe *P. falciparum* infection. In children in the endemic areas of sub-Saharan Africa, haemoglobinuria sometimes occurs in *P. falciparum* malaria, but it is rarely accompanied by renal failure. In some cases, haemoglobinuria is precipitated by a drug or dietary factor in an individual with glucose-6-phosphate dehydrogenase (G6PD) deficiency. Haemolysis in this condition usually only affects the older cells, so ceases when the haemoglobin has dropped to about 6 g/dL.

Bleeding disorder

A minor degree of disseminated intravascular coagulation (DIC) is common in *P. falciparum* malaria, and DIC severe enough to cause bleeding is an occasional complication in adults.

Malaria in pregnancy

All types of malarial infection can lead to abortion. In *P. falciparum* infection, even in normally immune women, pregnancy is associated with an increased likelihood of developing parasitaemia and with higher parasite densities, especially in the first pregnancy. Anaemia is a common consequence and many women enter labour with a low haemoglobin concentration making peripartum blood loss more dangerous. Organ complications such as coma and renal failure are rare in pregnant women living in endemic areas but among the non-immune, pregnant women are liable to the same complications as other adults.

P. falciparum in endemic areas is an important cause of low birth weight, especially in first-pregnancy babies, who are then at increased risk of dying in infancy from any of a variety of causes. Low birth weight because of maternal malaria presumably results from the fact that the placenta becomes packed both with late-stage parasites and host mononuclear cells, especially in the first pregnancy.

In endemic areas, it is common to find malaria parasites in umbilical venous blood; it is less common to find them in the neonate's peripheral blood and these usually disappear within the first 2 days of life. Illness brought about by congenital infection is rare in endemic areas, but may develop in infants born to non-immune mothers. *P. vivax* is a more common cause of congenital malaria than *P. falciparum*; the illness presents within a few days or weeks of birth with fever, haemolytic anaemia and failure to thrive.

Immunity in malaria

Immunity in malaria is most pronounced in *P. falciparum* infection. In areas of very high transmission, if a child survives to the age of 5 or 6 years, he or she is likely to have achieved a high degree of immunity to the lethal effects of the infection. This immunity has two main components: an ability to limit parasitaemia by the development of specific protective immunoglobulin (IgG) and cell-mediated immunity (antiparasitic immunity) and a physiological tolerance such that parasitaemia produces little or no fever or subjective illness (antitoxic immunity). In order to maintain this immunity, frequent re-exposure to infection is required. If re-exposure does not occur, the immunity wanes over a period of a few years. Although West African students living in the United Kingdom gradually lose their protective antibodies over a 5-year period, they rapidly regain immunity on re-exposure to infection, but the price may well be two or more attacks of malaria first on returning home. The development of a high degree of immunity in an entire population exposed to high levels of *P. falciparum* infection has an extremely important effect on the epidemiology of the infection.

As the CD4 count falls, an individual with HIV infection becomes increasingly susceptible to *P. falciparum* infection and is likely to develop a greater density of parasites in the peripheral blood than more immunocompetent people. It has not yet been shown that such individuals are susceptible to more severe malaria disease. HIV-positive pregnant women are more likely than others to have malaria in pregnancy and to fail to clear it with standard treatment. Conversely, malaria increases the plasma viral load in HIV-infected people, and there is evidence that placental malaria may enhance mother–child transmission of HIV.

Non-immune protective factors in malaria

There are several non-immune factors that affect susceptibility to malaria. *P. vivax* is unable to infect red cells lacking the Duffy blood group antigen. This is believed to account for the natural resistance of people of sub-Saharan African origin (who lack the Duffy antigen) to infection with this parasite.

Individuals with sickle cell trait (haemoglobin genotype AS) are resistant to the lethal effects of *P. falciparum* infection, but no more resistant to infection itself than those with normal (AA) haemoglobin. This is because the sickle trait prevents the development of high parasitaemia, probably partly as a result of parasitized red cells sickling in the circulation and being removed by the spleen before they can develop into schizonts.

Evidence that G6PD deficiency has a similar protective effect does exist, but is less striking. Sickle-cell anaemia itself is not protective, for malarial infection is disastrous in such patients. There is now good evidence that the beta-thalassaemia trait confers protection against *P. falciparum*. Malnutrition was once thought to protect against the lethal effects of *P. falciparum* infection, but recent case–control studies have failed to confirm this.

Immune disorders in malaria

Some complications of malaria are related to immune effects. *Malarial nephrosis* is an occasional complication of *P. malariae* infection in children. Antigen–antibody complex is bound firmly to the glomerular basement membrane. An intractable nephrotic syndrome results, with non-selective proteinuria and a bad prognosis. Neither treatment with corticosteroids nor eradication of the malaria seems to influence the outcome. The intractability of the condition seems to be determined by the permanence of the complex-binding mechanism.

A more tractable condition is hyper-reactive malarial splenomegaly (formerly known as tropical splenomegaly syndrome), in which marked splenomegaly in *P. falciparum* infection is associated with infiltration of the hepatic sinusoids with lymphocytes, with or without features of secondary hypersplenism. Serum IgM levels are very high. This condition usually resolves within a few months if the patient is given continuous, effective chemoprophylaxis (see Chapter 8).

There is good evidence that an acute attack of malaria has general immunosuppressive effects. The effects of chronic malaria are less well defined. Interventions against malaria (e.g. bed nets) have sometimes led to a fall in mortality from other causes, including respiratory infections, suggesting that malarial immunosuppression may increase susceptibility to other common pathogens. The immunosuppressive effects of malaria may account for the tendency of the Epstein–Barr virus to produce Burkitt's lymphoma in malaria-endemic areas.

Diagnosis

Direct diagnosis

The specific diagnosis of malaria is made by examining stained blood films. The thin blood film shows the undistorted parasites within the red cells (Figure 9.4). It is of most use in the detailed study of parasite morphology and species identification. Its disadvantage is that it requires a very prolonged search to detect a low parasitaemia, so its sensitivity is low. A patient may have a fever resulting from *P. falciparum* and yet have no parasites detected by searching the thin film.

The thick film, in which cells are piled upon each other 10–20 deep and lysed and stained at the same time, allows far more red cells to be examined. It has the disadvantage that the morphology of the infected erythrocytes—important in distinguishing between parasite species—can no longer be assessed. Parasite morphology is also

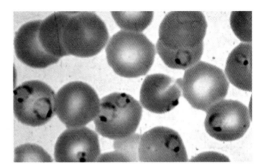

Figure 9.4 Thin blood film in a patient with severe *P. falciparum* malaria, showing ring-stage parasites in unaltered erythrocytes, some containing more than one parasite. This is an extremely high-density parasitaemia.

less clear than in a thin film. However, in experienced hands, the thick film is the best method to use for answering the question, 'Does the patient have malaria?'

Serodiagnosis

Serodiagnosis of malaria is of no use for diagnosis of the acute attack. It depends on finding specific antibodies, and most methods in common use are incapable of distinguishing between antibodies to the different species of parasite. Antibodies may be detectable for several years after the last attack of malaria. The main use of serodiagnosis is in excluding malaria in a patient suffering from recurrent bouts of fever who does not present during a bout. Serology may also be used in surveys as an approximate measure of exposure of a population to malaria. The most frequently used serological technique is the indirect fluorescent antibody test (IFAT).

New methods of diagnosis

Many new techniques for identifying malaria parasites are being developed. Rapid diagnostic tests (RDT) are 'dipstick' like tests that detect parasite enzymes or antigen in whole blood. They have the advantage of not requiring a microscope and require less training than microscopy. Most are sensitive and specific for the detection of *P. falciparum*; some can also detect other species, but may not be as sensitive. They are most useful where skilled microscopy is unavailable. Other techniques include the quantitative buffy coat (QBC) technique, which makes use of the fact that parasitized erythrocytes have a different specific gravity from unparasitized red cells, and can therefore be looked for in a particular segment of the blood in a centrifuged capillary tube. Polymerase chain reaction (PCR) tests can be used to detect parasite DNA. While these methods are useful in research studies, they have not replaced thick and thin films for routine clinical diagnosis.

Treatment

The treatment of a patient with malaria is supportive and specific. Supportive treatment may include the following:

1 Reducing the temperature if hyperpyrexia is present—especially common with *P. falciparum* infection. Oral or rectal paracetamol is the method of choice. If this is unavailable, tepid sponging and fanning offers temporary benefit.

2 Rehydration, especially when vomiting and diarrhoea have been prominent and in the patient with deep breathing suggestive of acidosis.

3 Monitoring renal output and taking corrective measures if necessary. First, rapidly correct any hypovolaemia; if oliguria persists, maintain careful fluid balance. Peritoneal dialysis or haemodialysis, if indicated, may be life-saving.

4 Monitoring the need for blood transfusion, which may be life-saving. However, blood should only be transfused when there are strong clinical indications; for example, when the haemoglobin concentration is <4 g/dL (haematocrit <12%) or when higher levels are accompanied by coma, acidosis or hyperparasitaemia. In most patients, the haemoglobin concentration rises rapidly when the attack has been terminated by specific chemotherapy.

5 Terminating convulsions with appropriate drugs—rectal diazepam or lorazepam, rectal or intramuscular paraldehyde, and intramuscular phenobarbital are some options. These should be used in a sequence, proceeding to the second or third option only when the others have failed.

6 Monitoring of blood glucose and correction of hypoglycaemia where necessary (10–40 mL of 50% dextrose diluted×3 with saline and infused over 5–10 min).

7 Reducing acidaemia. Rehydration, blood transfusion (when appropriate) and antimalarial therapy are usually sufficient for this purpose. The use of bicarbonate infusion is not of proven benefit, but may be attempted with care in severe acidosis, provided that due attention is already being given to correction of hypovolaemia, hypoxia and anaemia.

8 Treating DIC if this complication is severe enough to cause bleeding—fresh whole blood, platelet-rich plasma and fresh frozen plasma may be given according to availability.

9 Giving antibiotics is likely to be helpful:
- if the diagnosis of malaria is in doubt;
- in an unconscious patient in whom lumbar puncture is deferred; or
- in patient groups known to have a high risk of bacteraemia accompanying severe malaria.

This may vary geographically: at-risk groups identified have been children with cerebral malaria in coastal Kenya and young children with severe anaemia in southern Malawi.

Specific chemotherapy

Specific treatment is directed to terminating the parasitaemia as rapidly as possible. The drug of choice depends on national policy in the particular country, and on the likely place of origin of the patient's parasites. Drug resistance is an increasing problem throughout the world, and the picture changes with time. Many endemic countries now have a national programme that sets policy for first-line treatment of uncomplicated malaria, with other drugs for treatment of failures or of severe disease. In some countries, multidrug resistance threatens to make malaria untreatable and new additions to the armamentarium of drugs are urgently needed. In general national policy should be followed. Treat non-severe malaria with oral drugs if the patient can take them. Complicated *P. falciparum* malaria requires parenteral antimalarial drugs, at least until there is clinical improvement and the patient can swallow.

Drugs that prevent the development of the blood stages which are causing the illness are traditionally called schizonticides. Some of them also act against the gametocytes of some species, but this has no relevance to the clinical situation. Some of the schizonticides also have useful anti-inflammatory effects. The most widely used schizonticide has until recently been chloroquine, but the spread of parasite chloroquine resistance has limited the use of this drug in the recent years. Chloroquine remains the drug of choice for all non-falciparum malarias. *P. vivax* resistance to chloroquine is increasingly common, but as the disease is not life-threatening, it is reasonable to try chloroquine first.

Artemisinin drugs are now playing an increasing part in malaria treatment, both in combination with a partner drug in the first-line therapy of uncomplicated malaria (artemisinin combination therapy [ACT]) and in the treatment of complicated disease due to *P. falciparum*. Parenteral quinine remains in widespread use in Africa for the initial treatment of severe malaria.

Drug doses quoted in the following sections are for average-weight adults in a tropical setting.

The artemisinin drugs

These compounds are derived from the plant *Artemisia annua*, which has been used for thousands of years as a herbal remedy for fevers in China. The plant's active components, arte-ether, artemether and artesunate are highly effective antimalarials, active against chloroquine-resistant and multidrug-resistant *P. falciparum* and useful in the treatment of severe and complicated malaria as well as uncomplicated disease. Parasites are cleared from the circulation faster by artemisinins than by quinine or chloroquine as their action is parasite stage-specific. In the treatment of severe disease, artemisinins are less toxic and more convenient to use than quinine.

If used alone for treatment of *P. falciparum* infection, an artemisinin drug must be given for at least 5 and preferably 7 days; shorter courses are followed by recrudescence of parasites in over half of the cases. Artemisinins are therefore usually used in combination with other antimalarial drugs.

Oral, intramuscular, intravenous and rectal formulations of various artemisinins are available.

- *Artesunate* is available as tablets, suppositories and as powder for preparing an intravenous solution. Several studies now show that rectal artesunate and other artemisinins could play an important role in the treatment of severe malaria when parenteral treatment is difficult. Intravenous artesunate has recently been shown to reduce mortality when compared to quinine for the treatment of severe malaria in Asia. Ongoing trials will demonstrate whether this also applies to Africa, where most patients are young children.
- *Artemether* is an oil-soluble derivative suitable for intramuscular injection. In several studies, artemether has proved as efficacious as quinine in the treatment of severe malaria in children, although absorption from the injection site appeared to be impaired in a few very ill, acidotic children.
- *Artemisinin* can be used orally or rectally.

No important human toxicity of artemisinins has been detected after thousands of treatments. Brainstem damage has been observed in animals given more than 10 times the usual human doses of arte-ether or artemether, but careful examination has failed to reveal any neurotoxicity in clinical practice. Artemisinins reduce gametocyte production. This may in turn reduce the transmission of malaria locally, although probably not to an important degree in hyper- or holoendemic areas. The rapid killing of asexual blood-stage parasites is a property of artemisinin drugs that makes them particularly suitable for combination therapy.

Artemisinin combination therapy

For many decades in the mid-twentieth century, chloroquine monotherapy was the standard treatment for malaria. Then *P. falciparum* resistant to chloroquine began to appear and to spread, followed by parasites resistant to many other first-line antimalarial drugs. We now, belatedly, recognize the importance of combining drugs with different modes of action, as is usual practice in the treatment of tuberculosis, leprosy, cancers and HIV infection, in order to delay the development of resistance.

Various combinations of antimalarial drugs have been evaluated for their capacity to cure patients and to prevent the emergence of drug-resistant parasites. Artemisinin drugs are particularly useful as a component of combination therapy, because they lower asexual parasitaemia rapidly, leaving a much diminished parasite biomass; a second drug can then kill the remaining parasites, with a greatly reduced chance that a resistant mutation will occur and break through the treatment. ACT is therefore being strongly promoted worldwide as first-line treatment for uncomplicated malaria, with different ACTs incorporating various artemisinins and partner drugs. It remains to be seen whether the application of this global strategy will reduce the advance of drug-resistant *P. falciparum*.

Co-artem (artemether–lumefantrine)

This was the first commercially available ACT. It is currently being deployed as first-line therapy for uncomplicated malaria in a number of African countries. The standard adult dose is four tablets twice a day for 3 days. Absorption of the lumefantrine component is increased considerably by fat and therefore this drug should ideally be taken with food.

Amodiaquine-artesunate

Amodiaquine is a 4-aminoquinoline with a molecule that has some resemblance to chloroquine and some to quinine. The dose is the same (in terms of base) as for chloroquine. Toxic effects are also similar to chloroquine, but agranulocytosis has been reported.

Since amodiaquine is effective against some strains of chloroquine-resistant *P. falciparum* (both *in vivo* and *in vitro*), it has been incorporated into an ACT—amodiaquine-artesunate—that is currently being rolled out for first-line therapy in a number of countries, mainly in Africa.

Quinine

The main use of quinine is for treatment of severe *P. falciparum* malaria. Its isomer, quinidine, is equally effective but more cardiotoxic. Quinine is a natural alkaloid derived from cinchona bark, a bitter crystalline powder practically insoluble in water. It forms salts of varying solubility: the sulphate and bisulphate are used for oral preparations and the dihydrochloride or chloride for injection. It is a powerful schizonticide; it also has an anti-inflammatory action.

Toxic effects are diverse. The symptom complex of tinnitus, deafness, dizziness, nausea and vomiting, which is known as cinchonism, is almost inevitable with normal doses of quinine—therapy does not need to be stopped or changed on account of such symptoms unless they are severe. Others include hypoglycaemia (especially in pregnancy); hypotension (if excessive dose or if given too fast intravenously); thrombocytopenia (a rare idiosyncratic reaction); and erythematous rash. Overdose of quinine can cause deafness, blindness and severe hypotension. Quinine has a stimulatory effect on uterine muscle, and overdose can cause abortion. However, this is not a reason to avoid quinine in pregnancy, because the benefit of curing malaria greatly outweighs the risk of uterine excitation from therapeutic doses of the drug.

The following doses are expressed as dose of salt.

- Adults

Oral—600 mg 8 hourly for 7–10 days (usually as sulphate).

Parenteral—The intravenous route is preferred, but only where staff and facilities are available for the careful monitoring of infusions. First (loading) dose of 20 mg/kg (maximum dose 1400 mg) quinine dihydrochloride is infused over 4 h in an isotonic glucose–electrolyte fluid (e.g. half-strength Darrow's–5% dextrose); subsequent doses of 10 mg/kg are similarly infused over 2 h at 12-hourly intervals for children or infused over 4 h at 8-hourly intervals for adults. Change to oral therapy as soon as the patient can take it.

Intramuscular—Injection of quinine dihydrochloride may be given if intravenous infusion is impossible. It is usually well tolerated if given deep, with aseptic precautions. The provided ampoule (300 mg/mL) should be diluted fivefold with sterile water to reduce the pain of the injection. As with intravenous infusion, the first dose should be a loading dose of 20 mg/kg; to reduce the volume of this large dose, it may be divided between the two thighs and further divided by giving half at time zero and the remainder 4 h later.

Chloroquine

This is a synthetic compound of the 4-aminoquinoline group. It is a powerful schizonticide; it also has anti-inflammatory action and so helps to reduce the non-specific symptoms of malaria (malaise, headache, myalgia). Widespread resistance of *P. falciparum* to chloroquine has reduced its role in treatment of this infection. There is evidence that parasites may regain chloroquine sensitivity after several years, in a human population not exposed to the drug, so that chloroquine (in combination therapies) may prove useful again in the future.

Chloroquine is relatively non-toxic if properly administered in the correct dosage. The drug should be given orally when possible. Intravenous infusion must be over 2–4 h, and intramuscular or subcutaneous chloroquine should be divided into frequent small doses rather than given as a single large injection. The drug is taken up by the liver, so higher blood levels follow parenteral rather than oral administration allowing larger, less frequent doses than by mouth.

Main toxic effects include: gastrointestinal effects (nausea, vomiting, etc.); a fall in blood pressure; generalized itching (a common complaint in black-skinned people only); the hair may turn white with chronic overdosage; the vision may also be affected with prolonged use. Dosages are as follows, and all doses are expressed as dose of base as this is the active part of the drug.

- Adults

Oral—600 mg initially, 300 mg 6 h later, then 300 mg/day for 2 days (total dosage 1.5 g).

Intravenous—5 mg/kg (maximum 300 mg) infused over 3 h in saline, repeated every 8 h to total of 25 mg/kg.

Intramuscular or subcutaneous—2.5 mg/kg (maximum 150 mg) every 4 h to total 25 mg/kg.

When giving chloroquine parenterally, change to oral treatment as soon as the patient can take it.
- Children

Oral—The dose should be in proportion to the body weight (using the full dose at 60 kg).

Sulfadoxine–pyrimethamine (Fansidar)

This highly convenient, inexpensive single-dose therapy has been widely used as first-line treatment for malaria in many countries, but increasing resistance has greatly reduced its usefulness in recent years. The two-component drugs inhibit different enzymes required by the parasite for folic acid synthesis. Sulfadoxine (like other sulphonamides) competitively inhibits the enzyme dihydropteroate synthetase (DHPS), while pyrimethamine (like the biguanide proguanil) inhibits dihydrofolate reductase (DHFR). Resistance appears to be the result of mutations in the parasites' DHFR and DHPS genes, and the capacity to detect these mutations by PCR provides a useful means of monitoring and predicting the extent and spread of sulfadoxine-pyrimethamine (SP) resistance in different populations.

Mefloquine

This is a 4-quinoline methanol drug chemically related to quinine. It is bound to plasma, has a half-life of 21 days and is effective as a single adult oral dose of 750–1250 mg. No parenteral preparation is available. Naturally occurring low-level resistance has been reported. Toxic effects include headache, dizziness and disturbances of sleep. Occasional severe toxic effects are fits, psychomotor disturbances and psychoses. Individuals with a history of convulsions or neuropsychiatric disease are therefore advised not to use mefloquine. There have been many hundreds of well-observed cases in which the drug has been used in pregnancy without adverse effect on mother or fetus—nevertheless it is wise if possible to avoid the use of mefloquine in pregnancy on general grounds. Patients on cardiosuppressant drugs or beta-blockers should not take mefloquine because of its additional effects on the myocardium.

Mefloquine is much too expensive to be used on a large scale in malaria control programmes in endemic areas.

Atovaquone–proguanil (Malarone)

This is a recently licensed combination therapy for the treatment of uncomplicated *P. falciparum* malaria. The standard regimen is four tablets daily for 3 days. Its cost is prohibitive for use in national programmes.

Halofantrine

This is an effective antimalarial that has been used in some parts of Africa. However, it is cardiotoxic, prolonging the electrocardiographic QT_C interval and leading to arrhythmias. It is therefore no longer recommended for the treatment of malaria.

Classifying antimalarial drug resistance

Antimalarial drugs can be judged *in vivo* by their efficacy in patients with malaria. They can also be assessed *in vitro* by measuring their capacity to inhibit the growth of cultured *P. falciparum*. An *in vivo* assessment requires the identification of a number of individuals with malaria (fever, parasitaemia and no other cause of illness), who must be observed to take the correct dose of the drug being assessed. Parasitaemia is monitored on days 0, 1, 2, 3, 7, 14 and 28. A further sample on day 56 can provide useful additional information. When possible, blood samples from the time of the initial infection and any subsequent parasitaemia should be kept for later DNA analysis, so that a new infection can be distinguished from a recrudescence of the original infection (the latter indicating true drug failure).

Classification of resistance allows for the fact that a patient may be completely well, even though parasitaemic, after treatment. In this classification, patients are described as having the following:

• *Early treatment failure (ETF)*—if they develop severe illness with parasitaemia during the first 4 days after treatment; or if they remain febrile and parasitaemic throughout those 4 days.

• *Late treatment failure (LTF)*—if, having improved clinically, both fever and parasitaemia recur by day 14.

• *Adequate clinical response (ACR)*—if there was neither ETF nor LTF, and the patient does not develop febrile parasitaemia by day 28, that is, for an ACR, the patient may have either fever or parasitaemia by day 28 but not both.

• *Adequate clinical and parasitological response (ACPR)*—if there was neither ETF nor LTF, and the patient has no parasitaemia by day 28.

The problem of relapse

Relapse—the emergence of a new parasitaemia from hypnozoites that have been dormant in the liver since an earlier *P. vivax* or *P. ovale* infection—can usually be prevented by giving a course of primaquine, but some strains of *P. vivax* (e.g. from Papua New Guinea) are resistant to normal doses of the drug. Primaquine acts on hypnozoite forms of *P. vivax* and *P. ovale*. It also destroys gametocytes of all species—a function that is not relevant to the prevention of relapse. The principal danger of primaquine therapy is acute haemolysis that may occur if the drug is administered to an individual with G6PD deficiency. Since primaquine is never an emergency treatment, patients can first be tested so that the dosing schedule can be modified for those with G6PD deficiency.

For radical cure of relapsing forms of malaria, 30 mg base/day is given for 10–14 days for *P. vivax* and 15 mg base/day for 10–14 days for *P. ovale*. The dose may have to be doubled in some *P. vivax* strains. For subjects with G6PD deficiency, a single weekly dose of 45 mg base for 6 weeks is usually well tolerated and is preferable to daily dosing with a lower dose.

Primaquine can no longer be justified as a method for clearing gametocytes of *P. falciparum*. In the rare circumstances where such an objective might be justified, artemisinin drugs would achieve the same effect more safely. (The benefit of this anti-gametocyte property of artemisinin drugs in highly endemic areas is doubtful, because most transmission occurs from individuals who are not even known to carry the parasite).

Chemoprophylaxis

Chemoprophylaxis of malaria involves the regular administration of drugs to prevent clinical symptoms. Drugs taken for this purpose act in two ways: as *schizonticides*, so that when the parasites enter the red cells they are destroyed, and *causal prophylactics*, which prevent the development of the PE schizonts in the liver and may also have blood schizonticidal effects.

Currently, chemoprophylaxis is routinely advised only for non-immune travellers visiting endemic areas. The use of malaria prophylaxis requires a careful assessment of the malaria risk and potential benefit for each individual – this assumes a detailed knowledge of malaria transmission in the region to be visited. The choice of drug depends upon individual patient factors and the region visited, which defines the predominant malaria species and whether they are likely to be drug sensitive. Factors in the traveller that should be considered are the presence of health problems or medications, the length of stay, whether medical resources are available at the destination, and previous experience with antimalarials. For the few areas where there is little chloroquine resistance, such as parts of central America or the Middle East, chloroquine alone or in combination with proguanil can be used. For the rest of the world, one can choose between mefloquine, doxycycline and atovaquone-proguanil, although there are some limited areas of mefloquine resistance in South East Asia.

Something akin to chemoprophylaxis is recommended for pregnant women in endemic areas. It has been shown in some endemic communities that two or three doses of a drug such as SP, given during the second half of pregnancy (irrespective of maternal illness or parasitaemia), reduces placental malaria and low birth weight in first-born babies. This routine administration of antimalarials occasionally in pregnancy is more accurately termed intermittent presumptive therapy (IPT) rather than chemoprophylaxis. A similar approach to malaria in infancy is under evaluation.

Proguanil (Paludrine, Chlorguanide)

This is a synthetic biguanide. It is a bitter, white powder available as hydrochloride. Tablets are 100 mg proguanil hydrochloride, as well as a paediatric 25 mg preparation. It is a slowly acting schizonticide and a causal prophylactic. When a mosquito takes up gametocytes from a patient receiving proguanil, their development in the mosquito is inhibited, so the mosquito fails to become infective.

Proguanil is the safest of all antimalarials—no deaths have ever been recorded from overdose (up to 14.5 g). Occasionally, it can cause heartburn or epigastric pain, but this is minimized by taking the drug after food. Mouth ulcers are an unpleasant side effect in some people. Gross overdose may cause haematuria. It is safe in pregnancy in a normal dosage, but a folic acid supplement should be given.

The adult dose of proguanil is 200 mg/day. It is well tolerated by children who can take 25 mg/day from infancy; 50 mg/day from age 2; 75 mg/day from age 4; and 100 mg/day from age 6. When used as a prophylactic, proguanil should be combined with another drug. In the past, it was most widely used in combination with chloroquine as malaria prophylaxis for travellers to parts of the world with limited chloroquine resistance. Since such areas are now few, this use of proguanil has now diminished but the combination atovaquone-proguanil is currently an efficacious alternative.

Atovaquone–proguanil

This recently licensed drug combination is effective against chloroquine-resistant *P. falciparum*. It is a causal prophylactic, preventing development of parasites in the liver and, therefore, only needs to be continued for a week after leaving the malarious area. The standard dose is one tablet daily. Serious adverse effects are rare.

Doxycycline

This long-acting tetracycline is an effective prophylactic against malaria in a dose of 100 mg/day.

It is particularly useful in the areas of South East Asia where there is resistance to both chloroquine and mefloquine. It should not be used in pregnancy or lactation, nor in young children. An occasional toxic effect is a rash caused by photosensitization.

Mefloquine (for prophylaxis)

As a result of the spread of chloroquine resistance around the world, mefloquine (alone) is now the prophylactic drug of choice for many areas. Initial anxieties about drug accumulation have diminished, and it is now acceptable to recommend an adult dose of 250 mg/week for periods of a year or more. It can rarely cause neuropsychiatric side-effects and so should be avoided by some individuals (p. 67).

Chloroquine (for prophylaxis)

Increasing chloroquine resistance means that this drug is now no longer effective, either for treatment or prophylaxis, in most parts of the world.

Other drugs

No prophylactic regimen described can be completely depended on to suppress *P. falciparum* malaria, especially in non-immune people. Patients should be warned of this and advised to have an alternative drug available for treatment in case of failure. Similarly, a non-immune individual developing fever after return from an endemic area, even if he or she faithfully took prophylaxis, may have *P. falciparum* malaria. Nevertheless, if a patient develops malaria more than 4 weeks after leaving a malarious area, it is still most likely that it will be with one of the three non-*falciparum* species, all of which commonly have a long incubation period.

Recommendations for antimalarial prophylaxis in specific geographical locations are constantly changing. Authoritative up-to-date sources such as the WHO or UK guidelines are recommended (see Further reading).

Epidemiology

The epidemiology of malaria has been most studied in the case of *P. falciparum*. The two most important factors are
1 intensity of transmission (the number of infective bites per year);
2 the immune response of the host.

Measuring malaria in a community

Traditional methods

It has been customary in the past to characterize the epidemiological situation in a community by describing its malariometric indices. These are established by surveys that, by examining all age groups of the population, determine for each group
1 *parasite rate*—the proportion of blood films that are positive;
2 *spleen rate*—the proportion of the group with a palpable spleen.

Morbidity and mortality

It is now recognized that parasite and spleen rates are measures of malarial infection, reflecting the intensity of transmission, but they are not measures of the clinical impact of malaria on the community. It is the morbidity and mortality attributable to malaria that are important as the basis for designing a malaria control programme, and these indicators are equally important in monitoring the effectiveness of control.

Ways of estimating malaria-attributable mortality include hospital studies and 'verbal autopsies'. The latter technique makes use of tested questionnaires to enquire of mothers about the nature of the final illness in any children dying within a specified period before the survey. Unfortunately, the verbal autopsy technique cannot distinguish reliably between malaria and pneumonia or meningitis, and deaths caused by severe malarial anaemia may not be identified. Therefore, only an approximate measure of malarial mortality can be obtained.

Stable malaria

Transmission occurs for at least 6 months in the year and is intense. Malarial infection is acquired repeatedly. Children suffer repeated attacks of malaria from the age of a few months onwards. Very young children are partly protected by passive immunity acquired by transplacental passage of protective maternal IgG. This may modify the severity of the first few attacks, so allowing them to develop some active immunity while still partly protected. Children reaching the age of 5 or 6 years have substantial immunity, but the price of this immunity is that some children will die of malaria before immunity develops. The proportion who do so is likely to depend on many factors, including the intensity of transmission, the availability of drugs and the prevalence of parasite drug resistance. Data on the actual death toll in different populations are still rarely available.

When immunity has been established, older patients may still suffer attacks of malaria, but these take the form only of mild or moderate flu-like episodes lasting a few days. Severe and complicated disease rarely occurs. Nevertheless, in areas of stable malaria, malaria illness episodes in adults may be sufficient to cause absenteeism from work and thus to have an impact on the economy. There is little variation in the incidence of malaria from year to year (hence the word 'stable'), but there may still be pronounced seasonal fluctuations in new cases seen in children. In such an area, there is often a marked rise in the number of children seen with cerebral malaria about 2 weeks after the rains begin.

Unstable malaria

This situation is the antithesis of stable malaria. There are wide changes in transmission, not only throughout each year but also from year to year. This results in the tendency for epidemics to occur—hence the term 'unstable'. The transmission season is typically short and the mosquito population fluctuates widely. Infection is usually so infrequent that no member of the population has the opportunity to develop a significant level of immunity. For this reason, when transmission does suddenly increase (usually because of freak environmental conditions leading to an explosion in the mosquito population), people of all ages are equally susceptible to infection. This results in serious disease or even death, regardless of age. The health of the working community may be disastrously affected, and the economic effects of an epidemic can be dire.

Global malaria eradication

Attempts at global eradication of malaria in the mid-twentieth century failed and local eradication has only succeeded in a few areas, mostly islands. The main causes of failure were:

1 *Operational*—not all houses were sprayed. There are many causes for this, including lack of cooperation, poor mapping, accelerated destruction of thatched roofs (dichlorodiphenyl-trichloroethane [DDT] kills caterpillars and their predators; caterpillars soon reappear but predators do not) and resentment of intrusion into privacy.

2 *Technical*—resistance of mosquitoes to insecticide; behavioural resistance in which mosquitoes fly straight out of the house after feeding, and so do not rest on the sprayed surface; resistance of the parasite to antimalarial drugs.

3 *Political* (not a cause that was recognized by the WHO)—failure of countries to cooperate; civil war and severe political unrest; lack of a suitable infrastructure on which to build the control programme; political and administrative incompetence.

4 Ill-advised and unpopular pilot schemes.

5 Failure to convince the people of the need for the programme.

Malaria control at present

Global malaria eradication—the objective in the mid-twentieth century—was abandoned as unrealistic later in the century, the objective shifting to the control of disease and mortality that result from malaria. New tools are now available, and funds from many international sources are being increasingly mobilized. There are grounds for giving serious thought to the goal of eradication once again. Meanwhile, there is general agreement that malaria control requires a combined approach using several methods:

1 The provision of diagnostic and treatment services as close as possible to where the people live.
2 Simple, affordable, safe and efficacious therapy for uncomplicated disease.
3 Prompt recognition and treatment of severe disease, with systems of referral to hospital centres when necessary.
4 Education of the population about the features and dangers of malaria.
5 Drug prophylaxis or intermittent presumptive therapy for selected subgroups.
6 Antivector measures and water clearance, where achievable (and not elsewhere).
7 The use of permethrin-impregnated bed nets or curtains. Several randomized controlled trials in endemic areas have demonstrated that widespread use of insecticide-treated nets (ITNs) in a community can reduce child mortality and malaria-related morbidity. The use of ITNs has been hugely scaled up in many countries. Nets that do not require re-impregnation every few months are increasingly available.
8 Indoor residual spraying—the backbone of the original eradication campaigns—is being reassessed in many pilot programmes and may play an increasing part in malaria control in the future.

Vaccines may in the near future be added to the list of effective interventions. Several candidate vaccines have been evaluated or are undergoing trials, some of which have shown considerable promise in preliminary studies in endemic areas.

Individual precautions

Because the anopheline vectors of malaria are night biters, a high degree of protection is given by
1 covering up the exposed skin in the evenings (of limited value because most infective biting occurs between 10 p.m. and 2 a.m.);
2 the use of insect repellents such as dimethyl phthalate, dibutyl phthalate or diethyl toluamide;
3 the use of an efficient mosquito net over the bed, preferably impregnated with a synthetic pyrethroid such as permethrin or deltamethrin;
4 in the event of a febrile illness, testing for malaria and treating with minimal delay.

Further reading

Breman JG, Alilio MS, White NJ, eds. Defining and defeating the intolerable burden of malaria III. Progress and perspectives. *Am J Trop Med Hyg* 2007; 77 (Suppl): 1–327. [A series of articles about malaria today covering clinical, epidemiological, therapeutic, vectorial and immunological aspects and discussing prospects for worldwide control. All articles are available free on internet and on CD-ROM.]

Gilles HM, Warrell DA, eds. *Bruce-Chwatt's Essential Malariology*. London: Edward Arnold, 2001. [A convenient and erudite volume covering malaria from the point of view of numerous disciplines including clinical medicine, pharmacology, therapeutics, epidemiology, parasitology, immunology, entomology and public health.]

Health Protection Agency. Malaria prevention guidelines. http://www.hpa.org.uk/infections/topics_az/malaria/guidelines.htm. This source has also been published: Chiodini P, Hill D, Lalloo D, Lea G, Walker E, Whitty C, Bannister B. Guidelines for malaria prevention in travellers from the United Kingdom. Health Protection Agency, January 2007. [UK guidelines on prophylaxis.]

Snow RW, Guerra CA, Noor AM, Myint HY, Hay SI. The global distribution of clinical episodes of *Plasmodium falciparum* malaria. *Nature* 2005; 4330: 214–217.

Whitty CJM, Lalloo D, Ustianowski A. Malaria: an update on treatment of adults in non-endemic countries. *Br Med J* 2006; 333: 241–245.

World Health Organization. *Management of Severe Malaria*. WHO booklet, 2000. [A slim attractive book giving essentials of diagnosis and treatment. Useful for reference—fits easily into a coat pocket—and helpful as text for training seminars or for under- and postgraduate teaching.]

World Health Organization. Severe falciparum malaria. *Trans R Soc Trop Med Hyg* 2000; 94 (Suppl): 1–90. [A comprehensive review of clinical features, pathogenesis and management of severe falciparum malaria with an extensive list of references.]

Chapter 10

Visceral leishmaniasis

About 30 species of obligate intracellular protozoal parasites of the genus *Leishmania* are responsible for a variety of diseases in humans, collectively known as leishmaniasis. These diseases are further classified as visceral, cutaneous or mucosal according to their principal clinical presentations. A 'leishmaniac' is a person who is obsessed with these parasites.

Epidemiology

Visceral leishmaniasis (VL), also known as kala-azar (Hindi for 'black sickness'), is mainly caused by three species belonging to the *Leishmania donovani* complex, each with a characteristic regional distribution:

1 *L. infantum*—Mediterranean, Middle East, Central Asia, China

2 *L. donovani*—India, East Africa

3 *L. chagasi*—South and Central America.

VL may also be caused by *L. tropica* in the Old World and *L. amazonensis* in the New World.

Over 200 million people reside in endemic areas of more than 70 affected countries. There are approximately 600000 cases reported annually, 90% of which occur in Bangladesh, India, Nepal, Sudan and north-eastern Brazil.

Humans are the only known reservoir of *L. donovani* in Bangladesh, India and Nepal. Humans, and possibly rodents, are thought to be the reservoir in East Africa. Wild and domestic canines are important reservoirs of *L. infantum* and *L. chagasi*. Infection occurs following the bite of an infected female sandfly (*Phlebotomus* spp. in the Old World, *Lutzomyia* spp. in the New World). Transmission may also occur via blood transfusions, infected needles or syringes, and congenitally.

In some regions, such as north-eastern Brazil, expanding urbanization is associated with steadily increasing transmission of leishmaniasis. Globally, HIV is also contributing to the clinical re-emergence of leishmaniasis. Pathogen proliferation and disease progression are mutually enhanced in *Leishmania* and HIV coinfection. In regions of coendemicity, there is likely to be a dramatic shift from subclinical to clinical VL coupled with an increased rate of transmission of VL in the general population.

Parasite and life cycle

Leishmania amastigotes are spherical or oval bodies measuring 2–4 µm containing two distinct pieces of nuclear chromatin. The larger piece is called the nucleus, the smaller piece the kinetoplast. The sandfly becomes infected by taking up the amastigotes with its blood meal, the amastigotes being in the blood or skin of the infecting

Lecture Notes: Tropical Medicine, 6th edition.
By G.V. Gill and N.J. Beeching. Published 2009 by Blackwell Publishing, ISBN: 978-1-4051-8048-1.

host. The amastigotes are liberated in the stomach of the sandfly and begin to multiply by simple fission, eventually forming flagellated metacyclic promastigotes which are infectious to the new host. This process takes 1–2 weeks, depending on the species. The motile promastigotes migrate from the gut to the proboscis of the sandfly and are injected during feeding. Sandfly saliva inhibits the L-arginine-dependent nitric oxide killing mechanism of macrophages. The promastigotes are ingested unharmed by macrophages and metamorphose into amastigotes. These are distributed in the reticuloendothelial system where they lodge and multiply by binary fission.

Clinical features of VL

Clinical presentation ranges from asymptomatic or subclinical infection to acute, subacute and chronic presentations. The ratio of clinical:subclinical infections is in the range of 1:30–100. The incubation period is usually between 2 and 6 months but ranges from 10 days to more than 10 years. Males are about three times more commonly affected than females.

Onset is usually insidious with low-grade fever, progressive splenomegaly, hepatomegaly, lymphadenopathy (particularly in Africa), anaemia, anorexia, wasting and increased pigmentation in persons with dark skin (particularly in India).

The liver and spleen are usually firm, regular and non-tender on palpation. The spleen may reach enormous proportions, commonly extending beyond the midline and sometimes into the right iliac fossa. Patients may complain of a dragging discomfort or, less commonly, acute pain as a result of splenic infarcts. Other relatively common features include epistaxis and cough.

Patients with chronic VL may have visited traditional healers and have been subjected to medicinal cuts that subsequently become infected. Infection and ulceration of other superficial wounds is also common at the time of presentation. Intercurrent infections, such as pneumonia, bacillary or amoebic dysentery and tuberculosis, are particularly important in patients with long-standing disease and may be the main reason for

the patient seeking medical care. Other complications of VL include malnutrition, malabsorption, bleeding, nephritis and uveitis.

Some patients present acutely with an abrupt onset of high swinging fever and other symptoms resembling malaria. Specific cutaneous lesions are uncommon at the time of original presentation in VL. Rarely, a patient may be aware of a painless papule at the site of the infective bite. Post-kala-azar dermal leishmaniasis (PKDL) may occur following treatment and is discussed below.

Case fatality rates associated with VL range from 0–50% of treated cases to 85–90% of untreated cases.

Differential diagnosis of splenomegaly

Massive spleen

- Malaria or hyper-reactive malaria splenomegaly
- Portal hypertension, for example, caused by schistosomiasis, cirrhosis, etc.
- Lymphoma, leukaemia, myelodysplasia
- Haemoglobinopathies and hereditary haemolytic anaemias
- Splenic hydatid cyst
- Still's disease
- Glycogen storage and other metabolic diseases
- Amyloidosis

Moderate spleen

- Any of the above
- Bacterial endocarditis
- Brucellosis
- Cytomegalovirus
- HIV infection
- Infectious mononucleosis
- Leptospirosis
- Lyme disease
- Relapsing fever
- Syphilis
- Toxoplasmosis
- Trypanosomiasis
- Tuberculosis
- Typhoid
- Typhus.

Viscerotropic leishmaniasis

Splenomegaly and fever caused by *L. tropica* infection was noted in American troops involved in the Gulf War in the 1990s. None of these patients developed massive splenomegaly or other features typical of classical VL.

VL and HIV coinfection

Leishmania and HIV coinfection has been recognized since 1986. Most cases are thought to be caused either by reactivation of latent infection or associated with intravenous drug use (IVDU). IVDU-associated *L. infantum* infections are the most common *Leishmania* and HIV coinfections in southern Europe, where *Leishmania* and HIV coinfection accounts for 25–70% of all adult cases of VL and 1.5–9% of patients with AIDS develop VL. In north-west Ethiopia 15–30% of VL patients are coinfected with HIV. HIV and VL have a mutually adverse effect on disease progression and outcome.

Visceralization of *Leishmania* spp. normally associated with cutaneous or mucocutaneous disease is being increasingly reported among HIV-infected patients throughout the world.

Presentation of VL in HIV-positive patients is often atypical and may be a chance finding. Ninety per cent of cases have CD4 counts $<200 \times 10^6$/L. Atypical clinical features include dysphagia and cutaneous or mucocutaneous lesions. Nodular or ulcerative lesions may affect the tongue, oesophagus, stomach, rectum, larynx or lungs. The course varies from asymptomatic infection to rapidly progressive and fatal disease. Symptoms may be milder and more atypical as the CD4 count falls.

Prior to the use of ART, European studies indicated that 30% of patients died during or within 1 month of treatment. The mean survival was 12 months, and only 16% survived for more than 3 years. Relapses commonly occurred every 3–6 months. ART has reduced the clinical incidence of VL in HIV coinfected patients in southern Europe by up to 65%. Although ART may also delay relapse, 40% of patients taking ART will experience relapses unless receiving maintenance VL treatment, with a mean interval to first relapse of 7 months. Various regimens of antileishmanial drugs, such as pentamidine, liposomal amphotericin B and miltefosine, have been proposed to reduce relapses in HIV coinfected patients. Immune reconstitution inflammatory syndrome (IRIS) has been described in a small number of coinfected patients.

Investigations

Circumstantial evidence

Full blood count typically reveals anaemia, leucopenia and thrombocytopenia. This is partly explained by hypersplenism. However, a number of other factors may also be important, including possible autoimmune mechanisms and bone marrow depression.

Diagnostic work-up should include a coagulation screen or, if unavailable, at least an estimation of the bleeding and clotting times, particularly if a splenic aspirate is planned. Bilirubin and transaminases are (usually mildly) elevated in about 20% of patients, and the alkaline phosphatase is raised in about 40%. Serum albumin is low and globulins are raised, especially IgG. Albuminuria is common but urinalysis is otherwise normal in uncomplicated disease.

The formol gel test (FGT) is a simple test that is sometimes used to provide circumstantial evidence of VL. The FGT is not specific for VL and, when positive, indicates hyperglobulinaemia, whatever the cause. Add one drop of concentrated formalin solution (40% formaldehyde) to 1 mL of serum in a test tube. Shake to mix thoroughly. After 20 min at room temperature, the serum becomes a firm opaque jelly (like a cooked egg white) if the test is positive.

Serological evidence

IFAT and enzyme-linked immunoabsorbent assay (ELISA) have sensitivities and specificities above 95%. Although these tests may not be readily available in remote areas, it is possible to collect blood spots on filter paper, which can be sent elsewhere for testing.

The direct agglutination test (DAT) is also highly sensitive and specific, and easy to perform in the field. However, problems with stability of the antigen have led to unreliable results in some settings. A promising new version of the DAT is currently under development that uses freeze-dried antigen.

The K39 test is a commercially available immunochromatographic strip that uses recombinant leishmanial antigen. This has been shown to be 100% sensitive and 98% specific in India. However, when used to test clinically suspected VL in field conditions in Sudan and Nepal, K39 showed a lack of specificity. Serology may remain positive for years following successful treatment. Serology is unreliable in immunocompromised patients and is positive in only about 50% of patients with *Leishmania* and HIV coinfection.

Parasitological evidence

The gold standard for diagnosis of VL is identification of amastigotes of *L. donovani* spp. These are most readily found in splenic aspirates (>95% positive), bone marrow (>85%), buffy coat (>70%) and lymph node (>65%). In *Leishmania* and HIV coinfected patients, amastigotes may be detectable in peripheral blood (buffy coat) in 50%, bone marrow in 94% and in skin lesions and other affected tissues. Amastigotes are identified using a Giemsa or other Romanowsky stain. Aspirates may also be cultured on Novy, MacNeal and Nicolle's (NNN) medium.

PCR is capable of detecting infection with a single parasite and is being used increasingly for the diagnosis of VL and for monitoring relapse in HIV coinfected patients. PCR sensitivity is 82–100% for bone marrow and 72–100% for peripheral blood.

Urine antigen tests may prove useful in diagnosis and monitoring response to treatment. The detection of polypeptide fractions of K39 and K26 *Leishmania* antigen in urine of patients with VL has been shown to be 96% sensitive and 100% specific; these antigens were not detectable after 3 weeks of treatment, suggesting a good prognostic value. A latex agglutination test (KAtex; Kalon Biological, UK) that detects *Leishmania* antigens in urine has proved highly sensitive (86–100%) in two studies of HIV coinfected patients in Spain during clinical episodes when the parasite load was high. Furthermore, the test became negative following a satisfactory clinical response to treatment which may be helpful in monitoring the efficacy of treatment and the possible occurrence of relapses. Similar results have been found among HIV-negative patients.

Performing a splenic aspirate

Splenic aspiration is a straightforward procedure, relatively painless and safe, provided that one excludes patients with a bleeding tendency and those in whom portal hypertension, a splenic hydatid cyst or vascular abnormality is considered likely in the differential diagnosis. The patient should be comfortable and lying flat with the abdomen exposed. Select an area in the middle of the long axis of the spleen. Clean the skin with an alcohol swab or other antiseptic. Using a 21-gauge needle attached to a 5 mL syringe, insert the needle subcutaneously in line with the long axis of the spleen, draw back the plunger of the syringe to the 1 mL mark to create a negative pressure and swiftly insert the needle into the body of the spleen to a depth of about 2–3 cm at an angle of about 45° to the skin and withdraw immediately while maintaining negative pressure in the syringe. The entire procedure should take only a few seconds.

Having withdrawn the needle, there may be little or nothing visible in the syringe. This is not a problem. Disconnect the needle from the syringe and draw up 2 mL of air. Reconnect the needle and carefully squirt the contents of the needle onto one or more microscope slides and make a smear. The tiny amount of tissue that appears on the slide should be sufficient for diagnostic purposes.

It is probably safest to perform splenic aspirates in a setting where the patient can remain lying down and be monitored for a few hours and where facilities for transfusion are available if required. However, with experience, outpatient aspirates can be successfully carried out.

Management

Prior to embarking on specific chemotherapy with potentially toxic drugs, it is important to identify and treat intercurrent infections. Attention should also be given to improving the patient's nutritional status.

Pentavalent antimonials (SbV)

Sodium stibogluconate (Pentostam) and meglumine antimonate (Glucantime) are the drugs most commonly used as first-line treatment. These drugs are relatively expensive; however, an effective and cheaper generic version of sodium stibogluconate is now produced in India. The usual dose is 20 mg SbV/kg/day by slow intravenous infusion (the manufacturers of Pentostam recommend a minimum of 5 min) or intramuscularly for 20–40 days, depending on the geographical region. Side effects include arthralgia, nausea, abdominal pain and pancreatitis. Cardiotoxicity tends to occur with high-dose regimens, particularly with prolonged use, and includes ST segment inversion, prolongation of the QTc interval and fatal arrhythmias. Toxicity, particularly pancreatitis, is increased in HIV-positive patients. Furthermore, antimonials have been shown to stimulate HIV-1 replication *in vitro*.

Amphotericin B

Amphotericin B is currently regarded as second-line treatment and is used when antimonials are not appropriate, for example, in regions with high levels of resistance to SbV, such as Bihar, India. It is usually administered by slow intravenous infusion in 5% dextrose over 4–6 h, commencing at 0.1 mg/kg/day and gradually increasing to 1 mg/kg/day until a total dose of 20 mg/kg has been given. Studies in India have shown that there was no difference in infusion-related side effects if treatment was commenced at 1 mg/kg/day. Side effects include anaphylaxis, fever, chills, bone pain and thrombophlebitis. Hypokalaemia, renal impairment and anaemia may also occur.

Liposomal amphotericin B (AmBisome)

Amphotericin toxicity is reduced and efficacy enhanced by lyophilization, thereby enhancing distribution in macrophages and reticuloendothelial tissues. The most commonly recommended regimen for immunocompetent patients is 3 mg/kg/day on days 1–5, 14 and 21. Liposomal amphotericin B is very expensive; however, a recent study in India showed that administration of a single infusion (5 mg/kg) or five daily infusions of 1 mg/kg cured 92% of patients. If proved effective in larger trials, low-dose regimens could make the drug more affordable. In immunocompromised patients with HIV, the dose of liposomal amphotericin B is 4 mg/kg/day on days 1–5 followed by 4 mg/kg/day on days 10, 17, 24, 31 and 38. The relapse rate is high suggesting that maintenance treatment may be required.

Pentamidine

Pentamidine 4 mg/kg deep i.m. on alternate days for 5–25 weeks may be useful as second-line treatment in regions other than India where there is now significant resistance. Toxicity is common including sudden hypotension following injection, acute hypoglycaemia, renal impairment and arrhythmias. Long-term irreversible insulin-dependent diabetes occurs in more than 10% of patients treated. Pentamidine may have a role in preventing relapses in patients coinfected with HIV.

Miltefosine

Miltefosine is one of the most promising drugs to appear in recent times for the treatment of leishmaniasis. Originally developed as an oral antineoplastic agent, miltefosine is the first highly effective oral treatment for VL. Studies in India using 100 mg/day (or 2.5 mg/kg/day in children) for 4 weeks achieved 95% cure rates. Side effects include gastrointestinal upset, but this is rarely severe. However, miltefosine is abortifacient and teratogenic and may also reduce male fertility. Miltefosine has a long half-life (2–3 weeks) and a narrow therapeutic index, thus increasing the opportunity for the development of resistance. A reduced mortality was demonstrated among HIV–VL coinfected patients in Ethiopia when treated with miltefosine versus sodium stibogluconate. However, initial treatment failure and relapse rates were higher in HIV coinfected patients treated with miltefosine. Nevertheless, daily miltefosine may have a role in preventing relapses in *Leishmania* and HIV coinfected patients.

Combination treatment is now being investigated both as a means of mitigating against the development of resistance and also as a strategy for reducing the likelihood of relapse.

Aminosidine

Aminosidine (paromomycin) at doses in the range 15–20 mg/kg/day i.m. may be used alone for 21 days or synergistically with SbV or pentamidine, thereby allowing a shorter duration of treatment when used in combination therapy with these agents.

Post-kala-azar dermal leishmaniasis

PKDL occurs in about 10% of patients in India, 2–10 years after treatment for VL. Although PKDL is uncommon, an unusually high incidence (>50%) has recently been reported in southern Sudan, occurring at a mean of 56 days (range 0–18 days) following treatment. Initially, macules and papules appear around the mouth, which gradually spread over the face and sometimes more widely over the trunk and limbs. In time, nodules may develop resembling lepromatous leprosy. The papules and nodules in PKDL are usually packed with amastigotes and patients with this condition, which may persist for more than 20 years, may act as an important reservoir of infection. Prolonged treatment with SbV or other appropriate drug may be required to eliminate infection, although PKDL in Africa often resolves spontaneously without specific treatment. PKDL appears to be commoner and more severe in HIV coinfected patients.

Prevention

The stated aims of the WHO programme for the surveillance and control of leishmaniasis are 'to reduce the disease as quickly as possible to such a level that each country can integrate control surveillance activities at both technical and economic levels, into their overall health development activities'. To achieve this goal, WHO has set the following objectives:
- To provide early diagnosis and prompt treatment.
- To control the sandfly population through residual insecticide spraying of houses and through the use of insecticide-impregnated bed nets.
- To provide health education and produce training materials.
- To detect and contain epidemics in the early stages.
- To provide early diagnosis and effective management for *Leishmania* and HIV coinfections.

Achieving these objectives poses many problems. The methods that can be used to control VL depend on the epidemiological situation.

Eliminating or treating the reservoir host

Most success has been achieved where the domestic dog is the main reservoir—efforts being directed to catching and destroying infected dogs. Dogs with the infection look sick, lose their hair and have an enlarged spleen. France has been very active in controlling by this method. However, infected foxes invariably look healthy and are more difficult to control. Where humans are the main reservoir, active case-finding and treatment may be considered but is prohibitively expensive and likely to fail given that the majority of infections are subclinical. Detection and treatment of asymptomatic individuals carries additional cost and raises issues of individual risk–benefit, given the toxicity of available drugs.

There is no vaccine currently available for VL, although the future is brighter. Recent phase II trials in monkeys using alum-precipitated autoclaved *Leishmania major* with bacille Calmette–Guérin (BCG) have demonstrated protection against *L. donovani*.

Eliminating or avoiding the vector

Sandflies breed in dark moist habitats, such as cracks in masonry, piles of rubble, caves and in any dark protected sites such as holes in termite mounds or in outside latrines. Sandflies have a short flight range, seldom being found more than 200 m from their breeding place. They do not fly very high and are unlikely to reach people sleeping on the first floor of a building. They normally bite between dusk and dawn and are small enough to penetrate the mesh of standard mosquito nets. Insecticide-impregnated nets may be more effective but are relatively costly and do not prevent exposure in many epidemiological settings. Personal use of insect repellents or insecticide-impregnated clothing is generally not an option for people residing in endemic areas.

In India successful control was achieved during the period when widespread insecticide spraying of houses for malarial control was in use. The resurgence of infection on an epidemic scale has occurred in several areas many years after the spraying programme was abandoned.

In epidemics and localized outbreaks, residual insecticide spraying of houses and the immediate area around the house is the most effective immediate control measure. Sandflies usually succumb to DDT, and their hopping flight pattern renders them particularly vulnerable. DDT is cheaper than other residual insecticides, but it is losing popularity because of concern about the long-term environmental impact.

In regions where dogs are an important reservoir host (Latin America, Mediterranean basin and central and southwest Asia), the use of deltamethrin-impregnated dog-collars may be effective in reducing the burden of infection in both domestic dogs and children. (Note—the dogs wear the collars, not the children.)

Further reading

Alvar J, Aparicio P, Aseffa A *et al*. The relationship between leishmaniasis and AIDS: the second 10 years. *Clin Microbiol Rev* 2008; 21: 334–359. [Excellent review of emerging clinical and epidemiological issues related to HIV and leishmaniasis coinfection.]

Davies CR, Kaye P, Croft SL, Sundar S. Leishmaniasis: new approaches to disease control. *Br Med J* 2003; 326: 377–382. [Updated review of key aspects of control and annotated educational resource list.]

Guerin PJ, Olliaro P, Sundar S *et al*. Visceral leishmaniasis: current status of control, diagnosis, and treatment, and a proposed research and development agenda. *Lancet Infect Dis* 2002; 2: 494–501. [This article reviews the current situation and perspectives for diagnosis, treatment and control of visceral leishmaniasis and lists some priorities for research and development.]

Herwaldt BL. Leishmaniasis. *Lancet* 1999; 354: 1191–1199. [This review includes useful information on the clinical presentation, diagnosis and management of visceral, cutaneous and mucosal leishmaniasis.]

Lawn SD. Immune reconstitution disease associated with parasitic infections following initiation of antiretroviral therapy. *Curr Opin Infect Dis* 2007; 20: 482–488. [Interesting review describing 24 published cases of IRIS associated with parasitic infections.]

Murray HW, Berman JD, Davies CR, Saravia NG. Advances in leishmaniasis. *Lancet* 2005; 366: 1561–1577. [Comprehensive review that includes some excellent illustrations.]

Chapter 11

Cutaneous leishmaniasis

Cutaneous leishmaniasis is among the most important causes of chronic ulcerating skin lesions in the world. The organisms in the host tissues are mainly found in reticuloendothelial cells in the skin, where, as amastigotes, they multiply by simple fission. Microscopically, they cannot be distinguished from *Leishmania donovani*. The parasites, life cycles and vectors are similar to those described for species causing VL.

The clinical spectrum of disease may be classified as follows:

- cutaneous leishmaniasis (CL)
- diffuse cutaneous leishmaniasis (DCL)
- leishmaniasis recidivans (LR)
- mucocutaneous leishmaniasis (MCL), also known as mucosal leishmaniasis (ML).

It is common to attach the terms Old World or New World depending on the region in which the infection is acquired. The following species of *Leishmania* are commonly implicated:

- Old World: *L. tropica*, *L. major* and *L. aethiopica*; also *L. infantum* and *L. donovani*.
- New World: *L. mexicana* species complex (especially *L. mexicana*, *L. amazonensis* and *L. venezuelensis*) and *Viannia* sub-genus (most notably *L. [V.] braziliensis*, *L [V.] panamensis*, *L. [V.] guyanensis*

and *L. [V.] peruviana*); also *L. major*-like organisms and *L. chagasi*.

Ninety per cent of all cases of CL occur in Afghanistan, Brazil, Iran, Peru, Saudi Arabia and Syria, with 1–1.5 million new cases reported annually worldwide. Ninety per cent of all cases of ML occur in Bolivia, Brazil and Peru.

Clinical features

Cutaneous leishmaniasis

There is a variable incubation period, usually several weeks. Infections may be subclinical or clinical. Usually a papule develops at the site of infection, becomes a nodule and subsequently forms an ulcer with a central depression and raised indurated border. This may enlarge to a diameter of several centimetres and persist for months or years before eventually healing, leaving an atrophic scar. Some lesions do not ulcerate but persist as nodules or plaques (Figures 11.1 and 11.2). For differential diagnosis see Chapter 48.

Some patients have more than one primary lesion or may develop satellite lesions. A sporotrichoid-like nodular lymphangitis may occur (common with *L. [V.] panamensis* and *L. [V.] guyanensis*) in which there is thickening of the lymphatic channels draining the primary lesion with nodules at intervals along the path. Regional

Lecture Notes: Tropical Medicine, 6th edition.
By G.V. Gill and N.J. Beeching. Published 2009 by Blackwell Publishing, ISBN: 978-1-4051-8048-1.

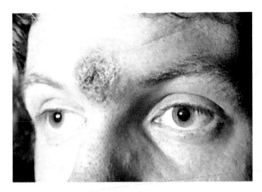

Figure 11.1 *L. tropica* lesion (Saudi Arabia).

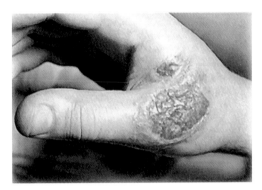

Figure 11.2 Cutaneous leishmaniasis lesion due to *L. mexicana* (Brazil).

adenopathy may occur and is sometimes bubonic in nature with *L. (V.) braziliensis*. Lesion pruritus or pain, and secondary bacterial infection may also occur. Koebner phenomena and 'seeding' at sites of skin trauma, including tattoos, also may occur.

Diffuse cutaneous leishmaniasis

The following species are usually involved:
- Old World: *L. aethiopica*—Ethiopia, Kenya
- New World: *L. mexicana*, *L. amazonensis*, *L. venezuelensis*

DCL closely resembles lepromatous leprosy. A single lesion gives rise to multiple diffuse soft fleshy nodules or plaques containing enormous numbers of amastigotes. Ulceration is unusual, probably because of deficient cell-mediated immunity. There may be extensive depigmentation in the areas of affected skin, increasing the resemblance to leprosy.

Leishmaniasis recidivans

This form is most commonly seen in Iran and Iraq and is also known as lupoid leishmaniasis. LR resembles lupus vulgaris and usually affects the face, sometimes invading mucous membranes. Lesions wax and wane, persisting for 20–40 years with scarring as they heal. The combination of scarring and signs of active inflammation is characteristic of the condition.

Mucosal leishmaniasis

Also known as espundia, ML is a dreaded complication of New World CL. Most cases are caused by the *Viannia* sub-genus, particularly *L. (V.) braziliensis*, *L. (V.) panamensis* and *L. (V.) guyanensis*. The onset is usually a few years after resolution of the original cutaneous lesion, but may occur while the primary lesion is still present or decades later. Haematogenous and lymphatic dispersal result in spread of amastigotes from the skin to the naso-oropharyngeal mucosa. Patients may initially complain of symptoms of chronic nasal congestion. The first perceptible lesion is often a nodule adjacent to the nostril. Granulomatous destructive lesions with chronic ulceration follow. After many years, the nasal septum, other nasal cartilaginous structures and palate may be destroyed, leaving a grotesque cavity in the centre of the face. The risk of mucosal disease following a primary cutaneous lesion is probably less than 5%. Rarely, destructive lesions may occur in the urinogenital region.

The differential diagnosis of ML includes:
- paracoccidiodomycosis
- histoplasmosis
- syphilis
- tertiary yaws
- leprosy
- rhinoscleroma
- midline granuloma
- sarcoidosis
- neoplasms.

Cutaneous leishmaniasis and HIV coinfection

A wide range of clinical presentations, sometimes occurring simultaneously, may occur in HIV coinfected patients, including papular, nodular, lepromatous, infiltrative, ulcerative, diffuse, psoriaform, cheloid, histioid and Kaposi's sarcoma-like. Visceralisation of cutaneous species may also occur. Similarly, VL species may present with cutaneous manifestations. Response to treatment may be problematic with delayed healing and increased likelihood of recurrences. Furthermore, CL may become clinically evident or deteriorate with improved immunocompetence following commencement of ART.

Investigations

Cutaneous and diffuse cutaneous leishmaniasis

Parasitological diagnosis is usually made by biopsy of the edge of the ulcer or other lesion. The specimen obtained can be divided in portions for
1 an impression smear (touch preparation) on a microscope slide that is then fixed with methanol and stained with Giemsa;
2 histopathology (less sensitive than impression smear);
3 culture on NNN medium; and
4 PCR. PCR is particularly useful as a relatively rapid way of distinguishing *Viannia* from non-*Viannia* sub-genus infections.

Other techniques that are sometimes used include needle aspirates and dermal scrapings.

Culture, isoenzyme and DNA sequencing techniques are available only in specialist centres. A promising new microcapillary culture technique using a monophasic medium is currently under development.

Leishmaniasis recidivans and mucosal leishmaniasis

Organisms are usually scanty in affected tissue, therefore PCR and culture are preferred for diagnosis. Serology is generally unhelpful but is

more likely to be positive in ML than in CL. The main use of serodiagnostic methods is when CL is suspected clinically but direct diagnostic methods have failed. In endemic areas a high proportion of the population may be seropositive. False-positive results may occur with lepromatous leprosy (LL), so the distinction between DCL and LL cannot be made reliably by serology. Fortunately, bacilli are always easy to find in LL.

Leishmanin test (Montenegro test)

This is a skin test using a killed promastigote suspension as antigen (area and species specific), injected intradermally and read at 48h, like the tuberculin test. In endemic areas, a high proportion of the population will be leishmanin test-positive and may also have healed scars. The test is positive in most cases of established CL and ML. It may be negative in some cases of CL caused by *L. aethiopica* and is usually negative in DCL. A strongly positive test may be useful in diagnosing LR cases, because the routine histology from these lesions is often indistinguishable from lupus vulgaris (cutaneous tuberculosis). The test is negative in active VL but may become positive after successful treatment.

With advances in other techniques for diagnosis, the leishmanin test is seldom used in clinical practice today.

Management

Before commencing treatment, the following issues should be considered:
- The number, size, evolution and persistence of lesions.
- The location of lesion(s) (e.g. on the face).
- Whether the patient is at risk of ML.
- Other features (e.g. the presence of nodular lymphangitis).

Treatment of cutaneous leishmaniasis

Cosmetically unimportant lesions caused by non-destructive and non-metastasizing species usually heal spontaneously and therefore may not require active treatment.

Local, topical and physical treatments

Various local, physical and topical therapies are sometimes used, including:
- heat treatment or cryotherapy;
- topical amphotericin B (*L. major*);
- intralesional antimony therapy; and
- paromomycin ointment (available in Israel).

Treatment with paromomycin may result initially in increased ulceration, so it is best avoided for ulcers on the face.

Oral Treatment

The following oral agents can be used for treating relatively benign cosmetically unimportant lesions.

Ketoconazole—modest activity against *L. mexicana, L. (V.) panamensis* and possibly *L. major.*

Itraconazole—better tolerated than ketoconazole but may be less effective against the *Viannia* sub-genus and *L. major.*

Fluconazole—variable effectiveness against *L. major.*

Miltefosine—currently being investigated for treatment of New World CL. Results against *L. (V.) panamensis* in Colombia were promising, however this was not so for *L. (V.) braziliensis* and *L. mexicana* in Guatemala. A recent non-randomized trial involving patients with ML caused by *L. (V.) braziliensis* in Bolivia showed that oral miltefosine was at least as effective as parenteral amphotericin B. In addition, the cure rate with miltefosine was approximately equivalent to historical cure rates using parenteral pentavalent antimony for mild and extensive disease in neighbouring Peru. The toxicity profile of miltefosine was superior to that of antimony and far superior to that of amphotericin B.

Parenteral treatment

Pentavalent antimony therapy (SbV) (i.v. or i.m.) is probably still the best option if optimal effectiveness is important. Short-course pentamidine has been shown to be effective in Colombia where disease is predominantly caused by the *Viannia*

sub-genus. Old World DCL is treated with a combination of SbV and aminosidine. Response may be poor in some parts of Ethiopia and pentamidine is used as an alternative; however, about 10% of patients are left with dia-betes mellitus following treatment. New World DCL is treated with SbV. LR may be treated with parenteral or intralesional SbV, or may respond to heat treatment.

ML treatment is of greater importance. Adequate systemic treatment of cutaneous lesions is assumed (but not proven) to decrease the already low risk of mucosal disease. ML is harder to treat than cutaneous lesions and becomes increasingly so as it progresses. Currently, the best treatment options are SbV 20 mg/kg i.v./i.m. for 28 days (achieves cure rates of about 75% for mild disease and 10–63% for more advanced disease) or conventional amphotericin B. Concomitant corticosteroids are indicated if respiratory compromise develops.

Choosing the most appropriate treatment for cutaneous leishmaniasis

The key questions are 'who needs parenteral treatment' and 'for how long'?

It is useful to classify clinical presentations as 'simple' or 'complex' based on the following criteria.

'Complex' : >2–3 lesions; >40 mm diameter; lymphatic/lymph node spread; cosmetic problems; functional problems; failure to respond to treatment as a 'simple' lesion.

Patients with complex lesions and all patients with *Viannia* sub-genus species or unidentified New World species should be offered parenteral sodium stibogluconate (SSG) as first-line management (Table 11.1).

Prevention

In general, the principles of prevention and control are the same as for VL. In the Middle East, it is customary for mothers to expose cosmetically unimportant areas of their infants to sandfly bites or to deliberately inoculate them with infected

Table 11.1 Summary of recommended first-line treatment for cutaneous leishmaniasis

Species	Clinical presentation	
	'Simple'	**'Complex'**
Old World species	Intralesional, topical, physical or appropriate oral treatment	SSG 20 mg/kg i.v. for 10–20 days
L. mexicana complex	As above	} SSG 20 mg/kg i.v. for 20 days (28 days for patients with ML)
L. Viannia sub-genus or unidentified New World species	SSG 20 mg/kg i.v. for 20 days	

Abbreviation: SSG, sodium stibogluconate.

Note: Clinical presentation 'Complex' if >2–3 lesions; >40 mm diameter; lymphatic/lymph node spread; cosmetic problems; functional problems; failure to respond to treatment as a 'simple' lesion.

material to render the child immune to that species. The development of effective vaccines is proving difficult. A vaccine using live attenuated *L. major* promastigotes has been produced which appears to be effective although its use carries a small risk of precipitating an aggressive lesion or the development of LR. There has also been some interesting work recently on the development of vaccines against sandfly saliva.

Further reading

Bailey M, Lockwood D. Cutaneous leishmaniasis. *Clin Dermatol* 2007; 25: 203–211. [Excellent recent review.]

Herwaldt BL. Leishmaniasis. *Lancet* 1999; 354: 1191–1199. [This review includes useful information on the clinical presentation, diagnosis and management of visceral, cutaneous and mucosal leishmaniasis.]

Murray HW, Berman JD, Davies CR, Saravia NG. Advances in leishmaniasis. *Lancet* 2005; 366: 1561–1577. [Comprehensive review that includes some excellent illustrations.]

Chapter 12

Tuberculosis

On 24 March 1882 Robert Koch demonstrated *Mycobacterium tuberculosis* to be the cause of the disease TB. Since then, advances in human understanding of the disease have been major catalysts in the development of modern medicine. In 1993 the WHO declared TB an international emergency, an unprecedented step, and interest and funding for TB control has increased since that time, leading to the establishment, in 2000, of the Global Partnership to Stop TB (Stop TB). As we approach the second decade of the twenty-first century, the full genome of *M. tuberculosis* is known, and the global number of new TB cases *per capita* has been falling slowly since 2003. Nonetheless, the total number of new TB cases continues to rise every year (an estimated 9.2 million new cases in 2006). Most of the world's 1.7 million TB deaths per year occur among poor adults and adolescents in the developing countries of the tropics. The main clinical and public health focus of this chapter is on TB as it manifests in adulthood, recognizing, meanwhile, that TB in childhood needs much more attention than it has attracted hitherto.

Microbiology

Of the mycobacteria, *M. tuberculosis*, *M. bovis* and *M. africanum* are now known to be genetically

Lecture Notes: Tropical Medicine, 6th edition.
By G.V. Gill and N.J. Beeching. Published 2009 by Blackwell Publishing, ISBN: 978-1-4051-8048-1.

very similar, have the highest pathogenicity and are together referred to as the *M. tuberculosis* (MTB) complex. They are anaerobic, non-spore-forming, non-motile bacilli with a large cell wall content of high-molecular-weight lipids. Growth is slow, the generation time being 15–20h, as compared to well under 1h for most common bacterial pathogens. Visible growth of yellow colonies in culture, usually on egg-based solid Löwenstein–Jensen medium, takes between 4 and 12 weeks.

Bacilli of the MTB complex are referred to as tubercle bacilli, acid-fast bacilli (AFB) or acid- and alcohol-fast bacilli (AAFB) on the basis of the ability of their lipid-rich cell walls to retain the red carbol-fuchsin stain in the presence of acid and alcohol during the Ziehl–Neelsen (ZN) staining process. Under oil-immersion light microscopy the stained bacilli appear as slightly bent rods, 2–4 µm long and 0.2–0.5 µm wide. Distinguishing between the three species is impossible by microscopy and difficult by culture. Furthermore, clinical presentations of disease caused by the bacilli are similar. Therefore, it is not possible to be precise about the relative contributions of the three species to the sum total of human TB disease. However, *M. tuberculosis* is globally the most prevalent and widely recognized to cause most of the global burden of disease, particularly in the tropics. This chapter therefore focuses on MTB and not on the other less pathogenic mycobacteria, often referred to as mycobacteria other than tuberculosis (MOTT). Examples of MOTT include the *M. avium–intracellulare* complex, *M. marinum* and *M. gordonae*.

Epidemiology

Magnitude of the problem

It is estimated that one-third of the global human population is infected with MTB, and the microbe is thought to cause one-quarter of avoidable adult deaths in developing countries. The geographical distribution of TB is shown in Figure 12.1.

Transmission

Although transmission of *M. bovis* from cattle to humans may be important in some parts of the tropics, humans are the only reservoir of MTB infection and transmission is possible only from individuals with disease. It occurs by droplet nuclei—infectious particles of respiratory secretions aerosolized by coughing, sneezing or talking, which are sufficiently small (around 10 μm, drying to <5 μm diameter while airborne) to remain suspended in the air for long periods and reach the terminal air spaces if inhaled.

Infection and immunity

Once MTB droplet nuclei reach alveolar level within the lungs, the bacilli are taken up by phagocytosis into air-space macrophages. Within these cells they are processed into phagosomes which fail to acidify. In this way, the bacilli avoid intracellular killing and may survive and multiply for long periods of time. Infected macrophages may therefore carry viable bacilli in the lymphatics to regional lymph nodes or in the bloodstream to any part of the body.

Both humoral and cell-mediated immune responses are mounted against MTB and are correlated with the development of detectable delayed-type hypersensitivity (DTH) reactions. Rarely, these are manifested clinically in the form of erythema nodosum or phlyctenular conjunctivitis. More usually, DTH to MTB is detected by intradermal injection of mycobacterial purified protein derivatives (PPD)—the basis of the Mantoux, Tine and Heaf tests. The extent of local skin erythema, induration and blistering (in vigorous responses) are measured 48 h after injection in order to grade responses. The release of interferon gamma (IFN-γ) by T lymphocytes in response to mycobacterial antigens has recently been exploited in the development of interferon gamma release assays (IGRA) for the detection of MTB infection (see later).

Although individuals clearly vary in their immune capacity to contain or eliminate MTB, it must be emphasized that immune responses to MTB—however generated—are generally not protective against further infection. A common misconception is that PPD skin responsiveness is correlated with the effectiveness of immunity to MTB. Although T-cell release of IFN-γ is now recognized as crucial, it remains unclear what combination of cell-mediated and humoral responses to MTB is most important in conferring protective immunity and those components responsible for DTH responses are not necessarily the most useful.

Progression to disease

In the usual course of events, somewhere between 5% and 10% of people will develop active TB after MTB infection. About 3% develop disease within the first year, with the remainder developing disease with ever-diminishing frequency thereafter. More than 90% of MTB infections therefore do not result in disease within a normal human lifespan.

The clinical manifestations of TB among those who develop active disease depend on two things: the state of the immune system and the location of the bulk of the MTB multiplication. In cases where disease occurs soon after primary infection, the bacilli multiply and spread in the context of a naïve immune system. Primary forms of disease therefore occur at common thoracic sites of initial multiplication—hence pleurisy extending from an alveolar focus and cavitation in hilar lymph nodes. They also tend to disseminate

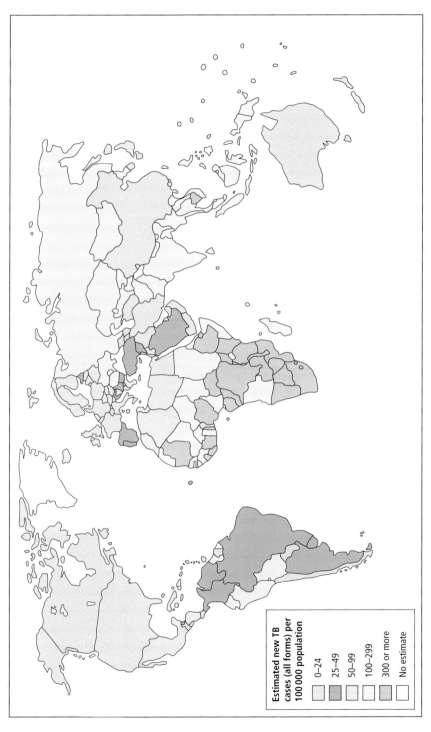

Figure 12.1 Estimated global TB incidence rates in 2006. (*Source*: WHO)

Estimated new TB
cases (all forms) per
100 000 population

0–24

25–49

50–99

100–299

300 or more

No estimate

to multiple sites including the central nervous system—hence tuberculous meningitis and 'miliary' tuberculosis. In disseminated disease, minigranulomas (tubercles) develop around small numbers of bacilli that are widely distributed within tissues.

In cases where disease occurs a long time after primary infection, either as reactivation of latent infection or as a result of reinfection with a new strain of MTB, the bacilli multiply in the context of a sensitized immune system. The associated DTH responses tend to lead to tissue destruction at the site of multiplication; hence cavitating caseous lesions in which large numbers of multiplying bacilli are contained by an encircling rim of giant cells and granulomas—the hallmark of tuberculous pathology. These 'postprimary' lesions are most commonly present in the apices of the lungs, the theory being that this location provides the most conducive combination of ventilation and perfusion for long-term latency. They may also occur at any site to which bacilli were seeded during initial multiplication around the time of primary infection.

Given sufficient time, postprimary-type disease in the lungs is likely to result in communication between the cavitating pathology and an airway.

MTB bacilli can then be aerosolized in droplet nuclei and expelled into the atmosphere when the affected individual coughs, sneezes or talks. Patients with cavitating lung disease are therefore the main sources of new MTB infections. The processes of infection and progression to disease are illustrated in Figure 12.2.

Risk factors for infection and disease

Risk factors for MTB infection fall into the following two broad categories:
1 Those which put people in an atmosphere where MTB-containing droplet nuclei accumulate in the atmosphere.
2 Those decreasing the ability of alveolar macrophages to incapacitate MTB once taken up.

The first category includes prolonged contact with a person or people with pulmonary TB (especially cavitating disease) and the environmental features associated with poverty. Overcrowded and poorly ventilated living and working conditions are clearly ideal for MTB transmission. As MTB is susceptible to killing on exposure to ultraviolet light, dark and humid conditions such as those found in mines and prisons also favour transmission. The second category includes anything

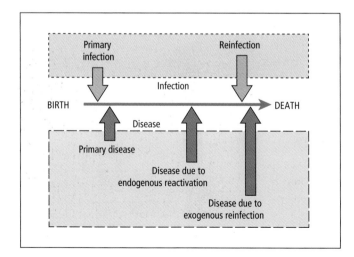

Figure 12.2 The processes of TB infection and progression to disease.

capable of compromising alveolar macrophage killing of MTB, such as corticosteroid therapy and HIV infection.

Risk factors for disease have in common their ability to impair cell-mediated immunity, particularly those functions dependent on T cells. Examples include HIV infection, malnutrition (particularly vitamin D deficiency) and corticosteroid therapy.

Effect of HIV on the epidemiology of TB

The superimposition of HIV infection in people with pre-existing MTB infection increases the risk of developing TB from 5% to 10% over a lifetime to around 15% per year. In addition to this increased risk of reactivation disease, HIV-infected people are at increased risk of acquiring new MTB infections which may also progress to disease. This has meant that in those parts of the world where the prevalence of MTB infection and HIV infection overlap geographically, there has been an explosive increase in the number of TB cases which has increased the annual risk of MTB infection for both HIV-infected and HIV-uninfected people. Both HIV infection and MTB infection tend to affect particularly adolescents and adults in the middle decades of life—their most economically productive years. In many developing countries in the tropics, particularly in sub-Saharan Africa, these two devastating infections overlap both geographically and socially, and the resultant impact on livelihoods has been appalling. TB not only arises in conditions of poverty, but it is itself a poverty-generating illness.

Clinical features

Pulmonary versus extrapulmonary disease

Pulmonary features predominate in around 85% of all TB disease presentations. Although in most instances pulmonary disease will be the only obvious pathology, it may be associated with tuberculous pathology in other organ systems. Parenchymal lung disease may extend and include pericardial disease or regional lymph node cavitation. Conversely, both pericardial TB and tuberculous lymphadenitis may occur in the absence of any concurrent pulmonary pathology and would then be classified as extrapulmonary disease manifestations. Counterintuitively, two forms of intrathoracic TB pathology may be classified as extrapulmonary TB when they occur in the absence of concurrent parenchymal lung disease: mediastinal lymphadenopathy and pleurisy. This serves to emphasize that any clinical presentation in which pulmonary parenchymal disease is present is classified as pulmonary, and only patients with pulmonary disease, not extrapulmonary disease, are capable of transmitting MTB to others.

Among extrapulmonary presentations, lymphadenitis (Figure 12.3) and pleurisy are the most common, each accounting for approximately 25% of the total. Genitourinary TB is next at around 15%, followed by miliary and bone TB at around 10%. Meningeal and peritoneal TB each account for less than 5% of extrapulmonary TB disease.

Systemic symptoms

The vast majority of TB presentations, whether pulmonary or extrapulmonary, are insidious in onset. Varying combinations of the chronic constitutional symptoms of fevers, night sweats,

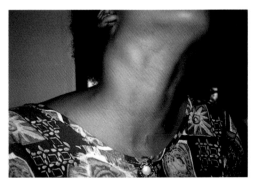

Figure 12.3 Solitary enlarged tuberculous cervical lymph node.

weight loss and malaise (perhaps secondary to an associated anaemia of chronic disease) are common but are neither universal nor specific indicators of TB.

Symptoms of pulmonary TB

Beyond the systemic manifestations, the symptoms and signs of TB depend on the site of the major pathology. As pulmonary disease, and not extrapulmonary disease, is the most common form of the disease in adults and adolescents and the priority target for public health intervention, it is the main focus for further clinical description here.

Persistent coughing of insidious onset is easily the most common symptom indicating pulmonary TB. As pulmonary pathology advances, the cough becomes more productive of mucopurulent sputum and chest pain may occur with severe coughing. However, it is important to remember that some patients with early pulmonary disease may not produce much sputum. The sputum may be streaked with blood in about 10% of cases, and this usually indicates that the cavitating pathology has led to local damage of small blood vessels. Frank or catastrophic haemoptysis can occur if the larger blood vessels become involved, but this is rare occurring in fewer than 1% of cases.

Signs of pulmonary TB

Patients with TB may be wasted. Other than this, the signs are dependent on the site and the extent of the underlying pathology. Much is often made of chest signs such as 'amphoric breathing' and consolidation. Certainly, the lung damage can be extensive and often includes signs of volume loss, including tracheal shift. The truth is that most patients with pulmonary disease have very few chest signs, and apart from detecting massive pleural effusions that need draining, the slavish pursuit of chest signs is of little use in guiding clinical management. Patients with advanced pulmonary disease in the tropics may have finger clubbing, a sign that is otherwise not often associated with TB in Europe and North America.

Clinical features of selected forms of extrapulmonary TB

Apart from tuberculous lymphadenitis (Figure 12.4), which usually presents as a unilateral chain of matted lymph nodes that may occasionally ulcerate and discharge, extrapulmonary TB is notoriously difficult to diagnose. This is because non-specific systemic manifestations predominate in the early stages, and these forms of the disease are not amenable to any investigations that come close to the immediacy and specificity of sputum smear microscopy for AFB. As pathology advances, more useful signs such as meningism, bone damage, serous effusions and fistulae may become apparent.

Effect of HIV on clinical presentations of TB

It is important to remember that there are exceptions to the simplified division of tuberculous disease into the 'primary' and 'postprimary' forms presented earlier. Postprimary disease may manifest itself as disseminated disease such as miliary TB if the immune system is very compromised by an additional factor such as HIV infection. Postprimary disease arising early in HIV infection, before significant immunocompromise is established, is likely to present with cavitating pathology that is indistinguishable from disease

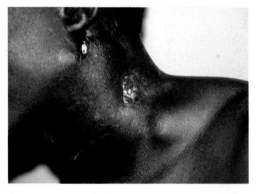

Figure 12.4 Cervical tubercuolous lymphadenitis with ulceration of some of the nodes.

arising in HIV-uninfected individuals. However, in the later stages of HIV infection, as underlying immunocompromise becomes more severe, postprimary TB disease becomes more likely to present in a disseminated or non-cavitating form resembling primary disease. This is why extrapulmonary 'primary-like' presentations of TB, such as pleural effusions, lymphadenitis, TB meningitis, miliary TB (Figure 12.5) and non-cavitating pulmonary TB, are more common among HIV-infected patients.

Differential diagnosis

The various types of pulmonary TB infections in the tropics have a wide differential diagnosis. Some of these, such as pulmonary paragonimiasis, nocardiosis, actinomycosis, coccidioidomycosis and melioidosis, are defined by their geographical distribution. Others, such as *Pneumocystis jirovecii* pneumonia (PCP) and pulmonary KS, occur in the context of HIV infection. The remainder, including bacterial pneumonias, lung abscess, atypical mycobacteria other than MTB, bronchial carcinoma, bronchiectasis, sarcoidosis,

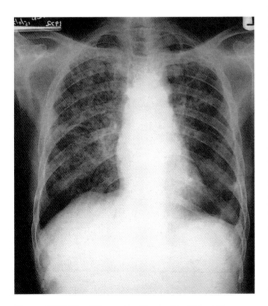

Figure 12.5 Chest X-ray of patient with miliary TB.

Wegener's granulomatosis and cryptogenic fibrosing alveolitis are more universal.

The differential diagnosis of the most common extrapulmonary forms of TB, lymphadenitis and pleurisy, is mainly from neoplastic processes such as KS, lymphoma and metastatic bronchial carcinoma.

Investigations

Isolation of MTB by culture from clinical specimens is the gold standard for the definitive diagnosis of TB. However, because of the slow generation time, mycobacterial culture takes between 2 (modern liquid-based culture techniques) and 12 weeks (more universal, solid-based culture techniques). This is clearly too long to be useful in guiding clinical decision-making. In addition, the laboratory infrastructure required to sustain quality-assured culture of mycobacteria is frequently unavailable in the poorer parts of the tropics.

Sputum smear microscopy for tubercle bacilli is therefore absolutely central to the diagnosis of TB. Approximately half of all culture-proven cases of pulmonary TB produce more than the threshold 10,000 organisms per mL of sputum required for detection by microscopy. These smear-positive cases tend to have more cavitating lung disease and are more infectious than smear-negative cases. Although smear microscopy is a specific test for pulmonary TB, it lacks sensitivity, particularly for early disease that has not yet cavitated. ZN staining of smears prepared direct from sputum and light microscopy remain the most universally available techniques. Systematic synthesis of existing evidence suggests that sensitivity of smear microscopy can be improved by between 2% and 30% if sputum specimens are concentrated using ordinary household bleach prior to smear preparation, but results are very variable, depending on the processing technique used. Using auramine-phenol staining and fluorescence microscopy can increase sensitivity more consistently by an average of 10% over that achieved by ZN staining and light microscopy. Neither approach is associated with a loss in specificity, but there is as yet no consensus on how or whether to operationalize these modifications in universal clinical and public health practice. Bleach concentration can require centrifuges or different lengths of sedimentation time and different bleach concentrations. Conventional fluorescence microscopes are expensive and costly to run because of the need for frequent bulb changes. However, new light emitting diode (LED) fluorescence microscopes look set to replace traditional halogen microscopes and can potentially be set up in most microscopy centres.

The main problem in the diagnosis of TB lies with patients who have clinical features suggestive of pulmonary TB but whose sputum smears are negative for AFB. Unless there are strong clinical indicators of an alternative diagnosis, the decision on whether or not to treat for TB lies with chest radiography. Unfortunately, chest X-rays of smear-negative TB cases are notoriously difficult to interpret as the features that are most specific to TB (such as cavitation) are frequently absent. The radiological features of pulmonary TB are also particularly difficult in HIV-infected individuals, where an increased proportion of culture-proven cases will have a variety of atypical radiographical manifestations, including lower lobe consolidation and patchy infiltrates. Films may even be normal.

PPD skin test positivity is used as a marker of MTB infection, and high-grade PPD responses are correlated with the presence of active disease. However, false-positives may occur with exposure to non-pathogenic environmental mycobacteria or BCG vaccination. Similarly, false-negatives are a problem when immune responses are blunted, for example by HIV, measles, drugs or severe malnutrition. PPD skin testing is mainly used in the diagnosis of TB in children, in whom most disease is of primary type and only rarely smear-positive. The IGRA techniques mentioned earlier are more specific and sensitive in detecting latent MTB infections than PPD skin testing. Nonetheless, they still have the following disadvantages which rule them out of routine tropical practice: their place in the diagnosis of disease (rather than infection) remains controversial; they require a level of laboratory functionality that is not

found in most tropical laboratories; and they are expensive.

A variety of laboratory tests indicating chronic inflammation, such as raised erythrocyte sedimentation rate and C-reactive protein, or anaemia of chronic disease may help in difficult cases but only have a limited role in the investigation of suspected TB cases in the tropics.

Management

Principles of TB chemotherapy

TB treatment aims to:
- cure the patient of TB
- prevent death from active TB or its late effects
- prevent relapse of TB
- decrease transmission of TB to others

These aims can be achieved while preventing the selection of resistant bacilli in infectious patients through the careful use of modern chemotherapy.

Antibiotic chemotherapy for TB has been built up over the past 40 years around five first-line drugs on the basis of several randomized controlled trials and cohort studies. Four of the drugs are bactericidal (streptomycin, isoniazid, rifampicin and pyrazinamide) while the remaining one is bacteriostatic (ethambutol). Each is referred to by a single capital letter in standard descriptions of different regimens (Table 12.1, which also details main side effects and doses). The bactericidal drugs act preferentially on slightly different populations of organisms (Table 12.2).

During the initial, intensive phase of chemotherapy, a minimum of three drugs should be administered concurrently to reduce the more rapidly dividing bacillary load. A minimum of two drugs can be used in the continuation phase aimed at sterilizing lesions containing fewer bacilli with slower generation times.

All modern drug regimens contain rifampicin, isoniazid and pyrazinamide and as yet there is no convincing evidence that regimens shorter than 6-months' duration will reliably cure TB. Monotherapy for TB disease should never be given as it will lead to the development of antibiotic resistance.

Table 12.1 First-line antituberculosis drugs, standard abbreviations, dosages and adverse effects

Essential anti-TB drug (abbreviation)	Mode of action	Main adverse effect(s)	Recommended dose (range) (mg/kg) Daily	Recommended dose (range) (mg/kg) Intermittent 3×/week
Isoniazid (H)	Bactericidal	Peripheral neuropathy	5	10
		Hepatitis	(4–6)	(8–12)
Rifampicin (R)	Bactericidal	Hepatitis	10	10
		Influenza-like syndrome and thrombocytopenia[a]	(8–12)	(8–12)
Pyrazinamide (Z)	Bactericidal	Arthralgia	25	35
		Hyperuricaemia leading to gout	(20–30)	(30–40)
Streptomycin (S)	Bactericidal	VIII cranial nerve damage—vestibular dysfunction; nephrotoxicity	15	15
			(12–18)	(12–18)
Ethambutol (E)	Bacteriostatic	Optic neuritis	15	30
			(15–20)	(25–35)
Thioacetazone (T)	Bacteriostatic	Exfoliative dermatitis	2.5	Not applicable

[a]More common with intermittent dosage.

Table 12.2 Different populations of *Mycobacterium tuberculosis* and their susceptibility to different drugs

	In cavities	In closed caseous lesions	In macrophages
Relative number of organisms per mL	10^7–10^8	10^2–10^4	10^2–10^4
Multiplication	Active/rapid	Slow/intermittent	Slow
Medium	Neutral/alkaline	Neutral	Acid
Most useful drugs	S R H	R H	Z R H

Abbreviations: H, isoniazid; R, rifampicin; S, streptomycin; Z, pyrazinamide.

All of the first-line drugs can be given orally except for streptomycin which requires intramuscular injection. Because of the requirement for needles and syringes, streptomycin is no longer recommended in the first-line treatment of new TB cases in areas of HIV seroprevalence.

Deciding which treatment regimen to use

It is important to follow national or regional guidelines for chemotherapy. Category I regimens are used for new patients who are unlikely to harbour resistant organisms. Category II regimens are reserved for patients who have previously received some form of antituberculous chemotherapy and are therefore more likely to harbour mycobacteria that have become resistant to one or more of the first-line drugs. It is therefore important to take a careful history about previous treatment before starting a patient on TB chemotherapy. Some examples of WHO-approved Category I and II regimens are shown in Table 12.3. A recent, large, multicentre trial in predominantly HIV-uninfected patients showed that the regimens using EH rather than

Table 12.3 WHO-approved antituberculosis regimens

TB treatment category	TB patients	Alternative TB treatment regimens	
		Intensive phase	Continuation phase
I	New smear-positive pulmonary TB or New smear-negative pulmonary TB with extensive parenchymal involvement; new cases of severe forms of extrapulmonary TB	2EHRZ (SRHZ)[a] 2EHRZ (SRHZ) 2EHRZ (SRHZ)	4HR 4H$_3$R$_3$ 6HE
II	Sputum smear-positive relapse; treatment failure; treatment after interruption	2SHRZE/1HRZE[a] 2SHRZE/1HRZE	5HRE 5H$_3$R$_3$E$_3$
III	New smear-negative pulmonary TB (other than in Category I); new less severe forms of extrapulmonary TB	2HRZ[a] 2HRZ 2HRZ	4HR 4H$_3$R$_3$ 6HE
IV	Chronic case (still sputum smear-positive after supervised retreatment)	Not applicable Refer to WHO guidelines on management of drug-resistant TB	

There is a standard code for TB treatment regimens. Each first-line anti-TB drug has an abbreviation (shown in Table 12.1). A regimen consists of two phases. The number before a phase is the duration of that phase in months. A number in subscript (e.g. 3) after a letter is the number of doses of that drug per week. If there is no number in subscript after a letter, then treatment with that drug is daily. An alternative drug (or drugs) appears as a letter (or letters) in brackets.
[a]Preferred option.

RH in the continuation phase were associated with significantly more unfavourable outcomes. An analysis of the outcomes amongst the subset of HIV-infected patients within this trial (none of whom received antiretroviral therapy [ART]) showed that they did particularly badly with the EH-containing regimens. There is, therefore, a global move towards universal adoption of the 6-month regimen with HR in the continuation phase. Some experts and countries remain concerned that allowing relatively unsupervised use of rifampicin in this way will lead to the increasing development of rifampicin resistance (see later controversy around direct observation of therapy and adherence, p. 97). The use of fixed-dose combination RH formulations should reduce this risk. Category III regimens have been recommended for use in less severe, smear-negative forms of disease, but for simplicity there has been a move towards the use of Category I regimens for all new cases, regardless of smear status.

A 'trial of therapy' as a way of confirming a TB diagnosis is not recommended, unless the situation is life-threatening. In some instances, non-TB infections may respond to the broad-spectrum antibiotic effect of drugs such as streptomycin and rifampicin. There is also an increased risk of chaotic ingestion of drugs and the consequent development of drug resistance.

Table 12.4 Recording standardized treatment outcomes in smear-positive pulmonary TB

Cured
Patient who is smear-negative at, or 1 month prior to, the completion of treatment and on at least one previous occasion

Treatment completed
Patient who has completed treatment but without smear microscopy proof of cure

Died
Patient who died during treatment, regardless of cause

Failure
Smear-positive patient who remained or became smear-positive again 5 months or later after commencing treatment

Defaulted
Patient whose treatment was interrupted for 2 months or more

Transferred out
Patient who has been transferred to another reporting unit and for whom the treatment outcome is not known

Monitoring treatment

Patients with smear-positive pulmonary TB should be monitored by sputum smear examination: once at the end of the intensive phase, once during the continuation phase and once at the end of the therapy. It is unnecessary and wasteful of resources to monitor using chest radiography. For patients with smear-negative pulmonary TB and extrapulmonary TB, clinical monitoring is the usual if somewhat unsatisfactory way of assessing response to treatment. Routine monitoring by mycobacterial culture of sputum is rarely feasible in developing countries in the tropics.

At the end of the intensive phase, most patients will have negative sputum smears. Such patients can then start the continuation phase of treatment. If sputum smears remain positive at this stage despite careful adherence to treatment, it may indicate that the patient had a particularly heavy initial bacillary load. Rarely, this is an indication of drug-resistant TB which will not respond to Category I treatment. Whatever the reason, the initial intensive phase should be prolonged for the third month. The patient then starts the continuation phase. If smears remain positive after a month of the continuation phase, this constitutes treatment failure and the patient should be restarted on a full course of a Category II regimen.

At the end of the treatment course, treatment outcomes are recorded according to one of six categories shown in Table 12.4. This allows for systematic cohort analysis and reporting of cure rates—an important part of TB control (see later).

The question of isolation

Routinely admitting smear-positive TB patients in order to 'isolate' them from the community is not an absolute requirement. In most cases, any onward community transmission of MTB from a smear-positive case will have occurred by the time the diagnosis is established, and modern chemotherapy will render such patients non-infectious by the end of the second week of treatment in more than 95% of cases, provided that the initial isolate is fully drug sensitive. Protecting others from infection is, on the whole, best achieved by careful chemotherapy rather than physical isolation. Admitting patients to hospital should be necessary only when the patient is severely ill and needs full hospital care, and it must be remembered that a TB case is more likely to come into contact with individuals who are vulnerable to MTB infection (such as those infected with HIV) in hospital than in the general community. If hospital admission is necessary, then this should be to a dedicated well-ventilated TB ward located away from other inpatients. Individual isolation rooms for TB patients are mostly unavailable in countries with high TB incidence. This will need to change with the increasing prevalence of drug-resistant TB (see later).

Adjunctive corticosteroid therapy

Many advocate the concurrent use of high-dose corticosteroids with TB treatment for large pleural and pericardial tuberculous effusions. There are some trials indicating that this is helpful for rapid relief of symptoms and for reduction in complication rates, but systematic reviews suggest that the evidence is not strong and is certainly not available for HIV-infected patients with TB. The potential disadvantages of corticosteroid therapy, including pharmacokinetic interactions with TB drugs and reactivation of other latent infections (such as *Strongyloides*), should be weighed carefully against potential benefits.

Prevention and public health aspects

The WHO-recommended DOTS strategy is the internationally recognized approach to TB control. BCG vaccination and isoniazid preventive therapy are mentioned briefly for completeness.

BCG vaccination

The BCG vaccine is the world's most frequently administered vaccine, and it has been available since the 1920s. It is a live attenuated vaccine that is given intradermally. Unfortunately, there is little evidence that it provides long-lasting protection against the development of pulmonary TB. This appears to be particularly true from the trials conducted in the tropics. Nonetheless, BCG is still included in the Expanded Programme of Immunization, mainly because there is some evidence that it protects against disseminated forms of TB in children. It has also been shown to be protective against leprosy and Buruli ulcer.

Isoniazid preventive therapy

The rationale behind preventive therapy is to eradicate latent infection in PPD-positive people before it develops into active disease. Several placebo-controlled trials in HIV-negative people infected with MTB have shown that isoniazid given daily for 6–12 months substantially reduces the subsequent risk of TB disease. However, preventive therapy has not been recognized as a cost-effective universal approach to TB control but instead has been focused on individuals at increased risk of developing active disease. Such individuals are usually identified by skin testing and are either contacts of known smear-positive index cases or people who are occupationally exposed to infection (such as nurses and doctors).

A series of randomized controlled trials have indicated that isoniazid preventive therapy also reduces the risk of subsequent TB in HIV-infected individuals with latent MTB infection—at least while they continue to take the isoniazid. Significant hurdles in operationalizing this as a TB control measure remain and are discussed in Chapter 13.

DOTS strategy for TB control

The objectives of TB control are to reduce mortality, morbidity and disease transmission and to prevent the development of drug resistance. The strategy recommended to meet these objectives is to provide standardized short-course chemotherapy under direct observation at least during the initial phase of treatment to, at least, all identified smear-positive TB cases (the sources of infection). The success of this strategy depends on the implementation of a five-point package.

1 *Direct* smear microscopy for case detection among symptomatic patients self-reporting to health services.

2 *Observation* of therapy for administration of standardized short-course chemotherapy to ensure adherence.

3 *Treatment* monitoring through a standardized recording and reporting system allowing continuous assessment of treatment results.

4 *Short-course* chemotherapy through a system of regular drug supply of all essential antituberculosis drugs, which should be free to patients at the point of delivery.

5 Government or non-governmental organization (NGO) commitment to ensure a sustained approach to policy and funding.

TB control activities should aim to meet two agreed targets: a cure rate of 85% and a case detection rate of 70%. Greatest emphasis has been placed on the cure rate target because achieving this will lead to less acquired drug resistance, which makes future treatment of TB easier and more affordable. The standardized outcome reporting categories described earlier make it possible to conduct quarterly cohort analyses of treatment outcomes and hence to report cure rates.

The controversy around direct observation of therapy and adherence

In recent years, there has been considerable debate over the extent to which direct observation of therapy (DOT) is required to ensure patient adherence to therapy. In its purest form, DOT (distinct from the five-point DOTS policy package) dictates that a healthcare worker should hold a given patient's TB treatment so that the patient can swallow every dose under the watchful eye of the healthcare worker—at least for the intensive phase. Many now accept that this system does not always make it easy for patients to adhere to every prescribed dose of treatment. If, for example, patients live far from the healthcare worker, they will inevitably incur considerable direct and opportunity costs in the daily travel required. Many innovative approaches to DOT have been piloted including DOT by grocery store keepers in rural areas, workplace DOT and DOT by respected family members. The guiding principle should be to make it as easy as possible for patients to stick with the therapy for the full course. The increasing use of three- and four-drug fixed-dose combinations to supplement the existing two-dose combinations of rifampicin and isoniazid should make it easier for patients to adhere and harder for drug resistance to emerge.

TB, poverty and the problem of case detection

Although TB transmission is reduced every time a smear-positive case is cured, overall reductions in prevalence and incidence depend on progress towards the 70% case detection target and this has proved more problematic than the cure rate target. Estimating the expected number of infectious cases in a given population conventionally relies on extrapolation from an estimate of the annual risk of infection (ARI). This is usually derived from PPD skin test surveys, but the reliability of these is diminished where HIV prevalence and/or BCG coverage is high. In addition, the relationship between the ARI and the expected number of cases where HIV prevalence is high is not known. A rough guide, in the absence of HIV, is to expect 50 infectious (smear-positive) cases every year from every 100 000 head of population when the ARI is 1%. In most developing countries in the tropics, the ARI is likely to be 2% (or more).

If reliable estimates of expected numbers of infectious cases are required, then full-scale community-based prevalence surveys or longitudinal cohort studies are required. These are expensive and time consuming, and most countries have not had the resources to undertake them. Overall, most countries do not yet have reliable data against which to measure their progress towards the case detection target or the means to measure the impact of TB control on overall TB burden of disease.

The process of case detection needs close attention, especially if it is to work for those who need it most, that is the poor. Smear microscopy is central in the DOTS strategy: no patients should start short-course chemotherapy unless they have had their sputum checked. The recommended approach is termed 'passive' case-finding; patients who are prompted by their symptoms to present to health facilities are then encouraged to submit a total of three sputum specimens. The process of sputum submission takes the patient a minimum of 24 h and three visits to the health facility, followed by another visit to collect the results and, usually, one further visit to start treatment. These repeat visits may be impossible for particularly disadvantaged patients such as the poor and women in some traditional cultures. It is therefore important to make adequately staffed, quality-assured microscopy facilities as accessible as possible in populations with high TB incidence. In some instances, this means establishing extra laboratory services (but no more than one such facility for 100 000 people, as the volume of work is then not sufficient for staff to retain skills). In other instances, this means ensuring excellent logistics for transporting specimens and results between microscopy centres and collection sites. The WHO has recently relaxed the requirement for three sputum specimens in order to categorize patients, accepting that two specimens are sufficient, provided the quality of the smear microscopy can be assured (see http://www.who.int/tb/dots/laboratory/policy/en/index.html).

There is increasing interest in improving case detection, including moves to re-examine the potential role of 'active' case-finding for certain high-risk populations, for example, in urban slums, prisons and military barracks. Mass screening of populations by radiography has not been thought cost-effective relative to opportunist 'passive' case-finding as described earlier but it, or related approaches (sometimes called intensified case-finding), may be appropriate in particular situations.

Multidrug resistant and extremely drug resistant TB

Wherever TB chemotherapy is delivered—especially if delivery is chaotic or disrupted—drug resistance develops, and some organisms accumulate resistance to successive drugs. When resistance to both isoniazid and rifampicin are detected *in vitro*, the isolate is categorized as multidrug resistant (MDR). Patients with disease caused by such organisms are unlikely to be cured by first-line regimens in Categories I, II or III. New guidelines exist for the programmatic management of such cases using the following principles:
• Use at least four drugs highly likely to be effective

• Do not use drugs for which resistance crosses over (e.g. kanamycin and amikacin, or rifabutin and rifampicin)
• Eliminate drugs that are not safe for the patient
• Include drugs from groups 1–5 choosing from hierarchy based on potency (Table 12.5)
• Be prepared to prevent, monitor and manage adverse events

The emergence of extremely drug resistant (XDR) TB in recent years is very worrying. It is defined as MDR plus resistance to (i) any fluoroquinolone and (ii) at least one of the three injectable second-line drugs (Table 12.5). This resistance pattern is virtually untreatable and has been associated with rapid progression to death in HIV-infected patients in South Africa.

The core message for all tropical practitioners is to work hard not to allow drug resistance to develop in the first place, by ensuring clinical practice within a public health framework that sits within the DOTS strategy.

HIV and TB

One of the challenges facing developing countries in the tropics is the management of TB in populations with high HIV prevalence. HIV-infected patients who develop TB are, on the whole, more difficult to diagnose in a timely fashion. Although their TB seems curable using short-course chemotherapy, they are at increased risk of dying during and after TB therapy. This mortality appears to be multifactorial and includes late initiation of treatment. This may be partly a result of the difficulties of diagnosis but stigma and other factors also contribute. Intercurrent HIV-related complications such as bacterial and fungal infections also contribute to mortality. One randomized controlled trial in West Africa from before the era of ART has suggested that administration of cotrimoxazole prophylaxis concurrently with short-course chemotherapy can help reduce mortality in HIV-infected patients with TB.

TB programmes in the tropics are now linking up with ART programmes to ensure that all TB patients are offered HIV testing and, where

Table 12.5 A hierarchy of potency for choosing drugs for the treatment of drug-resistant TB

Grouping	Drugs (abbreviation)
Group 1—First-line oral antituberculosis agents	Isoniazid (H); Rifampicin (R); Ethambutol (E); Pyrazinamide (Z)
Group 2—Injectable antituberculosis agents	Streptomycin (S); Kanamycin (Km); Amikacin (Am); Capreomycin (Cm); Viomycin (Vi)
Group 3—Fluoroquinolones	Ciprofloxach (Cfx); Ofloxacin (Ofx); Levofloxacin (Lfx); Moxifloxacin (Mfx); Gatifloxacin (Gfx)
Group 4—Oral bacteriostatic second-line antituberculosis agents	Ethionamide (Eto); Protionamide (Pto); Cycloserine (Cs); Terizidone (Trd); P-aminosalicylic acid (PAS); Thioacetazone (Th)
Group 5—Antituberculosis agents with unclear efficacy (not recommended by WHO for routine use in MDR-TB patients)	Clofazimine (Cfz); Amoxicillin/Clavulanate (Amx/Clv); Clarithromycin (Clr); Linezolid (Lzd)

From *Guidelines for the Programmatic Management of Drug-Resistant Tuberculosis.* WHO/HTM/TB/2006.361.

possible, access to ART. Several questions remain about how and when to add ART to first-line TB therapy. Pharmacological interactions between TB drugs (notably rifampicin) and ART, cumulative drug toxicity and side effects, and the risks of inducing immune reconstitution disease (IRD) are the key issues to take into account. The simplest programmatic approach is to wait, if possible, delaying adding ART to TB therapy until the intensive phase of TB therapy is complete.

Although improving access to ART for all HIV-infected patients is clearly important, it must be emphasized that the most significant gains for HIV-infected patients with TB in the tropics are likely to be found through strengthening core services to improve timely diagnosis and careful clinical care.

The Stop TB strategy

In recognition that DOTS is necessary, but not sufficient for global TB control, the Stop TB Partnership and WHO recommended a new approach in 2006, the Stop TB Strategy, to replace DOTS and to promote progress towards the TB-related Millennium Development Goals. The DOTS principles remains central to the new strategy which is summarized in Table 12.6, but makes explicit the need to engage more broadly, including approaches to drug-resistant TB and TB in the context of HIV as described earlier.

Table 12.6 The Stop TB strategy (2006–2015)

- Pursue high-quality DOTS expansion and enhancement
- Address TB-HIV, MDR-TB and other challenges
- Contribute to health system strengthening
- Engage all care providers
- Empower people with TB and communities
- Enable and promote research

Future developments

New diagnostics

There is clearly a need for a new diagnostic tool that is as robust and specific as smear microscopy, less dependent on laboratory skill and infrastructure, more sensitive and more immediate in readout. To date there are no obvious candidates for widespread use in developing countries.

New interventions

No new drugs look set to replace the current gold standard 6-month short-course chemotherapy in the short term, but there is interest developing around adding moxifloxacin to first-line regimens and suggestions that this may enable shorter treatment regimens to be developed. There is still no obvious replacement for the BCG vaccine.

Further reading

Enarson DA, Rieder HL, Arnadottir T, Trébucq A. *Management of Tuberculosis: A Guide for Low Income Countries*, 5th edn. 2000; IUATLD, Paris. [Available from International Union Against Tuberculosis and Lung Disease, 68 Boulevard Saint-Michel, 75006 Paris, France. See www.iuatld.org. Examples of model reporting forms are included, as well as a technical guide to sputum smear microscopy.]

Maartens G, Wilkinson RJ. Tuberculosis. *Lancet* 2007; 370: 2030–2043. [Useful up-to-date review.]

Steingart KR, Henry M, Ng V, Hopewell PC, Ramsay A, Cunningham J, Urbanczik R, Perkins M, Aziz MA, Pai M. Fluorescence versus conventional sputum smear microscopy for tuberculosis: a systematic review. *Lancet Infect Dis* 2006; 9: 570–581 (Review). Erratum in: *Lancet Infect Dis* 2006; 10: 628.

Steingart KR, Ng V, Henry M, Hopewell PC, Ramsay A, Cunningham J, Urbanczik R, Perkins MD, Aziz MA, Pai M. Sputum processing methods to improve the sensitivity of smear microscopy for tuberculosis: a systematic review. *Lancet Infect Dis* 2006; 10: 664–674.

WHO Stop TB Department. *Treatment of Tuberculosis: Guidelines for National TB Programmes*, 3rd edn. 2003. WHO/CDS/TB/2003.313 and *Guidelines for the Programmatic Management of Drug-Resistant Tuberculosis* WHO/HTM/TB/2006.361. [Available from the World Health Organization, Via Appia, Geneva, Switzerland and downloadable from www.who.int/gtb, a website that includes details of drug therapy as well as a full description of the Stop TB Strategy.]

Chapter 13

HIV infection and disease in the tropics

Over 90% of new HIV infections now occur in developing countries. Wherever HIV is prevalent, hospitals and clinics are faced with a large and escalating burden of disease. HIV and consequent AIDS are now the leading cause of death in sub-Saharan Africa and the fourth biggest killer worldwide, making HIV a major tropical disease.

Specific guidelines, current seroprevalence data, epidemiological reviews, summaries, reports and updates are published regularly by the WHO and The Joint United Nations Programme on HIV/AIDS (UNAIDS). These documents and many other useful resources are available on their websites—details of this are in the further reading.

Most countries have national AIDS programmes which provide management protocols relevant to local conditions and resources. These should be followed where available. This chapter will only consider HIV infection in adults.

The viruses

There are two distinct types, HIV-1 and HIV-2, as well as several closely allied species. These two viruses originated in the chimpanzee and sooty mangabey, respectively. It is likely that HIV-1 and HIV-2 infected humans as a result of

Lecture Notes: Tropical Medicine, 6th edition.
By G.V. Gill and N.J. Beeching. Published 2009 by Blackwell Publishing, ISBN: 978-1-4051-8048-1.

these primates being hunted for food. This probably happened many times before the social and environmental conditions were present to spark off the HIV epidemic. Theories linking the introduction of HIV into humans via polio vaccination campaigns in Africa in the 1950s have been disproved.

Differences between HIV-1 and HIV-2

There are clear differences between HIV-1 and HIV-2 in genomic structure and in the antibody response to infection. Although not always easy, the two infections can usually be separated serologically. HIV-1 is rapidly spreading round the world and is universally distributed, whereas HIV-2 is much less common and largely restricted to West Africa.

The two viruses are transmitted in the same way but HIV-2 seems less transmissible. Where HIV-1 and HIV-2 coexist, HIV-1 infection is rapidly overtaking HIV-2 in prevalence. Dual infections can occur and there is no evidence that one infection protects against the other. Both viruses cause the same immune defects and are associated with a similar disease. HIV-2 takes several years longer than HIV-1 to cause significant immunosuppression or death, and diseases such as Kaposi's sarcoma do not usually occur in HIV-2 infected individuals. The importance of HIV-2 in areas where it is prevalent is to ensure that the kits used for blood tests can detect both viruses. Differentiation is important with regard to antiretroviral drug efficacy. The rest of the chapter refers to HIV without differentiating between the two types.

Testing for HIV

Whom to test?

It is important to have a local policy on HIV testing that reflects local needs, resources and conditions.

In the past, health care professionals in developing countries may have taken a nihilistic view towards HIV testing, as there was nothing to offer the individual with a positive result. Now, with wide spread availability of antiretroviral therapy (ART), prevention of mother to child transmission (PMTCT) programmes and better management of opportunistic infections testing, should be offered as widely and to as broad a spectrum of people as possible.

The starting point should be voluntary counselling and testing (VCT) facilities. These should be easily accessible and provide a confidential service. They should be staffed by trained counsellors who can help clients decide on the pros and cons of accepting a test. Certain groups, such as commercial sex-workers and their clients, people visiting STI clinics (see Chapter 7), pregnant women, patients with tuberculosis and people working in high-risk occupations such as long-distance truck-drivers and soldiers, should be targeted. VCT facilities also act as centres for education on preventing HIV infection. Pregnant women should be encouraged to be tested to allow them to make informed decisions about this and future pregnancies. In many areas PMTCT programmes using single or dual ART are available to help prevent mother–child transmission.

Patients presenting to health care facilities for any reason in areas of high HIV prevalence should be opportunistically encouraged to test, as early diagnosis will almost certainly reduce the chance of future problems and allow ART to be started before the patient becomes critically ill. To this end programmes to offer testing to people

are available in many high-prevalence countries outside of health care facilities, such as in the work place. Certain large employers have introduced testing and treatment programmes aimed at keeping their workforce well and reducing the loss of highly skilled workers to AIDS, this makes both ethical and economic sense.

Hospital inpatients should also be tested, including patients with opportunistic infections; testing these patients allows ART to be started as soon as possible if appropriate, which may well aid the patients' recovery and prevent re-admission, thus reducing the burden on the health service as well as keeping the patient healthy and hopefully economically active. Patients with TB are another important group of patients to target. In high HIV–prevalence countries the majority of TB patients are also HIV infected. It can be argued that identifying these patients and starting ART when appropriate is a means of controlling TB as the patients will become less susceptible to TB.

Finally and very importantly, all blood donation programmes should do HIV testing on all donors. Also a comprehensive risk assessment of the donor should be undertaken to reduce the risk of using blood that may contain HIV. Table 13.1 defines various terms associated with HIV testing.

What test to use?

Some tests are specific for HIV-1 or HIV-2, whereas others can identify both types. All are highly specific and sensitive if the manufacturer's guidelines are followed correctly; the kits are as accurate as the laboratories using them.

The most widely used tests identify specific anti-HIV antibodies. This can be done by ELISA methods in the laboratory, a variety of rapid and/or simple colorimetric or agglutination tests that do not require a laboratory or electricity, and the Western blot. There is no single test that is suitable for all circumstances. ELISA testing is best suited for regular processing of large numbers of samples so that complete plates can be run. It is unsuitable for laboratories with limited facilities and fridge space, irregular electricity supply and inadequately trained or supervised technical staff.

Table 13.1 Terminology around HIV testing. The following terms are used interchangeably in the literature on HIV testing and counselling and are included here for reference and clarity

	Alternative wording	Alternative wording	Setting where performed
Provider-initiated means that the HIV test is at the request of the clinician	*Opt-out* means that patients can decline to be tested	*DCT* stands for diagnostic counselling and testing	Health facilities In-patient wards Out-patient clinics STI clinics TB clinics Antenatal care Home-based testing
Client-initiated means that the HIV test is at the request of the client	*Opt-in* means that clients volunteer to be tested	*VCT* stands for voluntary counselling and testing	Stand-alone sites in non-medical settings such as residential areas, institutions, churches and mosques Mobile services At home

Rapid and simple tests, such as particle agglutination or dot immunoassay tests, can be performed in less-sophisticated laboratories. Many are available as single kits and so can be efficiently used when small numbers of samples need testing. Some can be stored safely at room temperature. With central purchasing, unit costs can be kept quite low, depending on the kit.

Western blots are expensive and can be difficult to interpret and standardize. The WHO no longer recommends Western blotting for confirmation, suggesting instead that if it is necessary then the combination of laboratory ELISA with a simple or rapid assay is as reliable and much cheaper.

With ART available in many developing settings, tests for monitoring patients before and during ART are needed. CD4 counts are very useful to decide when to initiate therapy and to help monitor response. ART can be started on clinical grounds alone but a CD4 count should be done if possible. Viral load testing is expensive and currently quite technically demanding. Although not necessary to determine when to start treatment, a viral load estimation is very useful in assessing treatment response and detecting treatment failure before there has been clinical disease progression and the acquisition of multiple ART

resistance mutations. Cheaper and more accessible alternatives are being developed.

Many HIV/AIDS programmes will have specific protocols for HIV testing which should be followed. This may include a combination of tests such as a rapid test confirmed by a laboratory ELISA or a combination of two rapid tests.

Epidemiology

Surveillance

Surveillance is carried out in order to monitor the extent of HIV infection and disease in a given region or community. In developing settings, often few resources are available for epidemiological monitoring. At the start of the HIV epidemic in Africa, surveillance was only able to show gross changes in mortality and to monitor relatively crudely the arrival and subsequent spread of infection. With experience and institutional strengthening, surveillance is now much more accurate.

Specific at-risk groups include female sex-workers, clients at STI clinics, workers such as migrant labourers and long-distance lorry drivers and intravenous drug users. It is important to monitor these groups as they often drive the epidemic in certain areas. Other groups commonly monitored include pregnant women attending for antenatal care, blood donors, military recruits and newborn infants, although all these groups have inherent biases. Ideally, a population-based sample should be tested at regular intervals to accurately determine prevalence and incidence for a particular region. This provides the most valuable information but population-based testing is difficult and expensive to organize. Also, it may not be acceptable to the local population, as it involves testing people in their homes and collecting a lot of demographic information that individuals may find intrusive. It is important as a minimum to record age and sex in all surveys.

Disease surveillance is usually carried out in hospital and often concentrates on counting cases of AIDS as defined by the WHO in the provisional clinical case definition for Africa. HIV seroprevalence can be measured in specific groups such as hospital admissions, adults with active TB or pneumonia or cadavers in the hospital or district mortuary.

Seroprevalence

With rapid spread of infection (and delays in reporting and analysis) current figures quickly become out of date. By the end of 2007, WHO estimated 33.2 million people were living with HIV/AIDS worldwide (Table 13.2). During the same period around 2.5 million new infections occurred. About 2.1 million people died of HIV/AIDS in 2007. Seventy per cent of people living with HIV/AIDS reside in sub-Saharan Africa. Sub-Saharan Africa is the region hardest hit by HIV/AIDS, accounting for 68% of all new infections and 77% of all AIDS deaths. Table 13.3 shows the estimated number of cases by region.

Some of the largest increases in prevalence are occurring in former Eastern block countries, largely driven by injecting drug users. Latin America has seen a drop in mortality, partly because of the introduction of low-cost ART in some countries such as Brazil. This may act as a model for other areas, although it is sobering to

Table 13.2 Summary of global HIV/AIDS statistics (2007)

People living with HIV/AIDS	33.2 million (30.6–36.1 million)
New HIV infections in 2007	2.5 million (1.8–4.1 million)
Deaths due to AIDS in 2007	2.1 million (1.9–2.4 million)

Source: Adapted from UNAIDS report (December 2007).

note that in North America and Western Europe, where mortality has dropped considerably since the widespread use of ART, the incidence of new infections has been stable or is increasing.

Transmission

Sexual transmission

In nearly all developing countries the most important way HIV is transmitted is by heterosexual sex. The risk of acquiring HIV after sexual intercourse is hard to quantify. There are numerous factors such as the age and sex (young women seem more susceptible, perhaps because of an immature genital tract) of the individual as well as the factors mentioned below. However, it is thought that the risk is between 0.01% and 0.1% per sexual act.

Risk factors

There are several factors that markedly increase the risk of transmission, the most important being other STIs that cause ulceration, chancroid (*Haemophilus ducreyi*) in particular, as well as primary syphilis and genital herpes simplex. STIs that cause inflammation and discharge, such as gonorrhoea, *Chlamydia* and perhaps trichomoniasis also increase the chance of sexual transmission of HIV. In fact anything that disrupts the vagina's normal flora may cause increased risk of transmission. A recent study using nonoxinol '9', a vaginal spermicide, actually increased the incidence of HIV infection amongst the women using it. Cervical erosion may also be a risk factor in women.

Table 13.3 Number of adults and children with HIV/AIDS by region(2007)

Region	Number of adults and children with HIV	Adult prevalence (%)
Sub-Saharan Africa	22.5 million (20.9–24.3)	5
Middle East and North Africa	0.38 million (0.27–0.5)	0.3
South and South East Asia	4 million (3.3–5.1)	0.3
East Asia	0.8 million (0.62–0.96)	0.1
Latin America	1.6 million (1.4–1.9)	0.5
Caribbean	0.23 million (0.21–0.27)	1.0
Eastern Europe and Central Asia	1.6 million (1.2–2.1)	0.9
Western and Central Europe	0.76 million (0.6–1.1)	0.3
North America	1.3 million (0.48–1.9)	0.6
Oceania	0.075 million (0.05–0.12)	0.4
Total	33.2 million (30.6–36.1)	0.8

Source: Adapted from UNAIDS report (2007).

For a man, being uncircumcised may be a factor that increases risk; it certainly increases the risk of acquiring other STIs. Several recent randomized controlled trials in Africa have shown that male circumcision may protect against HIV infection.

Vertical transmission

In the developing world with no intervention, around 20–25% of children born to HIV-infected mothers may themselves become infected. Ten per cent will be infected transplacentally, 5% during delivery and around 10% as a result of breast-feeding. Factors associated with transplacental transmission include later stage of infection of the mother and high viral load. During birth the presence of an STI and prolonged labour will increase transmission. Breast-feeding does lead to HIV transmission and in the West, formula feeding is recommended to all HIV-infected mothers. In resource-poor settings, formula feeding is not practical. Even when formula is provided free, adequate facilities for its sterile preparation are rarely available. The benefits of breast milk in reducing infant mortality from pneumonia and diarrhoea probably outweigh the risk of HIV infection. There have been some confusing messages recently over whether to recommend

breast-feeding to HIV-infected mothers in developing countries and about what sort of breast-feeding. Some studies have shown that exclusive breast-feeding carries a reduced risk of HIV transmission compared to mixed feeding, which is commonly practiced in Africa. Exclusive breast-feeding for six months followed by rapid weaning is recommended where no alternative exists.

Transmission by infected blood

Two groups are at particular risk: patients receiving blood transfusions and people who inject drugs and share needles and syringes. Improperly sterilized injection equipment in hospitals and other health facilities is another (unquantifiable) risk.

Screening blood donors for HIV has greatly reduced the chance of HIV transmission through transfusion. Errors can occur in HIV testing and some donors may be in the 'window' phase with an acute infection that is not yet serologically recognizable. This can be a problem in areas of high incidence.

There is a small risk to health care workers exposed to HIV-infected blood. In a typical needlestick injury, where the skin is punctured but the inoculum is small, the risk of acquiring

HIV is about 0.3%; this figure is probably much lower where the health worker takes post exposure prophylaxis.

Control strategies

Control strategies need to be targeted at specific groups. Condom promotion and distribution is important for preventing new infections both in the community as a whole, as well as in sex workers and their clients who can be a core of HIV transmission in an area. Condoms are proven to be effective in preventing most STIs. They may not always be culturally acceptable and they rely on the male partner's cooperation. Provision of condoms at schools and in prisons may not be politically popular in some regions but targeting these areas is essential to prevent HIV transmission. Another difficult area is the provision of clean needles and syringes for intravenous drug users both in and out of prison; this may not be legally possible in many countries. Female condoms are also effective but are cumbersome to use and may not be accepted by some partners.

Treatment of STIs has been shown to reduce HIV transmission in some studies. There is debate over the likely benefits of mass STI-treatment campaigns; many areas are using syndromic management to simplify STI treatment and ensure that the important diseases are treated in a single visit (Chapter 7).

Targeting core groups such as commercial sex-workers and their clients is important but education for school children is also a high priority. Previously, sex education was not widespread in Africa and girls would not find out about contraception or STIs until they were attending antenatal programmes. Sex education and HIV awareness has to be tailored to the target audience as Western-style campaigns and materials are often inappropriate for developing countries.

Circumcision as mentioned above has been shown to reduce the chances of a male acquiring HIV. There are calls for the introduction of mass circumcision in southern African countries hardest hit by the HIV epidemic, as a means of reducing transmission.

Ensuring a safe blood supply is an important minimum standard in HIV prevention.

VCT can act as an entry point to HIV services and as a place for disseminating information about HIV prevention and risk reduction for those found to be HIV infected. Women found to be infected can be counselled about future pregnancies, and pregnant women can also be informed of ways to reduce transmission to their unborn child. PMTCT is a priority. Studies have shown that nevirapine (NVP) given as a single dose to the mother in labour and the child within 72 h of birth can reduce HIV transmission by over 50%, the use of two ARV's such as NVP and zidovudine (AZT) or triple therapy is even more efficacious, but not all PMTCT programmes are able to offer these interventions yet. The argument some governments have used for not implementing this strategy is that until ARV's can be provided for the mother, one risks creating a large group of orphans.

The current WHO recommendations for PMTCT are as follows:

1 Women who require ART for their health should have it initiated as soon as possible. Criteria for initiating ART are the same as for non-pregnant women, with the exception that it is recommended in WHO clinical stage 3 disease and with a CD4 cell count of $<350 \times 10^6$/L as opposed to $<200 \times 10^6$/L in non-pregnant persons. The recommended first-line regimen for pregnant women in need of treatment is AZT+lamivudine (3TC)+NVP as this has the best safety record in pregnancy.

2 For women for whom ART is not yet indicated it is recommended that AZT is given from 28 weeks of pregnancy, and single dose NVP and 3TC are given at onset of labour, with a 7-day trial of AZT plus 3TC in order to reduce the risk of NVP resistance; and for the infant, single dose NVP as soon as possible after birth with AZT for 7 days.

3 Infants born to HIV-positive women who had not received any ARV's should be given a single dose of NVP at birth plus AZT for 4 weeks. Alternative regimens are single dose NVP at birth and AZT for 1 week; or single dose NVP at birth.

For alternative regimens, specific indications with dosages and contraindications, consult either a country-specific programme or the WHO website given in further reading.

ART can be considered to be a method of preventing HIV transmission and is discussed in more detail later.

Other methods of prevention include vaginal microbicides, which have had a chequered past but are being evaluated in large prospective trials, and vaccines. Sadly, vaccines to prevent or control HIV infection appear to remain a long way off.

Cost and likely impact

There are few studies looking directly at the economic impact of HIV/AIDS on Africa. The data that are available show that HIV/AIDS is having a marked negative impact on GDP. It has been estimated that national average growth rates have been reduced by 2–4% per year across the continent.

Can ART reverse this? Targeting specific economically active groups (e.g. miners in South Africa) may be one strategy. It is hoped that by ensuring the people who generate the country's revenue and exports are kept productive, governments will be able to continue improving education and health services in an attempt to control the epidemic.

Until a few years ago, ART was beyond the budget of most developing countries and the individuals in those countries. But, due to a combination of international pressure on drug companies to reduce prices and the manufacture of good quality generic medication, as well as the advent of funding from international sources such as the global fund to fight AIDS, tuberculosis and malaria, the President's emergency plan for AIDS relief and the Bill and Melinda Gates Foundation, ART programmes are now well under way in many hard hit developing countries. Despite funding, these programmes still face enormous challenges in delivering medication and monitoring large groups of patients in rural and urban settings with little infrastructure, but huge strides have been made in getting thousands of people who need ART onto treatment. The organization and delivery of ART is discussed later.

Mechanisms of disease

Pathogenesis of HIV infection

The main cell population infected by HIV is lymphocytes that carry the CD4 antigen on their surface. This is because the CD4 molecule acts as the receptor to which the virus can initially attach before entering the cell. CD4 lymphocytes are T-helper cells. The key concept in understanding the pathogenesis of HIV infection is the selective loss of function and progressive depletion of T-helper lymphocytes. This is a dynamic process with millions of T cells being made daily and millions being killed daily by HIV. HIV slowly depletes the body's capacity to replace the killed T cells. The speed with which this process occurs can be predicted from the individual's viral load.

T-helper lymphocytes have an important role in the regulation of the cell-mediated immune response and also cooperate with B cells in the production of antibody. Loss of CD4 cells by HIV infection disrupts both cell-mediated and humoral immunity. This is shown by the loss of delayed hypersensitivity to such skin test (recall) antigens as PPD or tuberculin, *Candida* and mumps antigen; and by polyclonal B-cell activation with hypergammaglobulinaemia.

Other cell populations can be infected including macrophages, which may be important reservoirs of HIV outside the blood and may carry HIV to different organs, including the CNS. Cytokine secretion by infected macrophages is aberrant and may have a role in chronic fever, wasting and enteropathy. Active replication of HIV is evident in lymph nodes at all stages of infection and B cells may be non-specifically activated.

Different strains of HIV may differ in virulence in the cell types that are preferentially infected. A single HIV infection can generate many different antigenic variants, which escape the control of the immune system.

Progressive immunosuppression

With the progressive destruction of one part of the immune system, a distinct form of immunosuppression develops. As with other immune deficiency syndromes, a relatively limited number of organisms are able to exploit the specific immune defect and commonly cause disease in seropositive individuals.

It is unclear why some pathogens are so characteristic of HIV and others not. Different pathogens characteristically occur in the early and later stages of HIV disease. A few conventional pathogens cause clinical disease in the early as well as the later stages of HIV disease. The most common pathogens are *Mycobacterium tuberculosis, Streptococcus pneumoniae*, non-typhi *Salmonella* (NTS), *Cryptococcus neoformans, Toxoplasma gondii, Pneumocystis jirovecii*, human herpes virus 8, cytomegalovirus and the varicella-zoster virus are amongst the most important. Disease is caused by acute infection or by re-activation of a dormant or contained organism.

In the early stages of HIV, when immune function is relatively preserved, the main abnormality is a much higher attack rate with clinically typical disease presentation and a normal response to standard treatment. In later stages of HIV and in AIDS itself clinical presentations become atypical and there is a diminished response to standard therapy.

Opportunistic pathogens (relatively avirulent organisms that only usually cause disease in individuals with disrupted immune systems) are only seen in the later stages of HIV disease when much more severe immunosuppression has developed. Immune surveillance is also abnormal, and specific cancers can develop such as non-Hodgkin's lymphoma, primary CNS lymphoma and Kaposi's sarcoma. Cervical neoplasia is also more common in HIV-infected women. Some of these unusual infections and malignancies are so characteristic of (late) HIV disease that they can be grouped together and used to define AIDS.

Staging HIV disease

CD4 lymphocytes are found in peripheral blood and the normal count in a seronegative person is about $800–1500 \times 10^6$/L CD4 cells. The absolute CD4 count is a useful way of staging HIV infection and assessing the immune status of a patient. These tests are expensive but are becoming increasingly available in developing settings.

A count of $<200 \times 10^6$/L indicates severe immunosuppression and renders a patient susceptible to a wide range of opportunistic infections; at this level of CD4 count, ART is needed to prevent a person developing a life-threatening complication of HIV. Starting ART earlier when the CD4 count is $<350 \times 10^6$/L may have increased benefits for patients by not allowing their immune system to deteriorate to a point where they are very susceptible to infections. The WHO has developed a clinical staging system for HIV disease (2005) which can be used to guide clinical management of patients. Specifically, the stages can be used to identify patients in need of specific prophylaxis and ART. The clinical stages are as follows (for adults and adolescents):

Primary HIV infection:
- Asymptomatic or
- seroconversion syndrome

Clinical stage 1:
- Asymptomatic or
- persistent generalized lymphadenopathy (PGL).

Clinical stage 2:
- Weight loss <10% of presumed body weight
- Recurrent respiratory tract infections
- Herpes zoster
- Oral ulcers
- Seborrhoeic dermatitis
- Papular pruritic eruption
- Fungal nail infections
- Angular chelitis

Clinical stage 3:

Conditions where a presumptive diagnosis can be made
- Weight loss of >10% presumed body weight
- Unexplained diarrhoea for >1 month
- Unexplained fever for >1 month
- Oral candida
- Oral hairy leukoplakia
- Pulmonary tuberculosis in the last 2 years
- Severe bacterial infections (including meningitis, empyema, pneumonia, bone and joint sepsis)

Conditions for which confirmatory testing is needed
- Unexplained anaemia (Hb<8.0g/dl), and/or neutropenia (neutrophils $<500 \times 10^6$/L), Thrombocytopenia (platelets $<50 \times 10^9$/L for >1 month)

Clinical Stage 4:

Conditions where a presumptive diagnosis can be made

- HIV wasting syndrome
- Pneumocystis pneumonia
- Recurrent bacterial pneumonia
- Chronic herpes simplex infection for >1 month
- Oesophageal candidiasis
- Extrapulmonary tuberculosis
- Kaposi's sarcoma
- Cerebral toxoplasmosis
- HIV encephalopathy

Conditions for which confirmatory testing are needed

- Extrapulmonary cryptococcosis
- Disseminated non-tuberculous mycobacterial infection
- Progressive multifocal leukoencephalopathy
- Candida of trachea, bronchi or lungs
- Cryptosporidiosis
- Isosporiasis
- Visceral herpes simplex
- Invasive CMV e.g. retinitis
- Disseminated mycosis
- Recurrent NTS septicaemia
- Lymphoma (cerebral or B cell non-Hodgkin)
- Invasive cervical carcinoma
- Visceral leishmaniasis

Natural history

The following account of illness caused by HIV infection highlights those areas where the illness in the tropics differs from that reported in North America and Europe.

Acute seroconversion illness

Initially in acute infection, most adults develop a high viraemia and a marked fall in CD4 count; they are highly infectious. During seroconversion, neutralizing antibodies appear and viraemia is greatly reduced. A minority of adults experience an acute seroconversion illness which resembles glandular fever. A wide range of skin rashes are seen and with transient CD4 depletion, oral *Candida* and even opportunistic infections can occur. Because of the relatively non-specific features, the seroconversion illness may not be recognized unless severe.

The latent phase

After seroconversion the CD4 count rapidly rises to near normal and the individual feels well. Active viral replication is taking place in the reticuloendothelial system during this time, and viral load assays can be used to quantify this. Lymph node architecture is progressively disrupted and nearly 50% of adults develop PGL; this has no prognostic significance.

With time the CD4 count falls and immunosuppression slowly but inevitably progresses. The rate of progression is extremely variable but can be predicted from the viral load. It is during this latent infection that most onward transmission of HIV takes place and the individual feels well.

Early HIV disease

In the relatively early stage of HIV infection, when CD4 counts are only moderately reduced, many individuals start to experience specific symptoms of HIV or develop a disease typical of early HIV infection.

The HIV symptoms can be weight loss, night sweats, pruritic skin rash, unexplained fever or chronic diarrhoea. Early HIV disease can be; relatively trivial, such as oral *Candida* or oral hairy leukoplakia; painful and disabling but not life threatening, such as herpes zoster; or life-threatening bacterial or mycobacterial infections. This stage of disease is sometimes referred to as AIDS-related complex (ARC).

The serious early HIV diseases are pneumococcal infection (pneumonia and sinusitis), TB (pulmonary and lymphatic) and NTS infections (often bacteraemic). In general, clinical presentation is straightforward and the response to therapy good.

In many tropical regions, problems of early disease may cause significant morbidity, whereas it is of relatively minor importance in industrialized countries. This is because of the much higher exposure in poor, overcrowded tropical communities to respiratory and diarrhoeal pathogens.

Late HIV disease or AIDS

The important AIDS defining–opportunistic infections in tropical countries are cryptosporidiosis and isosporiasis in the bowel and cryptococcosis and toxoplasmosis in the CNS.

Extrapulmonary and disseminated TB (Figure 13.1), severe bacteraemic pneumococcal disease and disseminated salmonellosis are all common. Other Gram-negative septicaemia, including *Escherichia coli*, is increasingly being recognized. Mixed infections are also frequent.

Much early HIV disease, such as lobar pneumonia or pulmonary TB, is clinically typical and is only recognized as associated with HIV by serological testing. Studies that just focus on 'clinical AIDS' will fail to identify many early HIV disease cases.

There is intense exposure to TB, pneumococci and salmonellae. High mortality occurs in the early stages of HIV disease from clinical problems that are easily treated and cured in centres with better facilities and resources. The time from seroconversion to death in a patient not treated with ART is very variable but the average is around 8–10 years. Although there are no reliable data to show that there is a big difference between the time from acquiring HIV to death between developed and developing countries, it is now thought that untreated survival times may be similar.

Clinical problems

This section describes the common and important clinical presentations of HIV disease in the tropics

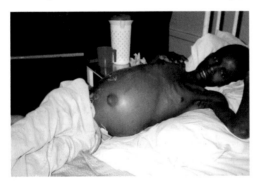

Figure 13.1 Gross ascites due to tuberculous peritonitis in a patient with AIDS.

and discusses simple investigations, management and treatment. It is assumed that therapy is limited to a range of cheap broad-spectrum antimicrobials, and that antibiotic sensitivity testing is not routinely available. ART and associated problems are discussed separately. A much more comprehensive description of problems and their management is available on the WHO website— known as the Integrated Management of Adult Illness (IMAI).

Skin problems

Skin problems are common in HIV-positive patients and cause considerable discomfort and morbidity.

Generalized pruritus

Many adults develop a chronic itchy maculopapular rash. In dark skin, many lesions become hyperpigmented and even nodular. Some cases are caused by scabies, for which treatment with benzyl benzoate is effective; it may need to be repeated and should include family members. The patient should be instructed to wash in warm water if possible then apply the benzyl benzoate and repeat the treatment a week later. In those who do not respond, antihistamines such as chlorphenamine are of limited use but may restore normal sleep. A topical corticosteroid sometimes eases itching. Extensive crusted or Norwegian scabies can be difficult to treat; ivermectin has been used successfully in some cases (Chapter 51).

Herpes zoster

Shingles is extremely common and is often the first recognizable HIV-related problem. Where HIV disease is widespread, lay people often recognize the implications of a zoster eruption and realize they are probably HIV-infected. Zoster affecting more than one dermatome is virtually diagnostic of HIV.

Adequate analgesia is important: codeine phosphate 30–60 mg every 6 h is usually effective. Persistent pain, post-herpetic neuralgia, may respond to amitriptyline or carbamazepine. Daily dressing may be necessary. If available oral aciclovir given early in the course of the eruption may shorten the duration of the rash and may prevent dissemination.

Skin infections

Minor wounds can develop into deep-seated and necrotic lesions which may cause bacteraemia. Poor wound healing or unusual skin infections can indicate underlying HIV infection. If antimicrobials are necessary, the best choice is a penicillinase-resistant penicillin such as flucloxacillin. Erythromycin or chloramphenicol may also be used.

Fungal nail infections and extensive tinea corporis, pedis and cruris are common. These may respond to a topical antifungal cream but often require an oral agent such as triazoles or griseofulvin, which may not be available.

Acute cough and fever

Acute respiratory infections are amongst the most important clinical problems that occur in HIV-infected adults in the tropics. Most patients who present with acute cough and fever have community-acquired bacterial pneumonia. This has always been an important disease in the tropics, but HIV has dramatically increased the incidence of bacterial pneumonia. *Pneumocystis jirovecii* pneumonia is uncommon in adults in Africa but is now recognized as a problem in HIV-infected infants.

There is usually a short history of cough, sputum (purulent, rusty or blood-stained), pleuritic pain, fever and rigors, marked toxicity and shortness of breath. Many cases will have had a previous episode. Examination reveals a sick and toxic patient, often lying on the side of the pneumonia. The patient is sweaty, taking rapid shallow breaths and coughing frequently. Some patients may be mildly jaundiced, have meningeal irritation, confusion and be shocked. Most will have lobar consolidation with bronchial breathing.

Nearly all infections are pneumococcal. *Haemophilus influenzae* is sometimes isolated but, in a series from Nairobi, this was usually co-infecting a primary pneumococcal pneumonia. Mixed bacterial and mycobacterial infections are relatively common in HIV disease.

Pneumonia can be confirmed by chest X-ray but this is wasteful if physical signs are definite. Gram-staining of sputum is useful. Pus cells confirm that a good specimen has been obtained; diplococci should be abundant. It is important to take a sputum specimen for acid-fast bacilli examination as TB often presents acutely and may mimic pneumonia. Treatment is the same as for HIV-negative patients: benzylpenicillin 0.6–1.2g parenterally 6 hourly for 5–7 days. An early switch to oral therapy is easier for the patient. If the patient is cyanosed, oxygen (if available) should be given by face mask; if shocked, intravenous fluids are vital.

The prognosis in HIV-related pneumonia is variable and depends on the underlying condition of the patient. When patients present late with extensive disease, mortality is high. If the patient is not responding there are several possibilities. There may be coinfection with NTS, *Haemophilus* or TB; an empyema is forming (especially with inadequate initial therapy); or the initial diagnosis is wrong and the patient has pulmonary TB. Changing to another antibiotic such as chloramphenicol or a cephalosporin, adding a macrolide or starting antituberculous therapy may be indicated. Also consider *Pneumocystis* pneumonia in a non-responding patient; this can be treated with high-dose cotrimoxazole. If an empyema is identified it must be drained. Remember that a liver abscess can present with fever and cough, as can malaria and typhoid. An abscess may be identified on ultrasound if available, or by noting a raised hemidiaphragm. These will most commonly be amoebic abscesses and will respond to metronidazole.

Chronic cough with fever

Chronic respiratory problems are common and highly associated with underlying HIV infection. Most patients have pulmonary TB. The main differential diagnosis is recurrent or partly treated bacterial pneumonia, which is common in late-stage patients. Pulmonary Kaposi's sarcoma can occur with skin lesions that are usually obvious although there may only be palatal lesions, which carry a very poor prognosis. Histoplasmosis can also present with a chronic cough.

Chronic cough and fever should be easy symptoms to identify; many patients will have weight loss, night sweats, weakness and haemoptysis; lower-lobe disease is frequent with widespread crepitations; effusions are much more common in HIV. TB frequently recurs so some patients will have had adequate previous therapy and re-present with sputum-positive disease within a few months.

The diagnosis of TB is more difficult to confirm by radiology or microscopy when there is underlying HIV infection. Classic upper-lobe cavitary disease is much less common and lower-lobe consolidation is more frequent. Fewer cases are smear-positive for acid-fast bacilli. TB culture is of little help for initial patient management because the result is so delayed, but it should be performed if possible especially in patients at high risk of multi-drug resistant TB, specifically patients who have been treated previously for TB, defaulters and certain risk groups such as prisoners. If a TB culture is taken, there must be a system in place for tracing the patient. Patients may need to be started on therapy on clinical suspicion alone; a combination of cough, chest pain and constitutional symptoms has a fairly high predictive value for TB. National treatment guidelines should be followed. Patients with TB/HIV-related disease respond well to short or standard-course therapy, unless they have end-stage overwhelming disseminated TB.

If bacterial pneumonia is suspected, a therapeutic trial of benzylpenicillin or ampicillin should be started. If a good response is seen then TB can be excluded. If not, TB therapy should then be initiated; one of the main challenges in therapy is to ensure good compliance.

High fever without focus

Fever is a frequent symptom in HIV-infected patients. Careful history and examination can sometimes reveal a focus, especially in the CNS, joints or soft tissue (pyomyositis is relatively common and requires drainage); or a cardiac murmur suggesting endocarditis. Patients may have chronic middle ear disease and sinusitis, which may be the cause of the fever. Patients can have chronic symptoms such as diarrhoea, dry cough or skin lesions and then acutely develop a high swinging fever but no additional focus.

Malaria must always be excluded. Usually a high fever without focus in the tropics in a patient with underlying HIV indicates a bacterial or mycobacterial infection. Again, remember the possibility of amoebic liver abscess.

In HIV-infected patients this clinical presentation is sometimes referred to as an enteric fever-like illness and is very common. NTS as well as S. typhi are important. Disseminated TB is increasingly recognized but M. avium less common. Without blood culture, salmonella bacteraemia cannot be reliably diagnosed. In Africa about 10% of all HIV-positive adults presenting to hospital will have NTS bacteraemia and a further 5% may have other Gram-negative sepsis (including E. coli and classical S. typhi). Disseminated TB may only be diagnosed at postmortem, therefore a high index of suspicion is needed.

The next problem is how to differentiate the two, and this cannot be done clinically. A positive blood culture will obviously identify Gram-negative sepsis but a negative culture can occur if antibiotic therapy has recently been given, or it may indicate disseminated TB. Many cases of disseminated TB are anergic with minimal pulmonary lesions. M. tuberculosis can take weeks to be positive in a blood culture, unlike M. avium.

How can these sick patients be managed without any microbiology support? Experience is that, with awareness of the possibility of NTS bacteraemia, prompt broad-spectrum antibiotic therapy backed up by intravenous fluids can reduce mortality. Knowing the antimicrobial sensitivity pattern can further reduce mortality.

The following strategy is suggested. For any patient with an enteric fever-like illness, exclude a pulmonary/pleural/pericardial/lymph node/abdominal/renal TB focus by a chest X-ray, urine microscopy, lymph node aspirate and, if possible, ultrasound. Then concentrate on the treatment of NTS bacteraemia. First-line blind therapy can be ampicillin and gentamicin or chloramphenicol. A quinolone would be the best choice but may not be available or affordable, but remember that oral ciprofloxacin has equivalent bioavailabilty to many intravenous antibiotics. It must also be remembered that fluroquinolones have some activity against mycobacteria; this is problematic if the patient has a partial response. If there is little or no improvement after 3 or 4 days (like typhoid itself, NTS bacteraemia can take several days to respond), drug resistance may be a problem. Switch to whichever first-line treatment was not used initially and consider empirical TB treatment.

Chronic diarrhoea

'Slim disease' is what many people equate with African AIDS. It was the first clinical problem specifically associated with HIV infection by Ugandan investigators in 1985, and named by the local patients and their carers, who recognized a new disease in their community.

Chronic diarrhoea with profound wasting is easy to identify and is associated with underlying HIV infection. Widespread metastatic disease, advanced TB (consumption), Addison's disease and untreated insulin-dependent diabetes present with wasting but not usually diarrhoea. While diarrhoea and wasting are the most obvious problems on the wards in Africa, if comprehensive studies of hospital admissions are carried out they account for only 10–20% of the HIV-related workload.

The diarrhoea is usually painless, watery and without blood or mucus. It can be variable or intermittent. Profound weight loss is clinically obvious and may be 20% or more of the premorbid weight. High fever is not typical and should suggest NTS septicaemia or disseminated TB.

Studies from various African centres have shown a variety of stool pathogens: about 15% will have *Cryptosporidium*, 15% enteropathic bacteria, 10% *Isospora* and 10% widespread TB with faecal mycobacteria. Amoebae, *Giardia* and helminths should be sorted and treated where possible. No pathogen is identified in many cases. The hyperinfection syndrome with *Strongyloides stercoralis* does not appear to be associated with HIV infection.

Specific treatment is very limited. Some salmonellae, *Shigella* and *Isospora* will respond to high-dose cotrimoxazole, so a trial of therapy may be indicated. Blind treatment with albendazole has also been shown to reduce diarrhoea but is very expensive. Nitazoxanide may be effective for *Cryptosporidium*. Disseminated TB may respond to anti-TB drugs if the patient is not too severely ill. Codeine phosphate 30 mg four times daily may offer some symptomatic relief. The current mainstay of management of patients with chronic diarrhoea is ART. This often leads to cessation of diarrhoea and rapid weight gain, although there are a number of patients who continue to have diarrhoea despite ART, often these individuals have to be managed palliatively.

Other specific problems

Many patients have painful oral *Candida*. Antifungal agents such as nystatin are effective where available but expensive; gentian violet mouthwashes may give some relief.

Oesophageal *Candida* presenting as dysphagia can be treated with a 2-week course of fluconazole, which is now available free in some African countries via a donation programme.

Kaposi's sarcoma

Only 4% of the first 5000 reported AIDS cases in Uganda had Kaposi's sarcoma (Figure 13.2). Although the cancer is endemic in East Africa, the high rates noted in homosexual men in the USA have not been seen, although Kaposi's sarcoma is now the most common cancer in many African countries. Kaposi's sarcoma is caused by human herpes virus 8, but in most cases immunosuppression such as HIV also needs to be present for Kaposi's sarcoma to occur.

It is usually easy to diagnose clinically. Unmistakable purple or violet raised plaques and sometimes nodular lesions can occur anywhere in the skin. The roof of the mouth is a typical site. The lesions are painless and do not itch. Lymphadenopathy is common and may occur in the absence of skin plaques. Lesions can disseminate, particularly to the lungs. Biopsy is not necessary unless the diagnosis is uncertain.

Some patients with few lesions progress slowly and will die from other causes. Other patients

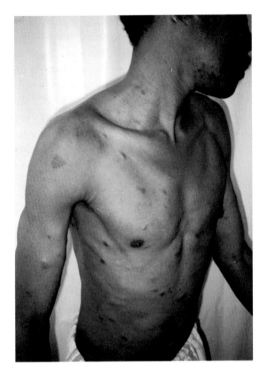

Figure 13.2 Multiple lesions of Kaposi's sarcoma in a patient with AIDS.

progress rapidly over several months. Widespread pulmonary disease is an ominous sign. The drugs used for chemotherapy are expensive and palliative only. Many patients with Kaposi's sarcoma respond to ART and this should be started immediately. If the patient has extensive disease that does not improve with ART, chemotherapy and radiotherapy remain an option if available.

CNS disease

Cryptococcal disease varies in incidence across Africa. It commonly presents as a headache with little neck stiffness, there may be behavioural change easily mistaken for psychiatric illness. Where available it can be diagnosed by India ink staining of CSF although this will miss over 30% of cases. Treatment ideally is with intravenous amphotericin B 1 mg/kg daily for 14 days. If this is not available then fluconazole can be used which may be available via donation programmes.

Headache should be treated with adequate analgesia, and may also respond to repeated lumbar puncture. ART should be initiated when the patient is well enough which will help prevent a relapse. Patients should be given secondary prophylaxis with fluconazole for life or until their CD4 count has risen to $>200 \times 10^6$/L for over 6 months.

Toxoplasmosis may present with a generalized encephalitis, but a relatively mild headache and an altered mental state are more common. Other signs include hemiparesis, ataxia, cranial nerve lesions, generalized incoordination, seizures and confusion. Fever is variable. Diagnosis is difficult with limited resources.

One autopsy study from West Africa found evidence of cerebral toxoplasmosis in 15% of HIV-infected cadavers and it was considered a prime cause of death in 10%. However, in Kenya the experience is that clinically obvious encephalitis is rare (less than 5%). Cerebral toxoplasmosis responds well to oral cotrimoxazole which is more readily available than sulphadiazine and pyrimethamine. As a stage 4 disease any patient with proven or suspected cerebral toxoplasmosis should be started on ART as soon as possible.

Reduced vision can occur in late stage HIV infection for a number of reasons. Cytomegalovirus retinitis is not uncommon, it occurs at low CD4 counts (CD4 $<50 \times 10^6$/L). This will present with fairly rapid painless loss of vision. The fundoscopic appearance is characteristic. Treatment with specific antivirals such as ganciclovir is very expensive and rarely available outside of major centres. ART may arrest visual loss and should be started as soon as possible.

A selection of simple protocols to manage common problems experienced by HIV-infected patients, for use by health care workers in primary health care clinics, is included in the chapter Appendix.

Prophylaxis

Antiretroviral prophylaxis

Prophylaxis for health care staff following accidental occupational HIV exposure is available in many places and is effective at reducing transmission.

Following an injury, the wound should be washed and encouraged to bleed. The source patient and the health care worker should be tested for HIV but if the test is not immediately available there should be no delay in giving prophylaxis. In areas where antiretroviral use is not widespread, a 4-week course of AZT plus 3TC is standard therapy. There are various risk assessment protocols which determine if the exposure was high or low risk, for example, an eye splash is lower risk than a needle stick with a solid needle, which is lower risk than a needle stick with a blood covered hollow needle. Also, if the source patient is taking ART, this may be considered high risk as the HIV may be resistant. Individuals with high-risk exposures may be advised to take triple therapy such as AZT, 3TC and lopinavir/ritonavir (Kaletra). Where available, protocols of the local institution should be followed.

TB chemoprophylaxis

A 6-month course of isoniazid has been shown to be effective chemoprophylaxis against TB. The main problems with this intervention are first proving that the patient does not have active disease and second, the logistics of identifying individuals and delivering the treatment to them. In many settings, prophylaxis is only provided to children who are still being breast-fed by mothers who have sputum-positive disease. There is an argument to give isoniazid prophylaxis to patients on ART who have completed TB treatment to prevent relapse but this is not widely practised.

Preventing pneumococcal disease

A recent study of 23-valent pneumococcal polysaccharide vaccine in Uganda showed a detrimental effect on survival in those receiving the vaccine. This study emphasizes the importance of testing interventions in the target population and not basing guidelines for Africa on studies conducted in the West.

Other infections

Following two studies in Abidjan, Côte d'Ivoire, cotrimoxazole prophylaxis is recommended for people living with HIV/AIDS in Africa. Cotrimoxazole has activity against several bacteria as well as *Isospora belli*, *Pneumocystis jirovecii* and *Toxoplasma gondii*. It also has some activity in preventing malaria. Although the Abidjan studies showed an improvement in survival and decreased morbidity in patients given cotrimoxazole, there is debate as to whether these findings are applicable to the whole of Africa, given different resistance levels to the drug across countries. Cotrimoxazole is generally given to all HIV-infected patients with CD4 counts $<500 \times 10^6$/L or with stage 2 or more advanced disease. Cotrimoxazole is also given as secondary prophylaxis to patients who have had previous cerebral toxoplasmosis or *Pneumocystis* pneumonia. There are no NTS vaccines licensed for human use. Fluconazole available through donation programmes can be used as secondary prophylaxis for patients who have had cryptococcal disease.

Antiretroviral therapy

Public health approach to ART

Combination ART has been in widespread use in developed settings since 1996. It has unequivocally been shown to extend patient's lives and reduce opportunistic infections and malignancies. The drugs initially were too expensive for widespread use but as mentioned above, prices have dropped dramatically and funding for large-scale ART programmes has been made available in many developing countries. The template for programmes delivering ART has been spearheaded by the WHO. The 3-by-5 initiative of the WHO (the aim to get 3 million patients on ART by 2005 in developing countries) recommended a standard first-line ART regimen followed by a second-line regimen if the first failed. This approach has been used and adapted by many developing countries and is known as a public health approach. In developed countries where there may be few patients with HIV, there are often very well-staffed health care facilities delivering and monitoring ART. Clinics are frequently run by specialist clinicians supported by

ART pharmacists, nurses, social workers and other health care professionals as well as well-equipped laboratories able to offer state of the art monitoring. This model of individually tailored ART delivery is not feasible in developing settings, where there are vast numbers of patients, but limited health care structure and very limited human resources. The public health approach to ART delivery aims to provide ART to large numbers of clients and monitor them effectively by using easy-to-follow, simple protocols that allow the limited number of non-specialized health care professionals available to safely deliver ART. Only patients with certain problems are referred to see clinicians or specialists. A limited number of ART regimens, often using fixed dose combinations of drugs, are used. Patients are screened, started on treatment and monitored using protocols based on the best available evidence. This approach allows the greatest benefit to be seen from ART in as many patients as possible. The approach is described in more detail below as well as in the further reading section.

The regimens

There are currently over 20 antiretroviral drugs licensed for clinical use and many more in development. The prices of newer drugs remain high, therefore the drug regimens used in developing settings tend to use older drugs that are either off patent or supplied at reduced cost. The three classes of drugs used in most regimens are nucleoside (or nucleotide) reverse transcriptase inhibitors (NRTI), non-nucleoside reverse transcriptase inhibitors (NNRTI) and protease inhibitors (PI), usually boosted i.e. combined PIs. ARVs are given in combination, and in many cases fixed dose combinations are given which aid compliance by reducing pill burden and lessening the chance of medication error and also are more cost-effective. Below is a list of the drugs most often used with a brief description.

Nucleoside reverse transcriptase inhibitors

Zidovudine (AZT)—One of the original ARVs. AZT has a long history or use and is relatively safe. One of the main side effects is anaemia which can be a problem in settings where many HIV-infected patients are already anaemic.

Stavudine (d4T)—Available in fixed dose combinations and widely used in developing countries. The main side effects are peripheral neuropathy and lactic acidosis.

Lamivudine (3TC)—Used in most first-line regimens. Few side effects but resistance develops very easily.

Emtricitabine (FTC)—Similar to 3TC.

Abacavir (ABC)—More expensive than AZT and d4T. Life-threatening hypersensitivity reaction can occur especially if a patient is rechallenged following an initial reaction.

Didanosine (ddi)—One of the original ARVs. Often poorly tolerated. Should not be given in combination with D4T. Can cause peripheral neuropathy and lactic acidosis.

Tenofovir (TDF)—The only nucleotide analogue reverse transcriptase inhibitor. Usually well tolerated. May cause renal impairment. Renal function should be measured before starting treatment and at regular intervals subsequently.

Non-nucleoside reverse transcriptase inhibitors

Efavirenz (EFV) —Well tolerated. May cause neuropsychiatric problems. Possibly teratogenic.

Nevirapine (NVP)—Available in fixed dose combinations. May cause severe rash and liver toxicity. If possible liver enzymes should be checked before starting NVP and shortly after. Interacts with rifampicin making concurrent administration of antituberculosis therapy problematic.

Boosted protease inhibitor

Lopinavir/ritonavir—Expensive but very potent boosted protease inhibitor combination. Well tolerated. High barrier to resistance. Used in second-line therapy.

To make the administration of ART as simple as possible and to preserve a patient's options for second-line therapy, the limited number of drugs available are given as set regimens which will vary from country to country depending on drug availability. Most programmes have a standard first-and second-line regimen. The first-line regimen may be two NRTIs and an NNRTI, for example, AZT or d4T (or TDF or ABC) plus 3TC or FTC plus EFV or NVP. A typical second-line regimen for a patient who had failed first-line treatment would be two NRTIs not used in the first regimen and a boosted protease inhibitor, for example, ddi or TDF plus ABC plus lopinavir/ritonavir.

When to start ART, monitoring and when to switch or stop treatment

The public health approach to HIV treatment uses simplified decision making based on the "four S's"
1 When to **S**tart?
2 When to **S**ubstitute for toxicity?
3 When to **S**witch treatment?
4 When to **S**top treatment and move to palliative care?

When to start therapy can be based on either WHO staging alone or a combination of WHO staging and CD4 counts if available. If CD4 counts are not available, all patients with WHO stages 3 and 4 disease should be started on therapy. If CD4 counts are available all patients with CD4 counts $<200\times10^6$/L should be treated, regardless of WHO stage. Patients with WHO stage 4 disease should be treated regardless of CD4 count (e.g. patients with Kaposi's sarcoma who have a high CD4 count). Patients with a CD4 count between 350 and 200 should be considered for treatment if they have a WHO stage 3 condition.

The level of monitoring depends very much on what is available. All patients should be monitored clinically, recording their WHO stage at initiation and subsequently. When on therapy patient's weight should be recorded and they should be clinically assessed at each visit for the development of opportunistic infections which may signal ART failure. Also compliance with therapy should be checked. Before ART is initiated patients undergo a series of education modules which ensure they understand the reason for therapy, how the drugs work, the importance of compliance, how to recognize side effects and the importance of continuing to practice safe sex.

CD4 counts (if available) are useful for helping decide when to start therapy and also at follow up every 6 months to see if the patient is responding immunologically. Viral load estimation remains expensive and difficult to organize logistically although dried blood spots can be used. Viral loads are not essential before starting therapy but are useful in assessing the success of therapy and deciding when to switch to second-line drugs.

Side effects of ART are common. These can range from mild rashes and gastrointestinal upsets to life-threatening complications such as lactic acidosis secondary to d4T, ddi or AZT. Simple easy-to-follow protocols should be in place in all ART programmes to help health care workers decide when patients should be referred or when drugs should be substituted. Common reasons for switching drugs are rash secondary to NVP, anaemia secondary to AZT or peripheral neuropathy or lactic acidosis secondary to d4T.

Treatment is switched when the first-line regimen has failed. Failure may either be clinical where CD4 or viral load monitoring is not available or immunological or viral. When the decision is made to switch to second-line therapy, the patient should be counselled again about adherence and it should be stressed that this may well be the last effective therapy that can be offered. Also a search should be made for opportunistic infections as these may make the second regimen less likely to succeed, and a check should be made if the patient is taking other medications including traditional remedies which may affect ART drug levels. Patients should not be rushed into therapy if they are unsure or unready to take it.

In developed settings, there are almost limitless ART regimens and often experimental drugs available meaning it is unusual for an individual to exhaust all therapeutic options. Sadly this is not the case in developing settings, where there may be no effective therapy when the second-line drugs have failed. Also some patients may be too sick to take treatment or have severe opportunistic diseases that progress despite ART. These patients should be palliated, often at home using a home-based care or outreach team. Palliative care resources are often very limited and availability of morphine outside of hospitals can be problematic. But every attempt should be made to ensure a patient can be cared for in the most humane and dignified manner possible, given available resources. Table 13.4 shows suggested screening tests before initiating ART and Table 13.5 shows a suggested format for follow-up visits.

Management of side effects

Side effects due to ART are not uncommon and should be anticipated. What is important is that both patients and health care workers are trained and prepared to recognize them and manage them appropriately. This is best achieved through education sessions for all patients about to start ART and having simple protocols in place for health care workers to follow about how to manage the adverse effects and when to refer the patient or stop therapy.

For example if patients are warned that when starting EFZ they are likely to develop vivid dreams they are less likely to default treatment. Other major side effects such as peripheral neuropathy due to d4T or ddi, anaemia due to AZT,

Table 13.4 Suggested screening tests before initiating antiretroviral therapy

Test	Comment
HIV serology	In patients diagnosed with HIV infection outside of the treatment centre it is prudent to confirm the diagnosis of HIV.
CD4	A CD4 count should be taken if possible to help stage the patient. Also subsequent CD4 counts can be related to the baseline count.
Viral load	Viral load is not essential before initiating therapy, but can be useful prognostically.
Full blood count	Assess and treat anaemia. AZT should be used with caution in patients with Hb <8.0 g/dl, who should be monitored very closely.
Renal function assessment	Renal function should be assessed by measuring electrolytes, urea and creatinine as well as urine dipstick. Patients with protein or blood on dipstick should be further evaluated if possible for treatable conditions. Patients with reduced glomerular filtration rate may need reduced doses of NRTIs.
Liver function test	Patients with raised liver transaminases should be further evaluated for its cause, such as hepatitis or alcohol. Patients given NNRTIs or PIs who have raised transaminases should be monitored closely for deterioration in liver function.
Tuberculosis screening	History and examination should be performed for signs and symptoms of TB. Sputum should be taken for AFB staining. Further investigation such as a chest X-ray maybe required in some cases. TB can be very difficult to diagnose in patients with low CD4 counts (<50).
Hepatitis B serology	Patients with hepatitis B will benefit from ART that includes agents active against the virus such as lamivudine and tenofovir. They are also at risk of deterioration in liver function if their ART is interrupted.
Syphilis serology	Syphilis and other STIs should be sorted and treated prior to starting ART.
Cervical smear	The incidence of cervical abnormalities is high in HIV-infected women. Screening should only be undertaken if referral pathways are available for the management of any abnormalities detected.

Table 13.5 Suggested format of routine follow visit for patients taking antiretroviral therapy

Component	Comment
General history and examination	General enquiry about patients' health and brief examination focussing on detecting opportunistic infections such as TB and STIs. This is especially important in the initial few months of therapy when side effects of therapy and immune reconstitution are more common.
Side-effect check	It is important to be familiar with the side-effect profile of the drugs in your formulary. Side effects may occur early or late. Several examples are: AZT—anaemia d4T—peripheral neuropathy and lactic acidosis ddi—lactic acidosis NVP—liver function abnormalities and rash EFV—vivid dreams and rash
Adherence check and counselling	This is vital; patients should be questioned about adherence and challenges they have faced. Pill counts can be performed. Patients should be supported and encouraged with adherence.
Safe sex and risk-behaviour check	It is important to reinforce these messages.
CD4	This should be checked every 6 months. A falling CD4 count may be the first indication of failing therapy.
Viral load	If available viral load estimation can show if ART is effective or not. A detectable viral load after 6 months of ART suggests either the patient is non-compliant or drug resistance has occurred and therapy needs to be changed.
Full blood count	This should be performed monthly in patients on AZT, which may have to be stopped if anaemia occurs or worsens.
Renal function assessment (Electrolytes, urea and creatinine measurement and urine dipstick.)	This should be performed monthly in any patient with pre-existing renal failure in case further dosage adjustment needs to be made. Also renal function should be checked in patients taking tenofovir.
Liver function assessment	This should be checked monthly in patients with pre-existing liver function abnormalities and in patients taking NVP.

Note: Frequency of visits should follow national guidelines. As a rule, following initiation of therapy a patient should be seen after 2 weeks to check for early side effects and to reinforce compliance. The patient should be seen again after a month and if there are no problems visit frequency can be increased to 3-monthly intervals. Patients experiencing problems or who need careful monitoring, for example anaemic patients taking AZT, should be seen more frequently.

lipodystrophy due to d4T should be checked for at each visit by health care workers. The dreaded side effect of lactic acidosis secondary to d4T, ddi or AZT may have an insidious onset and should be suspected in any patient on therapy for over 4 months who develops abdominal pain, breathlessness or who becomes non-specifically unwell. Cheap point of care lactate meters are available.

A frequent occurrence when patients start ART, especially if they have a CD4 count $<50\times10^6$/L is IRIS. The pathogenesis of this disorder is though to be due to the immune system recognizing pathogenic antigens of certain organisms such as *M. tuberculosis* and *C. neoformans* as it recovers. Patients can present with a paradoxical worsening of their clinical condition shortly after starting ART which can be at best discouraging or at worst life threatening. The most common IRIS events are skin reactions which often settle spontaneously or with symptomatic treatment only. IRIS involving TB or *Cryptococcus* should be treated by treating the causative organism first and frequently also using steroids to suppress the immune reaction. ART can usually be safely continued.

Organization of ART delivery

The organization of a country's ART programme should be undertaken by the national department of health which should produce country-specific protocols often based on WHO protocols adapted for local use. Before starting a programme it is important to ensure that there are adequately trained staff, provision has been made to deal with staff burn out, that a reliable and long-term source of medication is available and that all parts of the health service are aware of the programme and their role in it, for example, maternity services should be aware when and how to refer pregnant women for ART.

Monitoring needs to be in place to ensure that the programme is working well and to pick up deficiencies that can be corrected. Programmes tend to evolve at different rates for a variety of reasons; often monitoring may pick up a clinic or unit that is performing particularly well and the best practice from this area can be implemented elsewhere.

Further reading

Auvert B, Taljaard D, Lagarde E *et al.* Randomized, controlled intervention trial of male circumcision for reduction of HIV infection risk: the ANRS 1265 Trial. *PLoS Med* 2005; 2: e298. [The first trial to show the potential benefit of male circumcision in preventing HIV in Africa.]

Gilks CF, Crowley S, Ekpini R *et al.* The WHO public health approach to antiretroviral treatment against HIV in resource limited settings. *Lancet* 2006; 368: 505–510. [A description of the WHO's public health to large-scale provision of ART in developing countries with high HIV burden.]

McCarthy K, Meintjes G. Guidelines for the prevention, diagnosis and management of cryptococcal meningitis and disseminated cryptococcosis in HIV-infected patients. *South Afr J HIV Med* 2007; 3: 25–35. [Evidence-based guidelines for the management of cryptococcal disease in resource-poor settings.]

Dao H, Mofenson LM, Ekpini R, Gilks CF, Barnhart M, Bolu O, Shaffer N. International recommendations on antiretroviral drugs for treatment of HIV-infected women and prevention of mother-to-child HIV transmission in resource-limited settings: 2006 update. *Am J Obstet Gynecol* 2007; 197: S42–S55. [Up-to-date information on PMTCT.]

Sharp P, Bailes E, Chaundhuri EE *et al.* The origins of acquired immune deficiency syndrome virus: where and when? *Phil Trans R Soc Lond B* 2001; 356: 867–876. [A description of the probable origins of HIV.]

WHO. Antiretroviral therapy for HIV infection in adult and adolescents: recommendations for a public health approach. 2006 revision. Strengthening health services to fight HIV/AIDS. http://www.who.int/hiv/pub/guidelines/adult/en/index.html. [WHO HIV treatment guidelines.]

www.aidsmap.com. [A constantly updated HIV/AIDS resource that features current research articles and covers HIV/AIDS conferences, there is a focus on data relevant to developing settings.]

www.hivinsite.ucsf.edu/. [An extensive HIV/AIDS resource from the University of California, San Francisco.]

www.sahivsoc.org/. [Guidelines and articles on HIV treatment and prevention relevant to Southern Africa.]

www.unaids.com. [A comprehensive website with general information, technical reports and annually updated statistics of the global HIV/AIDS pandemic.]

1 Sore mouth

Patient complains of sore mouth
- Examine mouth with a torch
- Look for ulcers around lips and corners of mouth
- Look for white plaques on inside of cheeks and roof of mouth
- Look for purple growths on tongue

Ulcers around lips and corners of mouth

The patient probably has herpes
- Give them gentian violet and reassure

Ulcers on corner of mouth may be *Candida*
- Treat with nystatin
If there are ulcers on inside of cheeks, advise mouth washes with salty water. If this does not help, triamcinolone lozenges may help

White plaques seen

The patient probably has *Candida*
- Treatment with nystatin 1 ml qds for 7 days
- Regular mouth washes with sodium bicarbonate
- Ask patient to return if not better

Ask patient if they can swallow. If not, see **algorithm 2**
Can you easily scrape off/brush away the plaque? If **yes**: *Candida*

If white plaque cannot be scraped off, the patient probably has hairy leukoplakia.
This condition is not painful and will disappear after the patient has taken ART for a while

Red plaques seen or mouth sore
This may still be *Candida*
- Try nystatin 1 mL qds for 7 days

Purple lump on roof of mouth or tongue

The patient may have Kaposi's sarcoma
- Refer for review with regard to biopsy
- Look for skin lesions

Remember more than one condition can exist at the same time. Treat what you see. In all cases advise patients on maintaining good oral hygiene.

2 Difficulty swallowing

Patient complains of difficulty swallowing

Ask where the food sticks: in the mouth or further down?

Patient says food sticks in mouth

• Examine mouth with a torch
• Look for *Candida*, ulcers, Kaposi's sarcoma

Refer to **algorithm 1**

Patient says food sticks below mouth after swallowing or sticks in chest

• Examine mouth for *Candida* plaques. If present this may indicate that there is *Candida* in the oesophagus.
• Give fluconazole 200 mg for 2 weeks, then reassess patient.

If there is a lot of KS in the mouth, refer for further management

3 Skin rash or itchy skin

There are many causes of rash in patients with HIV/AIDS, some minor and others more serious
Ask: is the patient on antiretroviral therapy?

NO
• Ask if patient has started any other drugs recently. If so did the rash come on after the new medication?

• If the answer is **yes,** stop the medication and inform the medical officer

• Examine for scabies and treat with benzyl benzoate if the rash looks suspicious, for example burrows, rash on groin and hands

• Blistering rash may be due to Herpes zoster or in the genital area due to Herpes simplex. Treat with aciclovir

• Also remember fungal rashes on the feet and body which look scaly and red and also itch. The best treatment is with griseofulvin 10 mg/kg for 6 weeks

YES
• If the patient is on ART, ask which regimen and when therapy started

• Patients taking nevirapine or efavirenz who develop an itchy red rash within a few weeks may be having a drug reaction

• Often this is not severe and settles after a few weeks. If the rash is mild, reassure the patient and give antihistamines
Assess: is the rash severe or mild?

Mild rash
Patients on ART can still have scabies and other common causes of rash so check for these

Severe rash
If the rash is severe, for example covers most of the body, is very hot, weeping, blistering, involves the mouth or genital region *or* if the patient has jaundice or fever along with rash, then admit and refer for advice

Quite often patients starting ART get an itchy rash called folliculitis which is due to the immune system starting to function again. This usually settles after a few weeks and can be treated by using antihistamines

If you are still unsure about the cause of the rash, refer for advice

4 Headache

Patient complains of headache

Does the patient have fever?

YES

• Does the patient have a stiff neck?

• If yes, they may have meningitis. If they are very sick give 2 g ceftriaxone IMI immediately

• If there is no stiff neck, look for other causes of fever
Remember malaria if it is summertime

NO
Is the patient confused?
If **yes,** consider meningitis

NO
Search for a cause for the headache
Look at teeth, ears, ask about STI symptoms

If no obvious cause found:

Has the patient just started ART?
If **yes,** reassure. Headache is common in the first few weeks after starting ART and usually settles. Give paracetamol.

Refer if unsure of diagnosis

NO
• Think about a psychological cause also
• Ask about symptoms of depression such as difficulty sleeping, feeling low, crying for no reason, feeling tired all the time.

5 Cough

Patient presents with cough **Ask:** • How long has cough been present? (>2 weeks, think TB) • Does patient smoke? (if yes, how much?) • Is there sputum production? (if bloody, may be TB) • Is there chest pain? (common in TB) • Is there fever/night sweats? (if prolonged, think TB) • Is there weight loss? (common in TB) • Is the patient on TB treatment?	**Assess:** Don't forget to listen to the lung sounds (auscultate) and monitor the respiratory rate. Percussion, inspection and palpation may also provide valuable cues

If cough is present for under 2 weeks and the patient is not on TB treatment, then treat for chest infection. Only refer patient if they are unwell, for example breathless or in pain

If cough is present for more than 2 weeks then send a sputum for TB. TB is more likely if the cough is associated with chest pain, fever, weight loss, haemoptysis and if the patient has had previous TB. Refer patient if they are unwell for example in severe pain, breathless

If the patient is on TB therapy but not on ART,
• Ask how long they have been on therapy (new cough after 2 months is worrying)
• Ask if they have been taking their pills (compliance)
• Ask if the cough is new or worse than before (cough may take several weeks to settle after TB treatment is started)
• Ask if they feel breathless
There are many causes of worsening cough in patients on TB treatment. If the patient has a new-onset cough and this is severe, causes include pneumothorax, pneumonia on top of TB, resistant TB. These patients should be referred to the medical officer *either* urgently if the patient is distressed and breathless (RR>28/min) *or* at the next planned visit if the cough is not severe

Patient on ART and either on or not on TB treatment

• If the patient has just started ART, cough may be due to immune reconstitution. These patients should be referred to ART clinic as soon as possible, if they are unwell as defined above
• If possible a sputum sample should be taken for AFB in those patients not on TB treatment
• If the patient has been on ART for over 2 months, then use the protocols above

Obtain chest X-ray

Consult with specialist as needed when reviewing results and developing treatment plan

6 Breathlessness (see algorithm 5 for cough)

Breathlessness in patients with HIV can be caused by a number of conditions. Not all causes of breathlessness are due to problems with the lungs, other things can make a person breathless, such as anaemia or too much acid in the blood (lactic acidosis)
First, ask if the patient is taking ART

YES
- If the patient is on ART, ask how long they have been breathless
- If the breathlessness started since the ART began and is associated with feeling tired and generalized pains, then lactic acidosis is a possibility.
Measure serum lactate
Urgent admission and investigation is necessary

- If the patient had breathlessness before they started ART, look for other causes of breathlessness

- Examine the patient's lungs:
  Are there signs of infection?
  Is one lung dull to percussion?
  Are there crackles in the lungs?
  Are the patient's feet swollen?

- Look for signs of anaemia

- Note your findings and make a provisional diagnosis

If the patient is stable (pulse rate <100/min, RR <28/min), then refer to the medical officer at the next visit

If the patient is unwell (pulse rate >100/min or RR >28/min), **give the patient oxygen and refer to hospital**

NO

- Ask the patient how long they have been breathless
  Does it get worse on exertion?
  What makes it better?
  How many pillows does he/she use?

- Examine the patient's lungs (auscultation, percussion, etc.):
  Are there signs of infection?
  Is one lung dull to percussion?
  Are there crackles in the lungs?
  Are the patient's feet swollen?

- Look for signs of anaemia

Possible diagnoses may include:
  Pleural effusion
  Heart failure
  Anaemia
  COPD

- Note your findings and make a provisional diagnosis

If the patient is stable (pulse rate <100/min, RR <28/min), it may be possible to manage them as an outpatient

If the patient is unwell (pulse rate >100/min or RR >28/min), **give the patient oxygen and admit and treat as needed**

7 Diarrhoea

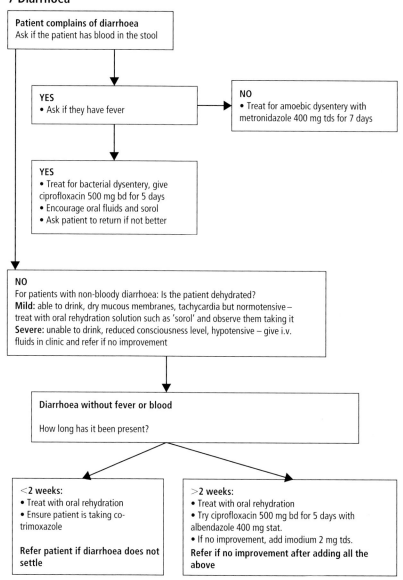

Patient complains of diarrhoea
Ask if the patient has blood in the stool

YES
• Ask if they have fever

NO
• Treat for amoebic dysentery with metronidazole 400 mg tds for 7 days

YES
• Treat for bacterial dysentery, give ciprofloxacin 500 mg bd for 5 days
• Encourage oral fluids and sorol
• Ask patient to return if not better

NO
For patients with non-bloody diarrhoea: Is the patient dehydrated?
Mild: able to drink, dry mucous membranes, tachycardia but normotensive – treat with oral rehydration solution such as 'sorol' and observe them taking it
Severe: unable to drink, reduced consciousness level, hypotensive – give i.v. fluids in clinic and refer if no improvement

Diarrhoea without fever or blood

How long has it been present?

<2 weeks:
• Treat with oral rehydration
• Ensure patient is taking co-trimoxazole

Refer patient if diarrhoea does not settle

>2 weeks:
• Treat with oral rehydration
• Try ciprofloxacin 500 mg bd for 5 days with albendazole 400 mg stat.
• If no improvement, add imodium 2 mg tds.
Refer if no improvement after adding all the above

8 Painful feet

Painful feet are common in patients with HIV due to neuropathy. Medication can make this worse in some cases.

Ask: is the patient taking TB treatment?
Ask: is the patient taking ART?

No   Yes

Patient not on TB treatment or ART
• Look for other causes of painful feet, for example diabetes, heavy drinking, poor diet
• Give analgesia (paracetamol 1 g qds followed by ibuprofen 400 mg tds)
• Patient may need amitryptiline 25 mg at night to help with pain, this can be increased every few weeks

Patient on TB treatment
• Look for other causes of painful feet as above
• Increase pyridoxine to 50 mg bd.
• Give simple analgesia
• Add amitryptiline as above

Patient on TB treatment and on ART
Carry out steps as above

Tell patient that when they finish TB treatment, their feet may improve

If the patient is on ART and the pain is severe and affecting their ability to walk/sleep/function in any other way, give analgesia as necessary and refer to ART clinic

9 Jaundice

Jaundice can be hard to diagnose by examination, unless it has progressed to a severe stage. However, there is at least one easy way of checking for this, and you may want to do this during each follow-up visit (especially for those patients who are taking regimen 1b).

With your finger gently press down on the patient's lower eyelid:
Jaundiced patients will often have a yellow tinge under the bottom eyelid.

If the patient reports they think their eyes have gone yellow, look carefully at the whites of the eyes; if there is jaundice they will be yellow all over, not just in small areas or streaks. Patients with jaundice may also have itchy skin, and may have dark urine.

Ask the patient: When did the jaundice start?
Also ask what medication they are on and when they started it.
Record these dates on the patient's OPD card.
Ask the patient how much alcohol they drink a week and record this on their OPD card.
Also ask if the patient has any nausea or vomiting, if they feel breathless and whether they have any abdominal pain.
Assess if the patient is drowsy, take their temperature and measure their blood glucose. Measure their blood pressure, pulse and count the respiratory rate.

There are many causes of jaundice. If the patient is not taking any medication, afebrile, and not drowsy they can be treated as non-urgent.

If the patient has developed jaundice after starting medication or shows danger signs, which are **drowsiness, fever, vomiting** or a **high pulse (>100/min)**, is **breathing fast (>20/min)**, or has **low glucose (<3.0)**, then they should be treated as urgent.

• **All pregnant patients should also be treated as urgent cases**

Non-urgent jaundice

This may be due to a number of reasons, such as hepatitis, alcohol, drugs the patient has forgotten to tell you about. If they are well, arrange basic investigations as an outpatient.

Urgent jaundice

This may be due to a reaction to medication, an infection, or alcohol. If the patient has any of the danger signs they should be **referred urgently to hospital. This is because jaundice can rapidly progress to liver failure and death if the underlying cause is not treated.**

10 Nausea and vomiting

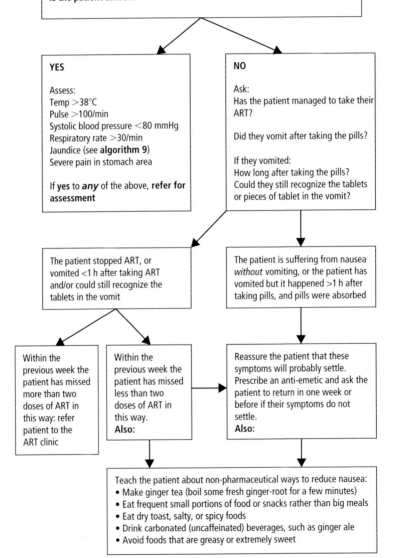

Nausea and vomiting are not uncommon in patients starting on ART. Usually the symptoms settle after a few weeks. Patients can be reassured and given an antiemetic such as metoclopramide 10 mg 8-hourly.
But it is important to recognize patients with severe symptoms that may indicate other more serious problems.

Is the patient unwell?

YES

Assess:
Temp >38°C
Pulse >100/min
Systolic blood pressure <80 mmHg
Respiratory rate >30/min
Jaundice (see **algorithm 9**)
Severe pain in stomach area

If yes to **any** of the above, **refer for assessment**

NO

Ask:
Has the patient managed to take their ART?

Did they vomit after taking the pills?

If they vomited:
How long after taking the pills?
Could they still recognize the tablets or pieces of tablet in the vomit?

The patient stopped ART, or vomited <1 h after taking ART and/or could still recognize the tablets in the vomit

The patient is suffering from nausea *without* vomiting, or the patient has vomited but it happened >1 h after taking pills, and pills were absorbed

Within the previous week the patient has missed more than two doses of ART in this way: refer patient to the ART clinic

Within the previous week the patient has missed less than two doses of ART in this way.
Also:

Reassure the patient that these symptoms will probably settle. Prescribe an anti-emetic and ask the patient to return in one week or before if their symptoms do not settle.
Also:

Teach the patient about non-pharmaceutical ways to reduce nausea:
• Make ginger tea (boil some fresh ginger-root for a few minutes)
• Eat frequent small portions of food or snacks rather than big meals
• Eat dry toast, salty, or spicy foods
• Drink carbonated (uncaffeinated) beverages, such as ginger ale
• Avoid foods that are greasy or extremely sweet

11 Symptoms and signs of STIs (see also Chapter 7)

All patients should be asked about STIs as part of each follow-up assessment.
Ask the patient if they have had unprotected sex since last seen. If so, record when.
Take the opportunity to give advice on safe sex and encourage the patient's partner to
attend for screening. Refer to counsellors where appropriate.

If a patient complains of symptoms of an STI, examine them and treat according to local
syndromic management protocols, as summarized below for male urethral
discharge, female vaginal discharge and genital ulcers (see bottom of page)

Male discharge
Penile discharge or swollen tender testis
Clinical features include penile discharge,
dysuria or swollen testis

• Treat with doxycycline 100 mg bd for 7
days and ciprofloxacin 500 mg stat
• Ask the patient to return after 2 weeks to
check cure; if still symptomatic, then refer
• Give safe sex advice and provide condoms
• Ask patient to refer partner for treatment

Female discharge
Vaginal discharge (non-pregnant)
Clinical features include excessive vaginal
discharge, dysuria, lower abdominal pain

• Carry out a vaginal examination
• If candidiasis is present, give
clotrimazole 500 mg pessary once at night
• Check if there is pain on moving the
cervix
• Carry out a pregnancy test

**Pregnant,
no pain on moving
cervix,** or

**pregnant,
pain on moving cervix**

• Refer for advice

**Non-pregnant,
no pain on moving cervix**

• Treat with doxycycline
100 mg bd for 7 days,
ciprofloxacin 500 mg stat
and metronidazole 400 mg
bd for 7 days

**Non-pregnant,
pain on moving cervix**

• Treat with doxycycline
100 mg bd for 14 days,
ciprofloxacin 500 mg stat
and metronidaole 400 mg
bd for 14 days

• Ask patient to return after 2 weeks to check cure, if still
symptomatic refer
• Give safe sex advice and provide condoms
• Ask patient to refer partner for treatment (if safe)

Genital ulcers (both male and female)

Examine the patient: multiple small recurrent painful ulcers are likely to be due to herpes, there
may also be tender nodes in the groin. Advise the patient not to have sex when the ulcers are
present and to always use condoms. Treat with aciclovir and teach about using aciclovir for
secondary prophylaxis. If the ulcers are severe or slow to heal, then refer.

Single or a few ulcers painful or painless maybe due to syphilis, chancroid, LGV or granuloma
inguinale. Treat with benzathine penicillin 2.4 MU. i.m., and erythromycin 500 mg qds for 7 days

12 Fever

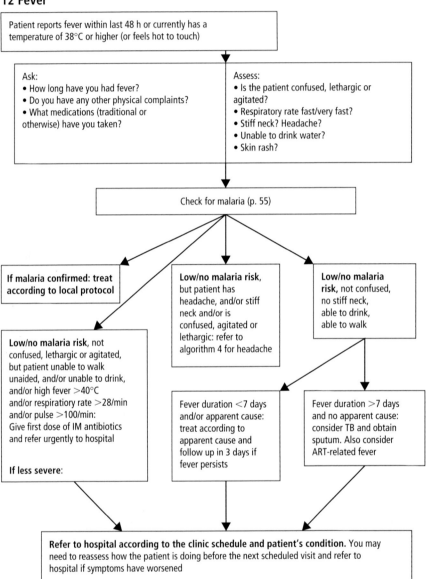

Patient reports fever within last 48 h or currently has a temperature of 38°C or higher (or feels hot to touch)

Ask:
• How long have you had fever?
• Do you have any other physical complaints?
• What medications (traditional or otherwise) have you taken?

Assess:
• Is the patient confused, lethargic or agitated?
• Respiratory rate fast/very fast?
• Stiff neck? Headache?
• Unable to drink water?
• Skin rash?

Check for malaria (p. 55)

If malaria confirmed: treat according to local protocol

Low/no malaria risk, but patient has headache, and/or stiff neck and/or is confused, agitated or lethargic: refer to algorithm 4 for headache

Low/no malaria risk, not confused, no stiff neck, able to drink, able to walk

Low/no malaria risk, not confused, lethargic or agitated, but patient unable to walk unaided, and/or unable to drink, and/or high fever >40°C and/or respiratiory rate >28/min and/or pulse >100/min: Give first dose of IM antibiotics and refer urgently to hospital

If less severe:

Fever duration <7 days and/or apparent cause: treat according to apparent cause and follow up in 3 days if fever persists

Fever duration >7 days and no apparent cause: consider TB and obtain sputum. Also consider ART-related fever

Refer to hospital according to the clinic schedule and patient's condition. You may need to reassess how the patient is doing before the next scheduled visit and refer to hospital if symptoms have worsened

Chapter 14

Onchocerciasis, filariasis and loiasis

Introduction

Onchocerciasis and filariasis are important para-sitic nematode infections, affecting over 200 millions of people living in the tropics and sub-tropics, that cause significant long-term mor-bidity resulting in physical and mental suffering, disability and economic hardship. Insect vectors are important in the transmission of these para-sites. Human infections occur when the insect vector feeds and introduces infective larvae which mature into adult worms and produce microfilar-iae, which in turn infect the insect vector.

Significant progress has been made in recent years in the community control of onchocerciasis and filariasis. A major challenge facing these pro-grammes is the elimination of adult worms which live for many years and are relatively unresponsive to standard antihelmintic agents. Recently, it has become evident that adult filarial worms depend on intracellular, endosymbiotic bacteria of the genus *Wolbachia* for their development, motility and fertility. It is also evident that *Wolbachia* play a significant role in the pathogenesis of disease associated with these filarial infections. The good news is that *Wolbachia* are susceptible to tetra-cyclines and several other antibiotics, offering

Lecture Notes: Tropical Medicine, 6th edition.
By G.V. Gill and N.J. Beeching. Published 2009 by Blackwell Publishing, ISBN: 978-1-4051-8048-1.

fascinating new possibilities in the management and control of filarial infections.

Loiasis affects about 25 million people—trans-mission mainly occurring focally in tropical for-ested regions of west and central Africa. Although most famous for dramatic appearances when the adult 'eye worm' journeys across the eye, loiasis is generally of less clinical importance than onchocerciasis or lymphatic filariasis (LF). However, co-endemicity of *Loa loa* is an important consideration in planning community control of these infections because of the risk that *Loa loa* encephalopathy may be precipitated by certain antihelminthic agents. *Loa loa* does not have a symbiotic relationship with *Wolbachia*, and thus is not susceptible to treatment with doxycycline.

Onchocerciasis

Onchocerciasis or 'river blindness' is caused by the filarial worm *Onchocerca volvulus*. It is a major cause of blindness in tropical Africa and of skin disease throughout its distribution in Africa, Yemen, and Central and South America (Figure 14.1).

Life cycle

Adult female *Onchocerca volvulus* worms are threadlike, about 40 cm long and live in human subcutaneous tissue, sometimes coiled within fibrous nodules, where they produce living

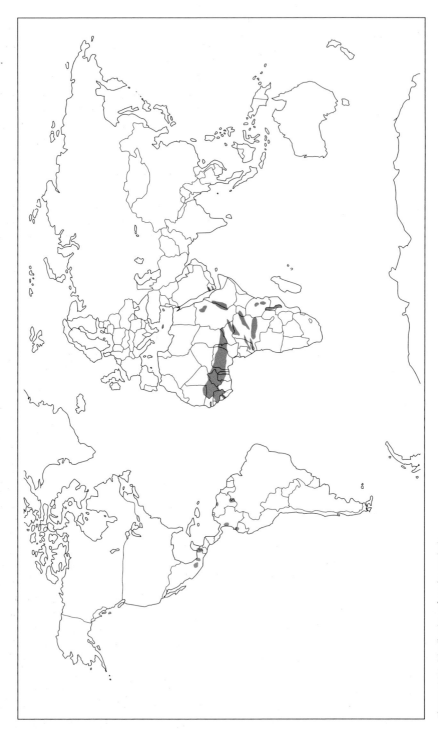

Figure 14.1 Distribution of onchocerciasis.

microfilariae. The microfilariae are about 350 μm long and migrate through the skin and often into the eyes. Microfilariae develop further only if they are taken up by biting blackflies of the genus *Simulium*. These flies can transmit infection after a week or more and deposit infective larvae as they bite another person. Adult *O. volvulus* live for 12 years on an average but sometimes up to 17 years, and microfilariae live for about 1 year.

Epidemiology

Because *Simulium* flies breed in rapidly flowing freshwater, onchocerciasis mainly affects people living or working near fast-flowing rivers. The *Simulium damnosum* complex contains the chief vectors in Africa and although they are found predominantly around rivers, some flies may be blown for great distances and may even reinvade other river systems that have been cleared of vectors in the past. *S. naevei* flies, which attach their eggs to crabs but do not fly far, were an important cause of onchocerciasis in Kenya in the past but this focus has been eradicated with insecticides. *S. ochraceum* and *S. metallicum* are vectors in the Americas and frequently breed in smaller rivers within coffee plantations.

Clinical features

Adult worms evade the host immune response and cause few symptoms. The pathology of onchocerciasis is almost entirely caused by immunological reactions to dying and dead microfilariae and their endosymbiotic *Wolbachia* which release bacterial mediators that trigger the innate immune system resulting in clinical pathology. In addition, activated eosinophils release cellular proteins that cause connective tissue damage.

The incubation period is usually about 15–18 months. Some people do not react to microfilariae and remain asymptomatic carriers for long periods. Onchocerciasis may increase the risk of seroconversion in HIV-1 infections and treatment of onchocerciasis appears to be associated with reduced HIV-1 viral replication. Onchodermatitis also appears to be more severe in HIV- positive patients.

Skin

Intense itching is the principal symptom and leads to excoriation and risk of secondary bacterial infection (Figure 14.2). Asymmetrical maculopapular rashes may be evident. Healing is associated with progressive depigmentation, or blackening and thickening of the skin (Figure 14.3). As time goes by, there is gradual development of degenerative skin changes and loss of elasticity giving the skin a wrinkled, prematurely aged appearance (presbydermia) (Figure 14.4). Sometimes, particularly in the presence of inguinal or femoral lymphadenopathy, this may give rise to the so-called hanging groin appearance. Patchy depigmentation, especially of the lower limbs, results in a characteristic 'leopard skin' appearance. Painless subcutaneous nodules may be palpable and are most obvious over bony prominences. It is

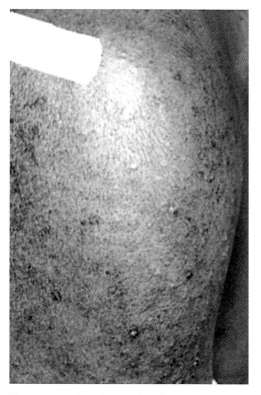

Figure 14.2 Early onchocerciasis with an itchy papular rash in a student from Cameroon.

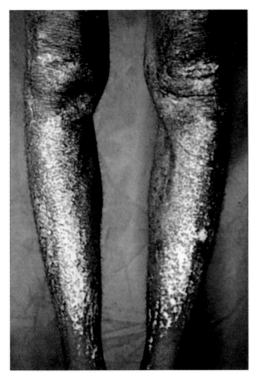

Figure 14.3 Onchocerciasis: typical depigmentation associated with grossly exaggerated skin fold pattern.

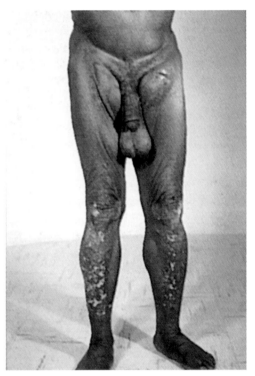

Figure 14.4 Advanced onchocerciasis (West Nigeria). There is depigmentation of the skin overlying the shins, enlargement of the inguinal lymph glands associated with laxity of the surrounding skin (hanging groins) and generalized presbydermia.

common to find several different skin manifestations occurring simultaneously.

A localized chronic papular dermatitis known as 'Sowda' is described in Yemen, Northern Sudan and West Africa. This is a hyperimmune response and microfilariae are scarce in skin snips.

Subcutaneous nodules

Adult onchocercal worms migrating subcutaneously are often arrested over bony prominences and enclosed in fibrous tissue. Nodules may measure several centimetres in diameter and enclose a number of live or dead coiled female worms. Nodules are firm and at first lie free, but may later become deeply attached (Figure 14.5).
• In Africa, nodules are found most readily over the pelvic brim, the sacrum, femoral greater trochanters and the medial aspects of the knees.
• In the Americas, nodules are more often found over the head.

Although nodules are likely to be clinically evident and diagnostically useful in patients with long-standing infections in highly endemic regions, this may not be the case elsewhere. In such a case, ultrasound examination may be helpful in demonstrating the presence of impalpable nodules.

Eye disease

Itching, redness and excess lachrymation are symptoms of early disease. Late disease leads to varying degrees of loss of vision and eventually to blindness. In Africa two epidemiologically distinct forms of ocular onchocerciasis have been described: a mild form occurring primarily in rain forested regions in which blindness is relatively rare, and a severe form occurring in savannah

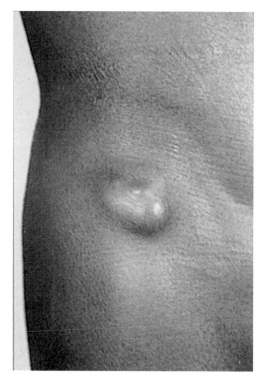

Figure 14.5 An *Onchocerca* nodule. The typical site in Africa. Many worms may be incarcerated in a multiloculated nodule.

regions where blindness is highly prevalent. *Onchocerca volvulus* strains in the savannah have a significantly higher *Wolbachia* DNA to nematode DNA ratio compared to forest strains, further implicating *Wolbachia* in the pathogenesis of onchocerciasis.

Anterior eye disease

- Punctate keratitis is caused by reactions to the death of microfilariae in the cornea. This may appear as a reversible, 'snow flake' opacity.
- Pannus forms as blood vessels invade the cornea from the sides and below. The pannus may cover the pupil—sclerosing keratitis—and cause blindness. This is particularly likely among heavily infected individuals in the African savannah.
- Iritis leads to a loss of the pigment frill and to synechiae that cause a deformed, often pear-shaped pupil. Secondary cataracts occasionally result.

Posterior eye disease

- May present as widespread chorioretinitis with pigmentary changes.
- Often accompanied by optic atrophy, which is sometimes the only finding.
- Various different forms of visual loss may result but a common presentation is with disabling 'tunnel vision'.

Eye disease is particularly likely when adult worms are near the eyes; therefore the risk tends to be higher with nodules on the head and upper body. Because disease progress is relatively slow, most people are blinded in middle life but with heavy infections or more virulent strains, blindness can occur in people in their twenties.

General health

Skin disease may be socially stigmatizing and resources spent on medication may cause significant economic loss. The unrelenting itch may result in chronic sleep disturbance, depression and precipitate suicide. Although onchocerciasis does not kill directly, blind people in village communities have a shortened lifespan and onchocerciasis has led to abandonment of fertile riverside ground in some areas. Very heavy infections in childhood can impair growth. An association with convulsions has been postulated from East Africa but the evidence remains inconclusive.

Diagnosis

Skin onchocerciasis is frequently misdiagnosed as scabies—the papular eruptions of HIV infection should also be considered. History of exposure in a known focus of onchocerciasis is helpful.

Finding microfilariae

Snips of skin should be taken without blood contamination. Take snips from the vicinity of subcutaneous nodules or in Africa from the lateral aspects of the calves, thighs, the hip region or the iliac crests. In the Americas, snips from the shoulder tip or outer canthus of the eye may be more valuable because microfilariae tend to concentrate on the upper part of the body. Up to six snips may be needed to be reasonably sure that infection cannot be detected.

Techniques

1 *Skin snip*—Clean skin with alcohol and allow it to dry; lift up a small piece of skin on a sharp sterile needle. Slice off a piece 1–2 mm^2 with a sterile scalpel or razor blade. The piece should be deep enough to show white dermis and capillaries should ooze blood into the site. Place the skin piece in 0.2 mL saline in the well of a microtitre plate. Fluid from the plate may be examined after half an hour to look for active microfilariae with the low power of the microscope. If microfilariae have not appeared, the plate should be covered with cling film, allowed to stand for 24 h at room temperature and re-examined for emergent microfilariae which will by then usually be immobile.

2 *Punch biopsy*—This technique is essentially the same but more elegant as it uses a Walser corneoscleral punch to obtain the snip. However these punches are expensive and difficult to keep sharp and sterilize.

Count the numbers of microfilariae in each skin snip. You may need to stain some to differentiate microfilariae of *Onchocerca* from other skin or blood microfilariae. PCR techniques sometimes demonstrate microfilariae in skin snips from which no microfilariae have emerged.

3 *Slit lamp*—Use a slit lamp to look for active microfilariae in the anterior chamber of the eye after the patient has spent 5 min in a 'face down' position to bring the microfilariae into view.

Other evidence

1 *Biochemical methods*—Skin-snip microscopy is less sensitive than newer biochemical methods, including skin-snip PCR, ELISAs, enzyme immunoassays (EIAs) and antigen detection. Recent advances include the development of a serum antibody test card using recombinant antigen to detect *O. volvulus*–specific IgG4 in finger-prick whole blood specimens. A triple-antigen indirect ELISA

rapid-format card test also appears promising. A highly sensitive and specific urine antigen dipstick test has also recently been developed.

2 *Surgery*—Subcutaneous nodules can be removed surgically to demonstrate adult worms, or aspirated with a needle to look for microfilariae.

Eosinophilia may be evident in early onchocerciasis.

One of the following two additional tests, now mainly of historic note, may be considered in patients with repeatedly negative skin snips, where other diagnostic techniques are unavailable.

The Mazzotti test is sometimes useful to detect lightly infected patients but is potentially dangerous. It consists of giving diethylcarbamazine (DEC) 6 mg orally and recording the development of an itching papular skin reaction within 24 h; this may be accompanied by fever, limb oedema and even hypotension or worsening of eye damage. This test should be used only for patients with negative skin snips and normal eyes. A safer variant of the Mazzotti test is the DEC patch test in which a 1 cm^2 filter paper soaked in a solution of DEC is applied to the skin of the patient. If positive, this will provoke intense localized itching and inflammation at the site of application. Rarely, a full-blown Mazzotti reaction may be precipitated by a DEC patch test.

Treatment

Ivermectin, a macrocyclic lactone drug originally introduced for veterinary purposes, is now in common use for individual and mass chemotherapy of onchocerciasis. The drug kills microfilariae by immobilizing them so that they are carried away from their usual locations via the lymphatics. Therefore, in contrast to treatment with DEC, microfilaria death following ivermectin is less immediate and is less likely to provoke irreversible inflammatory responses in vulnerable organs such as the eye. Mazzotti reactions are also rare following treatment with ivermectin. However, a temporary increase in itching, papular eruptions, limb oedema, headache and fever may sometimes occur. Ivermectin has little effect on adult worms other than reducing embryogenesis. Therefore, elimination depends on repeated doses over several years. A conservative estimate is that annual treatment with ivermectin alone would need to be sustained for at least 14 years to cover the estimated lifespan of the adult worm.

Ivermectin is administered orally at a dose of 150μg/kg body weight repeated every 3–6 months when treating individual patients, and at 1 or 2 year intervals when used in community control programmes in Africa or the Americas, respectively. Ivermectin should not be used in pregnancy or during breastfeeding although teratogenesis has not been demonstrated. Ivermectin should not be used in patients who also have heavy *Loa loa* infections as fatal cases of encephalitis have occurred.

Recent examples of persistent microfilaraemia despite multiple doses of ivermectin in Ghana have given rise to fears of ivermectin resistance. Although ivermectin-resistant onchocerciasis has not been demonstrated definitively, this may emerge soon. Given the genetic heterogeneity of *O. volvulus* and the likelihood that resistance alleles already pre-exist, concern is growing that mass treatment with ivermectin may be transforming the population genetics in favour of ivermectin-resistant *O. volvulus*.

Doxycycline has been shown to kill the endosymbiotic *Wolbachia* organisms in filarial species. A dose of 200mg daily for 6 weeks is effective in blocking embryogenesis and can maintain freedom from microfilariae for up to 2 years. Doxycycline also has a limited macrofilaricidal effect. In a non-randomized, placebo-controlled trial doxycycline 100mg/day for 6 weeks followed by a single dose of 150μg/kg of ivermectin resulted in up to 19 months of amicrofilaridermia, and complete elimination of *Wolbachia* species in worms excised for immunohistological testing.

DEC is no longer recommended in the treatment of onchocerciasis.

In the past, nodulectomy was advised for head nodules in an attempt to reduce the likelihood of eye disease. However, this is not a guarantee of eliminating risk of eye disease, because not all nodules are necessarily evident and remaining nodules would continue to produce microfilariae.

Improved drug treatment has significantly improved the outlook and has reduced the justification for therapeutic nodulectomy.

Treatment of individual patients

Currently, a combination of doxycycline 100mg daily for 6 weeks and a dose of ivermectin 150μg/kg on completion of the course of doxycycline and a further dose of ivermectin after 3–6 months is recommended for treatment of individual patients, unless contraindicated (age <9 years, pregnancy, breastfeeding).

Control

The control of onchocerciasis has progressed rapidly in the past 30 years, largely due to successful international public–private partnerships, sustained funding for regional programmes and technical advances.

Three landmark programmes have been implemented to date. They are as follows.

The Onchocerciasis Control Programme (OCP) (1974–2002): This programme eliminated onchocerciasis as a disease of socioeconomic and public health importance in 10 countries of West Africa. Initial efforts in vector control using the organophosphate larvicide temephos proved inadequate. A major breakthrough came with Merck's donation of ivermectin, following which larviciding was abandoned in favour of regular mass chemotherapy. OCP's achievements include the following: over 600000 cases of blindness prevented, 40 million people protected from eye disease, infection eliminated in 1 million cases, over 400 professional staff trained and 25 million hectares of riverine habitats and valleys have been made available for settlement making it possible to feed 17 million people. OCP has also played a major role in strengthening health systems in West Africa.

The African Programme for Onchocerciasis Control (APOC) (1995–present): The basis for this programme is a strategy of 'Community-Directed Treatment with Ivermectin' (ComDT), usually as a single annual dose, in 17 non-OCP countries where the disease remains as a serious public health problem and about 15 million people are infected. Communities select their own unpaid distributors who provide ivermectin to members of their community, creating a network that will ultimately cover 59 million people. In a few isolated foci, APOC also aims to eliminate the vector through insecticide spraying.

The ComDT approach has been highly successful and has been investigated in an expanded format that includes distribution of home-based management of malaria, insecticide treated bednets and vitamin A, detection of TB cases and provision of DOTS. Over a 2-year period, malaria home management coverage doubled, bednet coverage increased by two- to fourfold, vitamin A coverage increased significantly and the TB case detection rate doubled. Furthermore, ivermectin distribution also increased, probably due to the increased contacts distributors had with the community when dealing with other diseases.

The Onchocerciasis Elimination Programme for the Americas (OEPA) (1991–present): This programme has adopted an approach similar to that of APOC except that ivermectin is administered every second year.

The timescales required for onchocerciasis elimination using current strategies are vast. Annual treatment with ivermectin achieving 65% population coverage must be sustained for at least 25 years for elimination of infection in areas of medium or high endemicity. More than 35 years would be required if there is heterogeneity in exposure to *S. damnosum*. Significant reductions in these timescales may be possible with the development of strategies targeting *Wolbachia* using short-course antibiotics that can be safely administered to entire communities, without promoting the emergence of drug resistance among existing pathogens or damaging ecological systems.

High-risk foci of *Loa loa* are currently excluded from community ivermectin programmes because of the risk of encephalopathy in individuals with high *Loa* microfilaraemias. Table 14.1 summarizes individual and community chemotherapy of onchocerciasis.

Filariasis

Lymphatic filariasis

Filariasis caused by *Wuchereria bancrofti*, and in some areas of Asia by *Brugia malayi* or *B. timori*, affects about 120 million people and is endemic in at least 80 different countries in the tropics. More than 60% of those affected live in South-East Asia and over 30% live in Africa (Figure 14.6). Although many infections are asymptomatic, a

Table 14.1 Individual and community chemotherapy of onchocerciasis and lymphatic filariasis (LF)

Objective	Disease scenario	Recommended treatment[a]
Community control	Onchocerciasis	IVM 150 µg/kg once a year (APOC) or once every two years (OEPA)
	LF, Africa	IVM 150–400 µg/kg + ALB 400 mg once a year for 30+ years
	LF, outside Africa	DEC 6 mg/kg + ALB 400 mg, once a year for 20+ years
Individual treatment	Onchocerciasis	Doxycycline 100 mg/day for 6 weeks plus IVM 150 µg/kg once at the end of week 6, repeated 3–6 months later
	LF (+onchocerciasis or coinfection possible)	Doxycycline 200 mg/day for 6 weeks plus IVM 150 µg/kg once at the end of week 6, repeated 3–6 months later
	LF (onchocerciasis coinfection excluded)	Doxycycline 200 mg/day for 6 weeks plus DEC 6 mg/kg once at the end of week 6, repeated 3–6 months later

Source: Based on Hoerauf (2006).
Abbreviations: IVM, ivermectin; ALB, albendazole; DEC, diethylcarbamazine; APOC, African Program for Onchocerciasis Control; OEPA, Onchocerciasis Elimination Program for the Americas.
[a]See text for management of lymphoedema and discussion on therapeutic issues related to *Loa loa* coinfection.

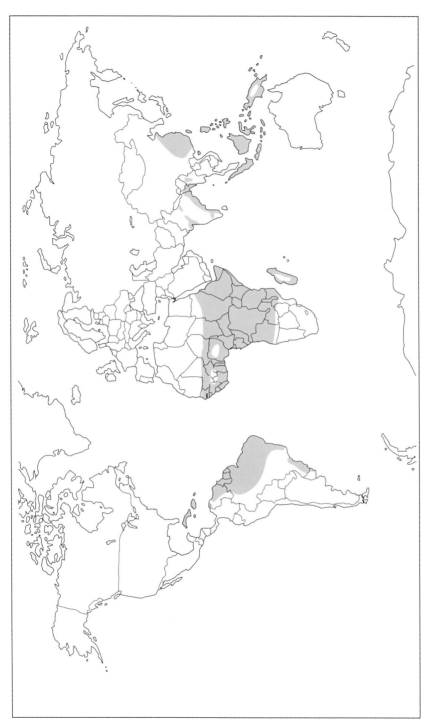

Figure 14.6 Distribution of lymphatic filariasis.

large number of people suffer acute or chronic illness including lymphoedema or elephantiasis (15 million), hydrocele or other genital disease (25 million), acute inflammatory attacks (15 million) and chyluria (5 million). WHO has targeted the elimination of filariasis by the year 2020, principally by means of community mass chemotherapy programmes using antihelmintic agents.

Bancroftian filariasis

Life cycle

Adult *W. bancrofti* are threadlike worms living in the lymphatics of the groin and scrotum or sometimes in those of the arm. Males measure about 4 cm long and females about 10 cm. They can live for more than 10 years and are actively reproductive for up to 4–6 years. Females release over 10 000 sheathed microfilariae daily. These have a lifespan of 1–2 years and appear in the peripheral blood periodically to synchronize with the biting habits of the predominant mosquito vector in the region. Nocturnal periodicity is the commonest—microfilariae are usually present only during the night and disappear into the pulmonary capillaries by day. In some Polynesian islands microfilariae are found in greater numbers in blood during daytime (diurnal subperiodic).

Many different mosquitoes including *Culex*, *Anopheles*, *Aedes* and *Mansonia* species may act as vectors, but the chief vector in towns is *Culex quinquefasciatus* which breeds in drains and polluted water and bites at night. Filariform larvae migrate to the mouth parts of the mosquito after 10 days or more and, in contrast to malaria, are not injected directly into the bloodstream but are deposited on the skin of the new human host during feeding. They then actively invade the new host via the biting area. Thus transmission is less efficient when compared to malaria. There is no multiplication of larvae in the mosquito.

Clinical effects

LF infections may produce a wide range of clinical effects that range from no clinical or microscopic

evidence of infection (asymptomatic amicrofilaraemia), asymptomatic microfilaraemia to filarial fever, chronic lymphatic pathology and tropical pulmonary eosinophilia (Chapter 30). Clinical symptoms may occur between 8 and 16 months following infection, although a first episode of acute filarial fever has been described more than 15 years following exposure. Acute episodes often recur several times a year. There has been considerable confusion and debate concerning the aetiology and classification of acute manifestations of LF. Recent developments, particularly with regard to the role of *Wolbachia*, have led to significant changes in our understanding of the pathogenesis of LF. Inflammatory episodes associated with LF are likely to be multifactorial involving responses to different stages of the parasite, secondary bacterial infection and inflammatory mediators associated with *Wolbachia*.

Clinical presentations include the following:

Acute filarial fever without lymphadenitis which must be distinguished from other acute febrile illnesses in the tropics.

Acute Filarial Lymphangitis (AFL). This occurs following the death of adult worm (whether spontaneous or post-treatment), resulting in a circumscribed inflammatory nodule or cord with centrifugal lymphangitis (i.e. spreading away from the affected node). The clinical course is usually mild and rarely results in residual lymphoedema. In severe cases, an abscess may develop at the site of an affected node and secondary bacterial infection may follow.

Acute dermatolymphangioadenitis (ADLA). ADLA is characterized by intense local inflammation resembling cellulitis or erysipelas, often associated with secondary bacterial infection in the presence impaired lymphatic flow. This results in diffuse subcutaneous inflammation which may be accompanied by ascending lymphangitis and is frequently associated with limb oedema.

Bacteria may enter through breaks in the skin. Stasis of lymph provides excellent conditions for rapid growth of bacteria. The sufferer may complain of high fever, pain, swelling, nausea and vomiting. An acute episode may last about a week. Inflammation leads to damage of small lymphatic vessels, and eventually to fibrosis and progression to elephantiasis. ADLA is commoner than AFL in endemic regions and is more important as a cause of lymphoedema and elephantiasis.

The possibility that a further distinct form of acute lymphangitis and lymphoedema may occur, triggered by filarial larval stages, has also been proposed. However, a case definition has not yet been agreed for this possible presentation.

Chronic LF may develop months or years after acute symptoms, or without a history of acute disease. Lymphatic obstruction leads to lymphoedema of the affected extremity and eventually to elephantiasis. Characteristically, in the initial stages there is reversible pitting oedema. This gradually becomes permanent and the skin thickens and becomes firm. Nodular verrucose skin changes follow. Sites most commonly affected are the legs, scrotum, arms and breast. Recurrent secondary bacterial skin infections, often streptococcal, may cause acute episodes of pain and fever and may be complicated by acute glomerulonephritis.

Other manifestations of LF include the following:
- Hydrocele, usually unilateral (commonest chronic manifestation of *W. bancrofti* filariasis).
- Lymph scrotum, lymphatic fluid seeps through the scrotal skin.
- Acute epididymitis.
- Funiculitis (inflammation of the spermatic cord).
- Monoarthritis.
- Glomerulonephritis.
- Chyluria, chylous diarrhoea and chylous ascites due to rupture of dilated lymphatics. Chyluria characteristically has a milky appearance, sometimes tinged pink because of the presence of red blood cells which can be seen to sediment if the urine is left to stand in a conical jar. Malabsorption, particularly of fat-soluble vitamins, may complicate chylous diarrhoea.

The differential diagnosis of filariasis is wide and depends on the clinical presentation. The following should be considered.
- *Filarial fever*—malaria, other acute fevers, other recurrent fevers, acute bacterial lymphangitis.
- *Groin swellings*—hernias, hanging groin of onchocerciasis.

- *Filarial lymph node enlargement*—chronic infection, HIV, TB, lymphogranuloma inguinale, lymphoma, leukaemia.
- *Filarial orchitis, funiculitis, hydrocele*—acute infection, brucellosis, TB, *S. haematobium*, 'surgical' causes.
- *Chyluria*—other causes of lymphatic obstruction, for example TB.
- *Elephantiasis*—chronic sidero-silicosis, Milroy's syndrome, leprosy (lepromatous), repeated streptococcal infection of feet.

Brugian filariasis

B. malayi is a cause of filariasis in certain rural areas of Asia. There are two main forms: the nocturnal periodic form in swampy areas from India to Korea and Japan, and the nocturnal subperiodic form in damp forests of South-East Asia. The subperiodic form has an animal reservoir in monkeys, cats, and pangolins. *Mansonia* species of mosquito are the major vectors although anophelines may also be involved. Clinically, brugian filariasis is less severe than bancroftian disease. Elephantiasis is usually limited to below the knees and scrotal involvement is less common.

Diagnosis of filariasis

Eosinophilia is common during the acute stages. Parasitological diagnosis can be made on peripheral blood by means of Giemsa stained thick blood films taken at the peak of microfilarial periodicity according to the species (usually 2200–0200 hrs for *W. bancrofti*). However, this is relatively insensitive unless microfilaraemia is high (>100 mf/mL). Concentration techniques greatly improve sensitivity (e.g. nuclepore filtration).

Staff and patients may be reluctant to undertake blood tests in the middle of the night, therefore the 'DEC provocative test' was introduced as a means of inducing parasitaemia during the day. This involved the administration of a single dose of DEC, which provokes microfilaraemia, and the collection of peripheral blood after 30–60 min for staining and examination in the standard manner. However, DEC may cause a severe Mazzotti reaction in patients coinfected with onchocerciasis and may precipitate an encephalopathy in patients coinfected with loiasis. With improved alternative diagnostics, the DEC provocative test is rarely necessary.

A variety of other diagnostic techniques are now available. These include complement fixation tests for circulating *W. bancrofti* antigen such as an ELISA (TropBio-test) and a rapid finger-prick immunochromatographic card test (Amrad ICT, Binax). These tests are very sensitive and specific, and diagnose adult worm infection as well as microfilariae, thus overcoming the problem of periodicity, and may well replace microscopy for diagnosis of *W. bancrofti*. IgG4 tests (Bm 14 test for both *W. bancrofti* and *B. malayi*; Bm-RM for *B. malayi*) may be used for monitoring control programmes and for screening travellers. PCR assays have also been developed for *W. bancrofti* and *B. malayi*. Scrotal ultrasound scanning may be useful for demonstrating live adult worms (the 'filarial dance sign') either for diagnostic purposes or for following up response to treatment.

Management of filariasis

A number of antihelminthic agents are effective.
• *DEC*—This has been the mainstay of treatment and prophylaxis for decades. The usual regimen is 6 mg/kg/day in two or three divided doses for 10–14 days up to a maximum total dose of 72 mg/kg. The side effects are less likely by starting with lower doses (1 mg/kg three times daily on days 1 and 2). The microfilaria count falls within a month and remains low for 6–12 months. If necessary the course of DEC may be repeated 1 month after completion of the initial course. DEC has limited effect in killing the adult worms. DEC should be avoided in areas endemic for onchocerciasis or *Loa loa* because of the risk of provoking a Mazzotti reaction or encephalopathy.
• *Ivermectin*—This kills microfilariae but not adult worms. It is mainly used in combination treatment with DEC or albendazole.
• *Albendazole*—This kills microfilariae and has some effect on adult worms if taken as a prolonged course.

The following general adverse reactions to antihelmintic treatment occur in decreasing order of frequency—headache, fever, dizziness, anorexia, malaise, nausea, urticaria, vomiting and wheeze. General reactions and fever are positively associated with the prevalence and intensity of microfilaraemia.

Local adverse reactions include scrotal nodules due to death of the adult worm, lymphadenitis, funiculitis, epididymitis, lymphangitis, orchitis, abscess formation, ulceration and, rarely, transient lymphoedema.

Combination treatment with antihelmintic agents is the basis for community control programmes.
• *Doxycycline*—Doxycycline 200 mg/day for 6 weeks has been shown to be highly effective in the treatment of filariasis, producing a 99% reduction in microfilaraemia at 12 months. The addition of a single dose of ivermectin after 4 weeks resulted in complete amicrofilaraemia. A subsequent trial of doxycycline 200 mg/day for 8 weeks achieved similarly impressive results with almost complete elimination of microfilariae at 8–14 months, and significant reduction in the adult worm burden and presence of filaria antigenaemia. More recently a similar macrofilaricidal effect has also been demonstrated using a 6-week course of doxycycline.

Doxycycline eliminates microfilariae gradually, thus avoiding adverse inflammatory events that may follow rapid destruction of parasites and release of bacterial symbionts. Adults are also gradually eliminated, avoiding the development of inflammatory nodules sometimes seen with rapid death of adult worms following treatment with DEC or ivermectin. In addition doxycycline eliminates *Wolbachia* surface protein, the inflammatory trigger for chronic disease. Use of doxycycline in the treatment of patients with LF has been shown to decrease plasma levels of lymphangiogenic factors, reduce dilation of lymphatic vessels, improve lymphoedema and reduce hydrocele.

Treatment of individual patients

If coinfection with onchocerciasis is present or possible, a combination of doxycycline 200 mg daily for 6 weeks and a dose of ivermectin

150 μg/kg on completion of the course of doxycycline and a further dose of ivermectin after 3–6 months is recommended for treatment of individual patients, unless contraindicated (age <9 years, pregnancy, breastfeeding).

In the absence of coinfection with onchocerciasis, a combination of doxycycline 200 mg daily for 6 weeks and a dose of DEC 6 mg/kg on completion of the course of doxycycline, and a further dose of DEC after 3–6 months is recommended unless contraindicated.

In either of the aforementioned situations, if coinfection with *Loa loa* is present, particularly if associated with a high *Loa* microfilaraemia, it is essential to reduce the microfilaraemia using albendazole prior to treatment with DEC or ivermectin. This is discussed in more detail in the section on *Loa loa*.

Prevention of morbidity

Lymphoedema management involves measures to assist lymph flow including elevation, massage, exercise and bandaging of affected limbs. Elevation of the limb with massage and compression bandaging to reduce oedema is useful, but is often not tolerated in the humid tropics.

Prevention of acute inflammatory episodes is focused on preventing secondary bacterial infection. Careful hygiene, use of disinfectant soap and water, and general skin care including early and effective treatment of any wounds or abrasions should be encouraged. Antibiotic prophylaxis with penicillin is useful if there are recurrent streptococcal infections. Surgical treatment of limb elephantiasis is not straightforward, leaves scars and is often unavailable to poor people.

Hydrocele requires surgical management.

Chyluria requires bed rest and attention to nutrition. Surgery may be required in some cases.

Control

1 Control of mosquito breeding is helpful, particularly in towns.
2 Insecticide-impregnated mosquito nets protect against night-biting mosquitoes and are important in areas of nocturnally periodic transmission.

3 Mass treatment of at-risk populations. The preferred strategy for a community programme will depend on the local epidemiology of LF and coendemicity of other filarial infections, as well as issues related to sustainable health systems, drug supply management, etc. Mass treatment programmes are now being implemented on an annual basis for community control of LF. Unfortunately, community control requires these programmes to run for 20–30 years.

Possible treatment strategies that may be used include the following:
1 Single-dose, once yearly two-drug regimen (albendazole + DEC or albendazole + ivermectin).
2 DEC-fortified salt for 1 year.
3 Combination of a single annual dose of albendazole + DEC and DEC-fortified salt.
4 Chemotherapy with single dose of albendazole + DEC followed by DEC-fortified salt.
5 DEC-fortified salt in islands or other areas where salt supply can be controlled.

The following two-drug regimens are currently recommended for community control programmes:

Outside Africa, DEC in single dose of 6 mg/kg given annually together with a single dose of albendazole 400 mg is effective in reducing microfilaraemia and longevity of adult worms. Annual treatment should continue for at least 20 years.

Within Africa, because of the risk of onchocerciasis and/or *Loa loa*, a single dose of ivermectin, usually 150 μg/kg (note that doses of up to 400 μg/kg have also been recommended) is given with a single dose of albendazole 400 mg. Annual treatment should continue for at least 30 years. Particular caution is advisable in regions where *Loa loa* is prevalent. Simultaneous administration of albendazole and ivermectin is unlikely to significantly reduce the risk of encephalopathy, and use of higher range doses of ivermectin may increase the risk. High-risk foci of *Loa loa* are currently excluded from ivermectin programmes.

The Global Alliance for the Elimination of Lymphatic Filariasis (GAELF), created in 2000, is an international public–private partnership that aims to eliminate LF as a public health problem.

GAELF coordinates activities of partners and concentrates on political, financial and technical support. Partners include national ministries, academic institutions, NGOs, WHO, UNICEF, World Bank, donors and development agencies. Two major drug companies have been instrumental in the development of this initiative. In 1997 GlaxoSmithKline (GSK) agreed to donate albendazole for as long as it is needed to eliminate LF as a public health problem. In 1998 Merck & Co. Inc agreed to provide ivermectin for LF in Africa in coendemic (onchocerciasis & LF) countries in association with GSK's albendazole donation for as long as necessary. Centred on the ComDT approach, the aim is to interrupt transmission by mass treatment of populations at risk using a treatment strategy appropriate to the target population. The strategy is based on the expectation that 70% coverage using two drugs (albendazole plus ivermectin in Africa; albendazole + DEC elsewhere) once a year for 4–6 years (the estimated reproductive duration of the adult worm) will suppress parasites in blood, prevent infection of mosquitoes and stop transmission. Table 14.1 summarizes individual and community chemotherapy of LF.

Loiasis

Loa loa (the 'eye worm') is transmitted by 'red' flies of the genus *Chrysops* that inhabit tropical forests of Africa. Larvae migrate subcutaneously, maturing into 3–7 cm long adult worms over the course of about a year. Adults may survive for more than 15 years. Female worms produce microfilariae which periodically appear in the peripheral blood and can survive for up to 2 years. Symptoms are mainly attributable to the adult worm and include urticaria, pruritis, arthralgia and malaise. Subconjunctival migration causes intense pain and inflammation. If local anaesthetic and suitable surgical instruments are immediately available (and you and your patient are feeling brave) the worm can be removed from the eye. Trauma to the migrating adult worm, most commonly on the extremities, may provoke a localized inflammatory reaction known as Calabar swelling. Neurological complications, including a potentially fatal meningoencephalitis, are more likely to occur in patients with high microfilaraemia, particularly following the administration of antihelmintics. Proteinuria is relatively common and haematuria may also occur. Pulmonary infiltrates, pleural effusions, arthritis, lymphangitis and hydrocele have also been described. Hypereosinophilia is common and *Loa loa* has been implicated in the aetiology of endomyocardial fibrosis (EMF), although EMF is also described in association with numerous other causes of hypereosinophilia.

Diagnosis and treatment

Diagnosis may be obvious from the history, particularly if an 'eye worm' has made an appearance. Dead, calcified worms may be incidental findings on X-ray. Peripheral blood microfilaraemia peaks between 1000–1500 hrs and the characteristic sheathed microfilariae measuring 250–300μm in length can be identified in thick blood films using Giemsa or Wright stains. Concentration techniques may be helpful if films are negative. A quantitative microfilarial load should be estimated as this may be useful in predicting the likelihood of an adverse reaction to treatment. Probable cases of *Loa*-related encephalopathy are defined based on threshold values for *Loa* microfilarial loads of >10000Mf/mL if measured before ivermectin treatment, or >1000Mf/mL if sampled after treatment. Patients with pre-treatment microfilarial loads >30000Mf/mL are at greatest risk of encephalopathy; however serious adverse effects may occur at lower levels and caution is advisable in all patients with pre-treatment microfilarial loads >2500Mf/mL.

Serological tests are available and may be helpful for diagnosis in travellers from endemic areas, but lack specificity and cross-react with other filarial parasites and *Strongyloides* spp.

Loiasis is commonly treated with DEC 2mg/kg orally three times daily for 7–10 days. DEC has an effect on both adult worms and microfilariae. Treatment is repeated every 2–3 months if symptoms remain. Ivermectin 150μg/kg as a single dose prior to treatment with DEC reduces the likelihood of a Mazzotti reaction in patients coinfected with onchocerciasis. However, treatment with DEC or ivermectin may be hazardous in patients with loiasis who have high microfilarial loads (>2500 Mf/mL) because massive release of antigens from dying microfilariae may precipitate meningoencephalitis or renal failure. In the past, plasmapheresis has been used to reduce heavy microfilarial loads prior to treatment with DEC under steroid cover. The currently preferred strategy for managing patients with high microfilaraemia is administration of albendazole 200 mg twice daily for 3 weeks to gradually reduce the microfilaraemia, followed by a course of DEC or ivermectin. Prednisolone 20 mg/day, given for 3 days before and for 3 days following the start of antihelmintic treatment, may reduce the risk of encephalopathy.

Rapid assessment procedures for loiasis (RAPLOA) have been developed to identify communities in Africa where individuals may be at high risk of severe adverse reactions to ivermectin. The Central province of Cameroon is the main focus for this problem. High-risk foci are currently excluded from ivermectin programmes for the control of onchocerciasis and LF.

Further reading

Addis DG, Brady MA. Morbidity management in the global programme to eliminate lymphatic filariasis: a review of the scientific literature. *Filaria J* 2007; 6: 2. [This review covers the major clinical manifestations of LF with specific reference to pathogenesis, epidemiology, economic and social impact, individual treatment and impact of mass treatment.]

Boatin BA, Richards FO. Control of onchocerciasis. *Adv Parasitol* 2006; 61: 349–394. [Detailed review describing epidemiological, biological, clinical and public health aspects of onchocerciasis.]

Hoerauf A. New strategies to combat filariasis. *Expert Rev Anti Infect Ther* 2006; 4: 211–222. [Comprehensive review including recent developments in the understanding of the pathogenesis of LF and onchocerciasis, and providing clear guidelines for treatment.]

Johnston KL, Taylor MJ. *Wolbachia* in filarial parasites: targets for filarial infection and disease control. *Curr Infect Dis Rep* 2007, 9: 55–59. [Recent work on *Wolbachia* has revolutionized our understanding of the pathogenesis of filarial infections and has opened the door to novel approaches to treatment using antibiotics.]

Molyneux D. Onchocerciasis control and elimination: coming of age in resource-constrained health systems. *Trends Parasitol* 2005; 21: 525–529. [Excellent description of the remarkable achievements in onchocerciasis control over the past four decades.]

Molyneux DH, Bradley M, Hoerauf A, Kyelem D, Taylor MJ. Mass drug treatment for lymphatic filariasis and onchocerciasis. *Trends Parasitol* 2003; 19: 516–522. [Summarizes progress towards control of LF and onchocerciasis focussing on mass drug administration programmes particularly those following the donation of ivermectin and albendazole.]

Chapter 15

African trypanosomiasis

African trypanosomiasis is caused by species of *Trypanosoma brucei*. There are three morphologically identical parasite species:

1 *T. brucei brucei* confined to domestic and wild animals.

2 *T. brucei gambiense* causing gambiense sleeping sickness in West and Central Africa.

3 *T. brucei rhodesiense* causing rhodesiense sleeping sickness in East and Southern Africa.

Transmission is by the bite of tsetse flies (members of the genus *Glossina*), which are only found in Africa. In general, the infected areas are found south of the Sahara and north of the Zambezi (Figure 15.1).

Parasites

The parasites are flattened and fusiform in shape, like slender pointed leaves, 12–35 μm long and 1.5–3.5 μm broad. They are actively motile using a thin fin-like extension from the main body, the undulating membrane, to propel themselves. The form of the parasite found in humans is the trypomastigote in which the kinetoplast is posterior to the nucleus and from which the flagellum arises. The flagellum runs along the free edge of the undulating membrane and usually projects

Lecture Notes: Tropical Medicine, 6th edition.
By G.V. Gill and N.J. Beeching. Published 2009 by
Blackwell Publishing, ISBN: 978-1-4051-8048-1.

in front of it, sometimes extending as far again as the creature's body (Figure 15.2).

Life cycle

This is the same for both species. Trypomastigotes from the infected host are taken up by the tsetse fly during a blood meal. In the stomach of the fly, the parasites multiply by simple fission, penetrate the gut wall and migrate to the salivary glands. There the morphology changes, the kinetoplast coming to lie just in front of the nucleus and the creatures are now called epimastigotes (crithidia). The infective trypomastigote (the metacyclic trypanosome) is found in the saliva about 20 days after the original infecting blood meal, and the fly remains infective throughout its normal lifespan of several months.

Disease

Local effects

Metacyclic trypanosomes injected during tsetse feeding multiply in the extracellular space and lymphatics before becoming disseminated by the bloodstream. This local multiplication may cause a marked inflammatory reaction—the trypanosomal chancre.

The trypanosomal chancre appears 3 or more days after the bite and typically increases in

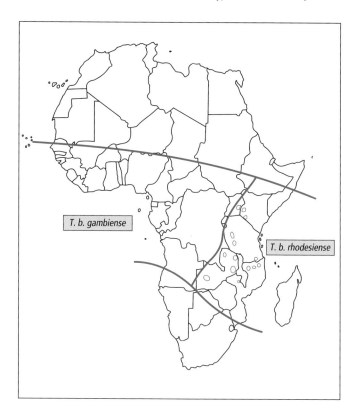

Figure 15.1 Distribution of human African trypanosomiasis.

size for 2 or 3 weeks, at the end of which time it begins to regress. The presence of a chancre is much more common in *T. b. rhodesiense* infection than in *T. b. gambiense* infection. Local lymphadenopathy may be found in the region of a bite.

Systemic effects

Multiplication of trypanosomes in the lymphatics leads to parasitaemia 5–12 days after the bite (haemolymphatic or early stage). Waves of parasitaemia are associated with fever. Parasites may then enter the CNS via the choroid plexus or by transcytosis across endothelial cells to cause a lymphocytic meningoencephalitis (late stage).

In general *T. b. gambiense* is better adapted to the human host than *T. b. rhodesiense*. *T. b. gambiense* is therefore relatively well tolerated; the illness it causes tends to be subacute or chronic and parasitaemia may even be asymptomatic. In contrast, *T. b. rhodesiense* is normally a zoonotic

infection which is transmitted to humans 'accidentally'. It causes pronounced systemic effects; parasitaemia usually causes severe incapacity and the course of the illness is relatively rapid.

Immune response and pathogenesis

The main response to trypanosomal infection is antibody production, particularly IgM. Antibody production initially controls parasitaemia, but antigenic variation in parasite surface antigens means that immune control is incomplete and this leads to successive waves of parasitaemia, which may explain the fluctuating nature of the illness. In the brain and other organs (e.g. heart or serous membranes), perivascular infiltration with lymphocytes, plasma cells and macrophages and characteristic morular cells occurs. Microglial and astrocyte proliferation may be associated with neuronal destruction and demyelination in the brain.

Clinical picture

Trypanosoma brucei gambiense

Early stage

Fever, headache and joint pains are the main early symptoms, sometimes accompanied by fleeting areas of cutaneous oedema. A small proportion of patients with parasitaemia are asymptomatic. Lymph glands become enlarged; they are often most prominent in the posterior triangle of the neck (Winterbottom's sign). Odd skin rashes sometimes occur (visible only in relatively unpigmented skins), usually taking the form of areas of circinate erythema. There may be generalized pruritus and characteristic thickening of the facial tissues giving a sad or strangely expressionless appearance. The spleen enlarges to a moderate size in many cases.

This early stage usually lasts many months, sometimes even over 2 years. Occasionally, patients with *T. b. gambiense* develop a rapidly progressive toxaemic disease that is fatal before the CNS is involved. However, most deaths occur after CNS invasion unless the patient develops an intercurrent infection.

Late stage symptoms and signs

Symptoms and signs of disturbed cerebral function predominate. Behavioural changes are common; a patient whose personal habits were previously fastidious becomes careless about appearance; his or her speech becomes coarse and temper becomes unpredictable and he or she may behave in a socially unacceptable way. Psychiatric manifestations of agitation or delusions may become severe enough to mimic mania or schizophrenia. Sleep becomes disordered in that the patient sleeps badly at night but falls asleep during the day.

In the early evolution of this change, the patient can be readily awoken and responds by conversing fairly normally. As time goes by, sleeping periods may become longer until the patient is sleeping most of the time and may even fall asleep while eating. At this stage, speech and motor functions in general are usually severely disturbed. Weight loss may occur because of inadequate nutrition unless the family makes strenuous efforts to help with feeding.

Focal CNS signs may develop, but there is usually more diffuse evidence of CNS disease, especially relating to extrapyramidal and cerebellar functions—widespread tremors involving the limbs, tongue and head; spasticity (mainly of the lower limbs); ataxia and sometimes choreiform movements. Convulsions are relatively uncommon. Kérandel's sign (delayed hyperaesthesia) may occur; following firm pressure on the tissues overlying a bone, there is a definite delay before the patient shows any sign of pain. In advanced cases, the tendon reflexes are often grossly exaggerated and the plantar responses may be extensor. Death usually occurs within a few months of CNS involvement becoming manifest but may be delayed for up to a year.

Trypanosoma brucei rhodesiense

Symptoms and signs

The parasite usually produces a more acute and virulent infection than does *T. b. gambiense*, with fever and systemic symptoms prominent. Serous effusions, especially pleural and pericardial, are common and myocarditis occurs. In the early stages, *T. b. rhodesiense* may cause hepatocellular jaundice and mild anaemia, and severe anaemia may soon develop. Both liver and spleen may be slightly enlarged, and lymph gland enlargement (seldom so prominent as in *T. b. gambiense*) is most common in the inguinal, axilliary and epitrochlear glands. *T. b. rhodesiense* may be fatal within a few weeks of the onset, often as a result of death from myocarditis before the CNS is involved.

The picture in the late stage of *T. b. rhodesiense* infection is much like that of *T. b. gambiense* but occurs early in the course of the disease and is more rapidly progressive. Clinical features of CNS involvement are similar to *T. b. gambiense*, but death is more rapid and neurological features are more pronounced than behavioural changes.

Diagnosis

Early stage disease

The diagnosis is usually made by demonstration of parasites. A number of methods may be used.

1 Examination of stained or unstained thick blood films: Films can be stained with a Romanowsky stain as for malaria or be examined wet (simply place a coverslip over a drop of blood) when the disturbance of the red cells produced by the movement of the trypanosomes can be detected using a dry 40× objective (Figure 15.2).

2 Concentration methods are used to detect scanty parasitaemia, including microscopy of the buffy coat following centrifugation using the microhaematocrit (MHCT), the more sensitive QBC technique and the minianion exchange column technique (MAEC). Microscopy is most useful for *T. b. rhodesiense* infection. The organisms may also be isolated by inoculation into special culture media or into animals.

3 Gland puncture: This is of most use in *T. b. gambiense*; posterior cervical lymphadenopathy is common and gland aspirates may be positive when there is no peripheral parasitaemia. A needle is inserted into an enlarged node held between thumb and finger. The flow of gland juice can be improved by massaging the gland while the needle is *in situ*. The juice is then expressed on to a slide, using a syringe containing air, and examined immediately.

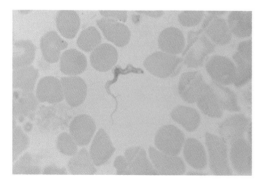

Figure 15.2 Parasite of *T. b. rhodesiense* in the blood film of a severely ill Zambian adult.

4 Bone marrow aspiration: This is useful in the early stages when other methods are negative.

5 The chancre: Trypanosomes can be recovered by aspiration from the chancre or from the regional glands draining the chancre if they are enlarged, before the blood is positive.

In *T. b. gambiense*, trypanosomes may be difficult to find in the blood, especially in late infections. The longer the duration of infection, the more difficult it is to find trypanosomes.

Late stage disease (CNS involvement)

This may be diagnosed clinically on the basis of neurological signs, but CSF examination should be performed in all patients following one or two doses of suramin or pentamidine to clear parasitaemia (and hence reduce the risk of parasites being introduced into the CSF from the blood). The deposit from 5 to 10 mL of centrifuged fluid should be examined as soon as possible for motile trypanosomes or should be made into a smear, dried, fixed and stained with a Romanowsky stain. Late stage disease is diagnosed by the presence of trypanosomes in the CSF or by a raised CSF cell count ($>5/mm^3$) or increased CSF protein level.

Immunological diagnostic methods

A number of serological methods are available. The card agglutination test for trypanosomes (CATT) is simple to carry out and gives good results in most areas of *T. b. gambiense* but is of no value in *T. b. rhodesiense*. It is a valuable test for screening populations as the results are obtained within 30 min. Disadvantages include limited sensitivity and specificity of the antigen, as trypanosomes share antigens with several other protozoa and bacteria. The card indirect agglutination test for trypanosomes (CIATT) which detects circulating antigens has been used for the diagnosis of both *T. b. gambiense* and *T. b. rhodesiense*. This technique may also be useful to follow responses after treatment. Positive serological tests should be confirmed parasitologically before treatment.

Routine laboratory findings

A mild normochromic anaemia is common. The WBC is usually normal, but the ESR is usually above 50 mm/h and sometimes over 100 mm/h. Serum and CSF IgM levels are usually very high.

Treatment

A number of different drugs have activity against trypanosomes. Most are relatively toxic and there is an urgent need for the development of new drugs for the treatment of sleeping sickness. Not all drugs penetrate the CSF, and different drugs are therefore used for the treatment of early and late stage disease. It is important to treat coexisting infections and anaemia prior to using specific treatment—many advocate routine antihelminth and antimalarial therapy.

Early *T. b. gambiense* and *T. b. rhodesiense* infections

Suramin is the drug of choice for treating first stage *T. b. rhodesiense* infection. It is also effective in *T. b. gambiense*, but pentamidine is now most commonly used to treat early *T. b. gambiense* infection. Neither of these drugs penetrate the CSF.

Suramin is administered intravenously. Following a test dose of 5 mg/kg, 20 mg/kg (maximum 1 g) should be given on days 1, 3, 10, 17 and 24. Suramin is usually well tolerated, but fever, nausea and proteinuria may occur. Infrequent idiosyncratic anaphylactic reactions also occur. Pentamidine can be given intramuscularly or intravenously; intravenous administration avoids painful local tissue reactions. Normal doses are 4 mg/kg/day for 7–10 days. The major reaction is syncope and hypotension; hypoglycaemia may also occur.

Late stage disease

Melarsoprol can be used for the treatment of late stage *T. b. gambiense* and *T. b. rhodesiense* infections. Eflornithine is only effective in *T. b. gambiense*.

Melarsoprol is a trivalent arsenic compound that is given intravenously and is active against blood, tissue and CNS trypanosomes. There are many different treatment schedules but it is normally administered as three or four series of three injections separated by 7 days at doses that range from 1.2 to 3.6 mg/kg (see Table 15.1 for commonly used schedule). Recent studies suggest that shorter 10-day courses (2.2 mg/kg daily) may be as effective for *T. b. gambiense*. Melarsoprol therapy is normally preceded by 1–2 doses of suramin to clear blood, lymph and tissue trypanosomes.

Melarsoprol is a toxic drug. The major side effect is a serious encephalopathy (reactive arsenical encephalopathy), which occurs with a frequency of 2–10% and a case fatality rate of up to 50%. The danger of severe toxic effects is minimized by improving the patient's general condition, as already described. Prophylactic corticosteroids reduce the risk of an encephalopathy in *T. b. gambiense*. Other side effects include peripheral neuropathy.

Eflornithine is used intravenously for the treatment of late stage *T. b. gambiense* infection at a dosage of 400 mg/kg/day in divided doses for 14 days. It is relatively expensive and difficult to administer but less toxic than melarsoprol. The common side effects (gastrointestinal symptoms and anaemia) do not usually require treatment to be stopped.

Table 15.1 Treatment schedule for an adult with late stage *T. b. rhodesiense*

Day	Drug	Volume (ml)	Dose (mg/kg)
1	Suramin	2.5	5
3		5.0	10
5		10.0	20
7	Melarsoprol	0.5	0.36
8		1.0	0.72
9		1.5	1.1
16	Melarsoprol	2.0	1.4
17		2.5	1.8
18		3.0	2.2
25	Melarsoprol	3.0	2.2
26		4.0	2.9
27		5.0	3.6
34	Melarsoprol	5.0	3.6
35		5.0	3.6
36		5.0	3.6

Nifurtimox has traditionally been used in Chagas' disease. There is emerging evidence of its efficacy for treating *T. b. gambiense* in combination with eflornithine or melarsoprol.

Monitoring cure

Patient symptoms should resolve after treatment. Despite the severity of the symptoms in advanced late cases, the degree of functional recovery after successful chemotherapy is remarkable. It may take 6 months or more for the CSF cell counts to fall below $5/mm^3$ and for normal protein concentrations to occur. Failure of these parameters to reach normal may be the first indication that treatment has been unsuccessful. Full cure cannot be assumed unless a 2-year follow-up has been completed. If treatment of patients with CNS involvement has been delayed, a variable degree of neurological defect will persist. This most commonly takes the form of intellectual impairment.

Relapse

Treatment of relapse can sometimes be difficult. Relapse in *T. b. gambiense* following treatment with suramin or pentamidine is often treated with melarsoprol; eflornithine can also be used. Relapse in *T. b. rhodesiense* is usually treated with a second course of melarsoprol.

Epidemiology

Approximately 40 000 cases of sleeping sickness are notified to the WHO each year; although it is estimated that between 300 000 and 500 000 individuals are infected. Over 90% of cases are due to *T. b. gambiense* infection. A lack of resources and civil conflict in many of the heavily affected areas has led to an increase in cases as previously successful control programmes have broken down.

T. b. gambiense infection

Humans are the most important reservoir of infection, although the pig and other animals are naturally infected in some parts of West Africa. Infection is spread from human-to-human by the bite of riverine tsetse flies (*G. palpalis* group), which breed along the banks of rivers and lakes. Infection tends to occur where human activities bring humans into contact with the fly, such as at river crossings and sites used for the collection of water and when fishermen come into contact with flies on the river or lake shores. Village-sized and larger outbreaks occur, sometimes amounting to epidemics. The spread of epidemics tends to be linear, following the distribution of flies along the course of rivers or affecting islands in lakes.

T. b. rhodesiense infection

T. b. rhodesiense is usually a zoonotic infection in members of the antelope family, especially the bushbuck. It can be maintained as a zoonosis in the animal population in the absence of human cases and is transmitted by tsetse species dwelling in savannah and woodland habitats (*G. morsitans* group). It is a particular hazard to those who spend long periods in enzootic areas in pursuit of their livelihood, such as hunters and honey-gatherers. Rarely, infection can occur in tourists visiting game parks.

Although *T. b. rhodesiense* cases tend to be sporadic, epidemics do occur especially in East Africa around Lake Victoria. In these epidemics, tsetse populations build up adjacent to human populations containing active cases. Domestic cattle that are infected develop a chronic parasitaemia and act as a reservoir host. The current epidemic in south-east Uganda is caused by peridomestic breeding *G. fuscipes* in thickets of the exotic plant *Lantana camora*.

Sleeping sickness control and surveillance

There are two major components of sleeping sickness control.
1 Detection and treatment of cases.
2 Vector control.

In *T. b. rhodesiense* areas, patients who present with symptoms of early parasitaemia (passive surveillance) can be treated at local rural centres; in epidemics, rapid deployment of active surveillance using blood film screening and the establishment of effective local treatment centres is important. In *T. b. gambiense* areas, limited clinical symptoms in the early stages require active surveillance. Individuals can be screened using gland aspiration or rapid antigen tests (e.g. CATT).

Vector control is best achieved using insecticide-impregnated traps and targets. Sterile insect release methods may also be useful in reducing vector populations. Residual insecticide application to *Glossina* resting sites, insecticide spraying and the clearing of riverine habitat have been used in the past but resource and environmental considerations means that these can no longer be considered. In epidemic situations, treatment of the cattle reservoir by cattle trypanocides may also be a strategy for prevention of human-sleeping sickness.

In all endemic areas, the disease should be made notifiable to a central trypanosomiasis control unit. Specialized staff can then be sent promptly to the area and steps can be taken (such as active case-finding and treatment) to prevent the development of an epidemic. This strategy has proved very effective in the past in Ghana, Nigeria and Uganda.

Further reading

Blum J, Schmid C, Burri C. Clinical aspects of 2541 patients with second stage human African trypanosomiasis. *Acta Trop* 2006; 97: 55–64. [A comprehensive clinical description.]

Fèvre EM, Picozzi K, Jannin J, Welburn SC, Maudlin I. Human African trypanosomiasis: epidemiology and control. *Adv Parasitol* 2006; 61: 167–221. [A recent comprehensive review.]

World Health Organization. *Control and Surveillance of African Trypanosomiasis*. Technical Report Series no. 881. Geneva: World Health Organization, 1998. [Advice on treatment and surveillance.]

Chapter 16

South American trypanosomiasis—Chagas' disease

Parasite, life cycle and pathogenesis

South American trypanosomiasis occurs in humans and a large number of wild and domestic animals and is widespread in Central and South America. It is caused by *Trypanosoma cruzi*, which differs from trypomastigotes of the *T. brucei* group in having a large kinetoplast. Trypanosomes in the blood of the mammalian host are taken up by triatomine bugs (reduviid, 'assassin bugs', 'kissing bugs'), which bite at night. All stages feed on blood but only adult bugs can fly. Organisms multiply in the hindgut of the bug as epimastigotes and develop into metacyclic trypanosomes which are excreted in the faeces of the bug during feeding. Infection is acquired by rubbing faeces of the bug into a wound or conjunctiva; infection can also be acquired by transfusion, congenital infection, or by drinking sugarcane or fruit juice contaminated with triatomid bugs.

In the host, trypomastigotes multiply at the site of the bite, enter the bloodstream and enter a variety of tissue cells, particularly neuroglia and muscle cells. Parasites develop as intracellular amastigotes and form pseudocysts; rupture of these pseudocysts causes inflammation, tissue damage and further dissemination. Most pathological effects are chronic, probably related to a combination of tissue damage, neuronal loss and an autoimmune response.

Clinical features

Acute Chagas' disease

This is most common in children but may occur at any age—only one-third of individuals are symptomatic. Penetration and local multiplication of the parasite at the site of entry may cause an area of cutaneous oedema (chagoma) or orbital oedema (Romaña's sign) if entry is via the conjunctiva. A febrile reaction may occur 1–2 weeks later with the development of lymphadenopathy, hepatomegaly and splenomegaly. Rarely, death may occur at this stage as a result of cardiac damage or meningoencephalitis, especially in children. If symptomatic, the acute phase lasts for 1–3 months and resolves spontaneously.

In untreated patients, asymptomatic low-level parasitaemia may continue for many years (indeterminate phase); 15–40% of patients will develop chronic Chagas' disease.

Chronic Chagas' disease

Chronic disease normally occurs 10–20 years after initial infection. Classical manifestations are as follows:

1 *Cardiac disease*—Biventricular cardiomyopathy or cardiac rhythm disturbance (often heart block).

Lecture Notes: Tropical Medicine, 6th edition. By G.V. Gill and N.J. Beeching. Published 2009 by Blackwell Publishing, ISBN: 978-1-4051-8048-1.

2 Mega-oesophagus or megacolon as a result of destruction of the intramural parasympathetic nerve plexus. This presents as aspiration pneumonia or intractable constipation and abdominal distension.

3 Similar mega disorders of other hollow muscular viscera such as small bowel and ureter may occur resulting from nerve damage.

Immunocompromise

HIV infection or the use of immunosuppressive drugs may lead to the reactivation of latent infection causing severe myocarditis or neurological problems.

Diagnosis

Parasitological techniques

1 *Microscopy*—In the acute phase, parasites can usually be easily found on thick or thin films; centrifugation techniques increase the sensitivity.

2 *Culture*—Parasites can be cultured, but specific media and expertise are required.

3 *Xenodiagnosis*—Low-level parasitaemias can be detected by allowing uninfected bugs to feed on patients. Three to four weeks later, the bugs are dissected to look for gut infection.

4 *Biopsy*—Amastigotes may be demonstrated in pathological specimens.

Other techniques

IgM and lifelong IgG responses may be detected by a number of techniques, including complement fixation test and ELISA. Cross-reactivity with other parasitic diseases and autoimmune disorders leads to poor specificity, and diagnosis should be based upon at least two positive techniques. Serological tests often remain positive after parasitological cure. PCR is effective in acute infection but has have limited utility in chronic disease.

Treatment

Acute stage

Nifurtimox and benznidazole suppress parasitaemia, shorten the course of the acute illness and prevent acute neurological and myocardial complications. Benznidazole is better tolerated. However, elimination of parasites and prevention of chronic disease only occurs in 50–80% of patients.

Indeterminate and chronic phase

Although treatment has traditionally been thought to have little effect in the intermediate phase, there is emerging evidence that benznidazole may be of benefit in clearing parasitaemia in some patients and may prevent progression to chronic disease. The value of parasitological treatment in chronic disease remains uncertain but may prevent progression. Cardiac complications require symptomatic treatment and insertion of pacemakers is often necessary.

Epidemiology and control

T. cruzi is found in a large number of mammalian species, but the most common wild hosts are rodents or small marsupials. Many species of triatomine bugs simply maintain infection amongst wild animals, but some species have become adapted to living in human dwellings, leading to human infection when infection is transmitted from domestic animals. A single adobe dwelling can harbour thousands of bugs and up to 50% of bugs may be infected. Chagas' disease can also be transmitted by transfusion and congenital infection occurs in up to 10% of seropositive women.

Control of the disease can be achieved by the use of seroprevalence surveys to determine areas at risk and spraying of pyrethroid insecticides. Improvement in the standard of housing is also important. Elimination of cracks in mud walls or replacement of natural material roofing with iron sheets reduces available habitats for the bugs. In a number of South American countries, such activities have reduced the incidence of Chagas' disease by between 60% and 99% over the past 20 years.

Further reading

Bern C, Montgomery SP, Herwaldt BL, *et al*. Evaluation and treatment of Chagas disease in the United States: a systematic review. *JAMA* 2007; 298: 2171–2181. [A systematic review of the evidence in Chagas.]

Prata A. Clinical and epidemiological aspects of Chagas' disease. *Lancet Infect Dis* 2001; 1: 92–100. [Good general review of South American trypanosomiasis.]

Rassi A, Rassi A, Little WC. Development and validation of a risk score for predicting death in Chagas' Heart Disease. *N Engl J Med* 2006; 355: 799–808. [Describes clinical risk score for the severity of Chagas' heart disease.]

Chapter 17

Schistosomiasis

Schistosomiasis is often known as 'bilharzia' or 'bilharziasis' after Theodor Bilharz who first described the parasite in humans and found the adult flukes in a human post-mortem in Egypt in 1851. Schistosome eggs have been recovered from both Chinese and Egyptian mummies, showing that the infection was present in both of these early civilizations. Today schistosomes remain distributed throughout the tropics and flourish wherever freshwater bodies, both natural and man-made, create habitats for the appropriate snail vectors.

Three main species of schistosome affect humans with different geographical distributions (Figure 17.1).

1 *Schistosoma haematobium* causes urinary schistosomiasis. It is scattered throughout Africa, parts of Arabia, the Near East, Madagascar and Mauritius.

2 *Schistosoma mansoni* is mainly found in Africa and Madagascar. It was exported by the slave trade to parts of South America and the Caribbean and Arabia, where permissive snail vectors were present.

3 *Schistosoma japonicum* is found in China, the Philippines and Sulawesi. There is a small focus in the Mekong river on the east border of Thailand. *S. mansoni* and *S. japonicum* cause disease of the bowel and liver. *S. intercalatum* is a minor species

confined to West Africa. It inhabits the veins of the lower bowel and produces terminal-spined eggs. *S. mekongi* is emerging as an important human pathogen in the Mekong delta alongside *S. japonicum*, and also affects bowel and liver.

Parasitology

The adult flukes causing human schistosomiasis are worm-like creatures 1–2 cm long which inhabit parts of the venous system of humans. The male worm resembles a rolled leaf in having a groove on his ventral surface in which the longer, more slender female is held *in copulo*. Both sexes are actively motile. The worms sometimes live for 30 years, but their normal lifespan is probably 3–5 years.

Life cycle

Fertilized adult females lay eggs in the terminal venules of the preferred host tissues (Figure 17.2). Their bodies obstruct the vessel and so impede the escape of eggs into the circulation. Most of the eggs penetrate the vessel wall and enter the tissues. Movements of the walls of the hollow viscus involved (as well as other factors) propel the eggs towards the lumen from which they escape to the outside world—in the urine in the case of *S. haematobium* and in the stools in the case of the other four species.

Lecture Notes: Tropical Medicine, 6th edition.
By G.V. Gill and N.J. Beeching. Published 2009 by Blackwell Publishing, ISBN: 978-1-4051-8048-1.

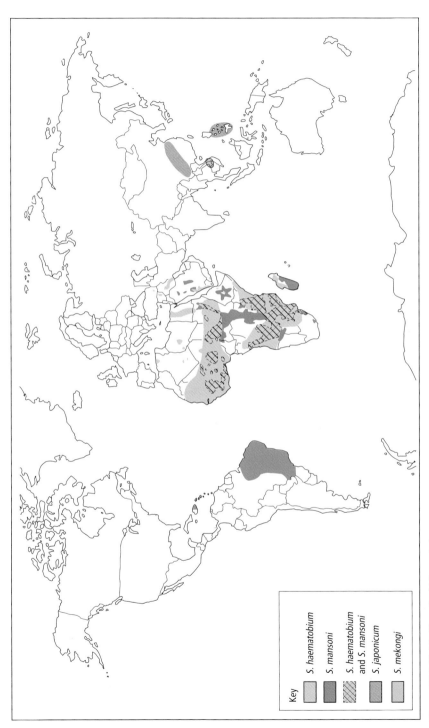

Figure 17.1 Distribution of schistosomiasis.

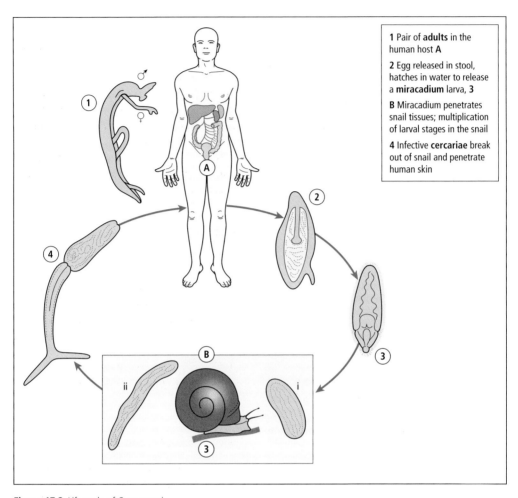

1 Pair of **adults** in the human host **A**

2 Egg released in stool, hatches in water to release a **miracadium** larva, 3

B Miracadium penetrates snail tissues; multiplication of larval stages in the snail

4 Infective **cercariae** break out of snail and penetrate human skin

Figure 17.2 Life cycle of *S. mansoni*.

The shapes of the eggs of each species are distinctive, and each contains a ciliated miracidium. This hatches out in freshwater and swims in search of a suitable snail intermediate host. Many species of snail host are known, but in general:
1 *S. haematobium* requires an aquatic sinistral turretted snail of the genus *Bulinus*;
2 *S. mansoni* requires a flat aquatic 'ramshorn' snail, most commonly of the genus *Biomphalaria*; and
3 *S. japonicum* requires a small amphibious operculate turretted snail, usually of the genus *Oncomelania*.

The miracidium penetrates the body of the snail and begins a complicated asexual replicative cycle that results, a few weeks later, in the release of minute fork-tailed cercariae into the water. As cercariae are about 200–500 μm long; they are just visible to the naked eye. They emerge from the sporocyst inside the snail in response to light. A snail may shed cercariae for many weeks. The cercaria is infective to the definitive host. If it finds no suitable host within 24–48 h it dies. If it contacts human skin, however, the cercaria penetrates, sheds its tail and body, and enters circulation with the new name—a schistosomule. The schistosomule reaches the liver through the lungs by passive intravascular migration. Once in the liver, it begins to feed and grow, and in

1–3 months develops into a mature fluke in an intrahepatic portal vein. The mature males and females couple and then migrate to their final habitats. It is easy to understand how *S. mansoni* and *S. japonicum* find the way to their homes in the lower mesenteric veins as they have only to travel straight down the portal vein. However, it is a mystery how *S. haematobium* reaches the vesical plexus.

The time elapsing between cercarial penetration and the passage of eggs is the prepatent period. It can be as short as 4 weeks with *S. mansoni*, usually 12 or more weeks with *S. haematobium*, and somewhere in between with *S. japonicum*. The prepatent period is sometimes very prolonged in light infections; perhaps if there are few worms in the liver, the sexes have difficulty finding each other.

Epidemiology

Magnitude of the problem

Some 300 million people are infected with schistosomes throughout the tropics wherever freshwater bodies (particularly lakes, dams and irrigation systems) support large snail populations near concentrations of human habitation.

Requirements for transmission

1 Contamination of water with viable eggs from a reservoir host.
2 Presence in the water of susceptible snail intermediate hosts.
3 Suitable environmental conditions for development in the snail.
4 Human exposure to water containing cercariae.

Reservoir hosts

In the three common schistosomes, humans are the main reservoir. Rodents and baboons may be able to maintain *S. mansoni* infection sometimes. Many animals are susceptible to *S. japonicum* infection, including domestic animals such as the horse and dog.

Epidemiological patterns

In most infected communities, infection is most common and heaviest in children between 10 and 15 years old. Because children have the highest egg output and are more likely to contaminate water, they are usually the most important reservoir of infection. Exposure may be occupational, such as occurs among workers on irrigated farms and fishermen. Transmission is often focal, and neighbouring villages may have greatly differing endemicities because of this.

Exposure and immunity

There is evidence that some degree of immunity to superinfection develops in schistosomiasis. It is certainly incomplete and may depend for its maintenance on the continued presence of some living schistosomes in the body. It does not seem to be antibody mediated and is probably directed against the schistosomule stage. The survival of adult worms in the circulation may be partly related to their ability to incorporate host antigens in their integument (surface).

The log–normal distribution

In a population apparently exposed to a uniform risk of infection, some people will be found to be very heavily infected and others very lightly infected. If egg output is accepted as being related to the number of adult worms present, the distribution of worms in the population is not 'normal'. It will always been found that some of those infected have an infection with perhaps 100 times as many worms as those with the most common level of infection. If a frequency–distribution plot of egg output is carried out, the usual Gaussian curve will be seen to be distorted by having a greatly extended 'tail' to the right of the graph. The curve can be made to resemble a 'normal' curve if, instead of the egg count, the logarithm of the egg count is plotted on the *x*-axis. This sort of distribution is called a log–normal distribution and applies to the abundance of almost all non-replicative parasites in humans and animals.

There is no generally accepted explanation, but it could be related to the host's first exposure to infection. If the initial challenge was with a large number of parasites, at a time when no immunity existed, a large population could become established in the absence of immune opposition. However, if the first exposure was to a small number of parasites, the subsequent development of immunity could resist further infective challenges, and the total number of parasites would then remain low.

Infection in children

In hot countries, children naturally play in water. This recreational exposure is sometimes the most important source of infection. At puberty, exposure often diminishes as modesty develops at the same time as sexual awareness. However, infection may still be acquired during activities such as personal bathing, washing clothes and utensils, and in the pursuit of irrigated farming. This change in behaviour is one factor in the tendency of the infection to diminish after puberty but it is not the only one. Acquired immunity also appears to reduce the likelihood of a given exposure to cercariae leading to an established infection.

Progression to disease

Most people infected with schistosomiasis die of an unrelated disease. In many parts of the world, although the prevalence is high, the adverse effects of the infection are difficult or impossible to demonstrate. The notion that the infection always causes general debility and malaise, in the absence of more specific effects, is wrong. In the absence of reinfection, the tendency is for most of the worms to die within a few years and for pathology related to the eggs (see later) to resolve. In only a small proportion of cases will progressive pathology develop. These are mainly those with heavy infections and re-exposure to infection over a period of many years. Treatment can certainly modify the natural history of the infection and even advanced cases may show a surprising degree of improvement after chemotherapy.

Clinicopathological features

Effects of cercarial penetration

Cercariae may cause an itchy papular rash ('swimmer's itch' or 'fisherman's itch') as they penetrate the dermis. This is seldom seen in endemic areas. A conspicuous cercarial rash is more often caused by avian or other schistosomes not otherwise pathogenic in humans. It is quite common in northern Europe, North America and South-East Asia.

Initial illness: acute schistosomiasis

An initial febrile illness is sometimes recognized following the first exposure. It does not develop in very light infections and is seldom recognized in residents of endemic areas. It is mainly a problem in immigrants or visitors encountering a large cercarial challenge for the first time.

The illness comes on 4 or more weeks after infection and is usually self-limiting. The theory is that as the worms begin to lay eggs, soluble antigen (Ag) leaks out of the eggs and enters into the circulation. While antibody (Ab) production lags behind antigen release, moderate antigen excess prevails. This favours Ag–Ab complex formation with the development of generalized immune complex disease. Because the antigen is soluble and distributed by the bloodstream, the effects are more general than local. The immune complex disease hypothesis probably also explains why acute schistosomiasis has been reported more frequently in *S. japonicum* where egg production per worm pair is heavier than in *S. haematobium* and *S. mansoni*.

Features of acute schistosomiasis

The condition is sometimes called Katayama fever, after the prefecture in Japan where it used to be common. Some or all of the following may occur.
- Fever
- Urticaria
- Eosinophilia
- Diarrhoea
- Hepatomegaly

- Splenomegaly
- Cough and wheeze
- Cachexia.

Perhaps it is seldom recognized in children in endemic areas because immune tolerance develops *in utero* because of transplacental passage of antigen. Spontaneous recovery may be related to restoration of Ag–Ab balance as the infection matures and antibody production increases.

Importance of the eggs: those that get away

Eggs that escape from the body enable the life cycle to be completed. Their passage through the bladder in *S. haematobium* typically causes terminal haematuria, the cardinal symptom of the infection. In heavy infections, irritation of the bladder may cause dysuria. In *S. mansoni* and *S. japonicum* corresponding effects may occur in the bowel—diarrhoea and blood. More commonly the presence of a little blood is noticed in an otherwise normal stool. In most infections, no bowel symptoms are noticed. Through these mechanisms of blood loss, schistosomes may contribute to the development of iron-deficiency anaemia in some individuals.

Importance of retained eggs: the main pathology

The serious mischief in humans arises from tissue reaction to retained eggs. This reaction, which follows sensitization to egg antigens, is a circumoval granuloma. It results from combined humoral and cell-mediated attack on the egg, and the granuloma occupies several hundred times the volume of the egg itself. Its characteristics are epithelioid and giant cells, as well as lymphocytes and eosinophils, arranged in concentric fashion around the egg. The cellular content diminishes with time to be replaced by fibroblasts and a collagenous scar. Precipitation of Ag–Ab complex on the egg surface helps activate inflammation.

The duration of the vigorous cellular response to a single egg lasts a few weeks. If egg laying is stopped by chemotherapy, the cellular component of the granuloma usually resolves in 2 or 3 months. Not all granulomas lead to scars (Figure 17.3). These pathological processes occur, with variations, in all the schistosome infections. They help to explain the specific features of each of the species described next.

Clinical features of *S. haematobium*

Bladder pathology and squamous cell carcinoma

Eggs become deposited in the bladder and nearby organs, not singly but usually in clutches. This is because a female schistosome may occupy the same site for long periods, during which time she lays several hundred eggs a day. The eggs give rise to a granulomatous lesion up to several centimetres

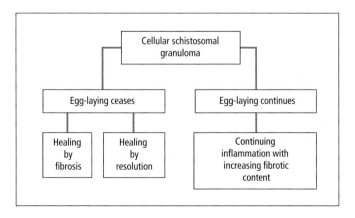

Figure 17.3 The fate of the granuloma.

in diameter. Most commonly these fleshy lesions form in the bladder mucosa where they simulate tumours and are called pseudopapillomas. They may be sessile (flat) or pedunculated (on stalks). Smaller deposits of eggs cause lesions a few millimetres in diameter, resembling tubercles. If bladder inflammation due to *S. haematobium* is very persistent and prolonged over many years, it is associated with the development of squamous cell bladder carcinomas.

Bladder calcification

This is common in *S. haematobium* because of calcification of the eggs, not of the bladder itself. A calcified bladder outline on X-ray is fully compatible with normal bladder function.

Obstructive uropathy

When granulomas form near the ureteric orifices or in the ureters themselves, the ureters may become obstructed. This is the cause of early obstructive uropathy. The secondary effects are hydroureter in which the ureter becomes dilated and elongated with varying degrees of hydronephrosis. In the most severe cases, kidney drainage may be so impaired as to cause uraemia. It used to be thought that all the changes of obstructive uropathy were irreversible. It is now known that in the early cellular phase of the granuloma, complete resolution may follow effective chemotherapy. Longitudinal follow-up has shown that, provided reinfection does not occur, spontaneous resolution without significant scarring may also occur.

Genital schistosomiasis

Eggs from *S. haematobium* may be deposited at various sites throughout the urogenital system. Urethral papillomatous lesions have been reported in men and boys, and some men report changes in ejaculate consistency with or without blood in the semen. Semen microscopy in these cases often reveals eggs, but the effect on sperm counts, function and fertility have not been systematically investigated. Female genital schistosomiasis is increasingly recognized to include inflammatory lesions arising around deposited eggs in the vulva, vagina, cervix and fallopian tubes. The lower lesions can sometimes be mistaken for malignancies while the higher lesions are associated with sterility.

S. haematobium and the lung: schistosomal cor pulmonale

Eggs escaping from the pelvic veins into the caval circulation reach the lungs. In heavy prolonged infections, granuloma formation may cause obstruction in pulmonary arterioles. Pulmonary hypertension, right ventricular hypertrophy and congestive heart failure may follow. Cyanosis develops from vascular shunting in the lungs.

Clinical features of *S. mansoni*

Most patients with *S. mansoni* infections have few or no symptoms: the liver is often enlarged, the spleen only in the presence of portal hypertension or during the initial illness. Severe clinical effects, except those caused by ectopic worms (see later) are only seen in heavy infections.

Pseudopolyposis of the colon

In severe *S. mansoni*, granulomas in the large gut may develop into papilloma-like outgrowths of the mucosa. They may ulcerate and bleed and cause symptoms of dysentery. There is no proven causal relationship to colonic carcinoma, and strictures do not form.

S. mansoni and the liver: schistosomal liver fibrosis

Severe long-standing *S. mansoni* infections cause a characteristic liver disease, 'Symmer's pipestem fibrosis'. Large numbers of eggs escaping from the lower mesenteric veins and reaching the periportal regions cause a granulomatous response that leads to gradual occlusion of the intrahepatic portal veins. Portal hypertension follows, but liver cell function is not disturbed until very late in the pathological evolution. The clinical features are:

- enlargement of liver and spleen and
- bleeding from oesophageal varices.

Patients tend to survive their bleeds much better than patients with true cirrhosis (e.g. caused by hepatitis B or alcohol) because of the well-preserved hepatocellular function. Also, because the serum albumin level is well maintained, ascites is not typical until the terminal stages of the disease. In late cases, hepatic perfusion may be so impeded that peripheral liver ischaemia occurs. Then, features of true cirrhosis may develop. When portocaval shunts are well established, the eggs of *S. mansoni* may bypass the liver in large numbers and so reach the lungs. In some cases, they may be numerous enough to cause schistosomal cor pulmonale.

Clinical features of *S. japonicum*

This resembles *S. mansoni* but, for an equal number of worms, the infection is more severe. The parasite is less well adapted to humans, the circumoval granuloma is very large, and the egg output of each female worm is greater than that in *S. mansoni*. The initial illness (Katayama fever) may be prolonged and sometimes fatal. Many Chinese workers believe that *S. japonicum* can cause carcinoma of the colon, but most other experts consider the case is unproven.

Neuroschistosomiasis

Some worm pairs wander from their usual habitats and take up residence elsewhere. The chances of this happening are increased in heavy infections. The most important site for ectopic worms is the CNS, such as in the paravertebral venous plexus or the cerebral cortical veins. All three species may occasionally be found at these sites but this is, by comparison with pathology associated with worms in their usual sites, a rare occurrence.

In the paravertebral plexus, egg laying leads to the development of a granuloma in the constricted space of the spinal canal. The clinical syndrome is spinal cord compression or a cauda equina lesion. If treated promptly, full functional recovery may occur. When it does not ischaemic injury may be the cause. In the brain, large localized granulomas produce symptoms and signs indistinguishable from a cerebral tumour.

Schistosomiasis pathology at unusual sites

Schistosomiasis cases that do not have overt antemortem pathology have been shown at postmortem to have schistosome eggs in virtually all organs but without associated inflammation. The relation of eggs found in the brain in this way to symptoms such as epilepsy and neurosis remains speculative. The factors that lead to damaging granuloma formation in some instances but not others are not well understood. Despite this conundrum, pathology associated with schistosomal eggs has been reported on rare occasions in diverse sites including skin, peritoneum and even bone.

Investigation

Direct diagnosis

This is the only approach that can lead to a definitive diagnosis. The adult worms are inaccessible, so the aim is to find living eggs. The miracidium inside the egg dies within 4 weeks.

S. haematobium

Something about bladder wall activity means that most eggs are voided around midday. Specimens collected between 10 a.m. and 2 p.m. are most likely to contain eggs. For quantitative surveys, it is very important to standardize urine collection times. Exercise has no demonstrable effect on egg output. There is no significant or reliable concentration of eggs in any part of the urinary stream. The methods for finding eggs depend on their high specific gravity (sedimentation) or their size (filtration).

Urine sedimentation

Eggs are sedimented by natural gravity (30 min in a conical glass; the sediment is then aspirated by Pasteur pipette and examined under coverslip using lens power 10×) or by artificial gravity (10 mL urine in 15 mL centrifuge tube, spun for 3 min at 1500 r. p.m. (revolutions per minute), arm radius not critical; the deposit is then examined as before).

Living eggs are translucent, and the miracidium is recognizable. Flame cells can be seen flickering. The viability of the eggs can be checked by adding them to boiled (cool) water in a flask. Emerging miracidia are visible in light shone across the neck. Normal-looking eggs usually hatch. Opaque (calcified) eggs do not, and do not themselves signify active infection (live worms).

Urine filtration

Urine is passed through a filter by vacuum or pressure. An entire 24-h urine collection can be filtered. There are several variants of this method including a miniature membrane version that allows the eggs to be detected unstained. Advantages of the method are that it is sensitive, accurate for counts and a permanent record is available. Disadvantages are cost and time.

Schistosoma mansoni and Schistosoma japonicum

Direct smear examination is not sufficiently sensitive (e.g. for an output of 100 000 eggs per day; a stool of 200 g; a smear of 2 mg; the average count is 1 egg per smear). There is a 1 in 3 chance of finding no eggs in a patient who could be harbouring about 1000 *S. mansoni* worm pairs. Instead, more sensitivity is achieved through concentration techniques such as formol-ether; thiomersal, iodine and formol (TIF) glycerol sedimentation (the simplest) or a modified Kato smear.

Biopsy techniques for all schistosomal infections

A small piece of rectal mucosa can be removed by biopsy forceps or curette under direct proctoscopic vision. It is placed on a slide under a coverslip and examined under lens power (10×). *S. haematobium* eggs are often trapped in the rectal mucosa, but may be calcified. It can be difficult to identify living eggs. Histology is not used for diagnosis as a routine. Serial sections are often needed as only

the central slices of a granuloma will contain parts of the egg.

Indirect diagnosis

As less toxic drugs have become available, the imperative of making a definitive diagnosis before therapy has been reduced. Although all the indirect means of diagnosis suffer more or less from a lack of specificity, treatment is increasingly based on this approach.

Immunodiagnostic tests for all species

There are numerous tests for detecting circulating antischistosomal antibody including CFT, IFAT, ELISA and several others. Although the better ones correlate well with the results of direct diagnostic methods, they all suffer from the following disadvantages to a greater or lesser extent:

1 They give no indication of the intensity of infection.

2 They do not distinguish between past and present infection.

3 They are not species specific.

4 Most require high technology and are often 'in-house' in academic institutions rather than commercially available for widespread use.

5 They do not reliably become positive until 3 months after infection.

Immunodiagnostic tests capable of detecting the presence of circulating antigen would be of much greater use to the clinician and epidemiologist. Unfortunately, this field has not progressed to the point where tests are available for routine clinical use in the tropics.

Approaches to diagnosis of different schistosomiasis clinical syndromes

Acute schistosomiasis

In the initial illness, the association of fever and eosinophilia with the other symptoms should raise the question of worms, as should the patient with diarrhoea and eosinophilia, although other worms such as *Strongyloides stercoralis*, *Capillaria philippinensis* and *Trichuris trichiura* can cause the same symptoms. In the differential diagnosis of these, direct diagnosis by examination of the stools is paramount.

Eosinophilia is not always prominent in acute schistosomiasis. In addition acute schistosomiasis occurs at the onset of initial egg production, so eggs are rarely found in urine or stool and the antibody detection tests are not reliably positive at this stage of infection. For these reasons, the diagnostic process includes elimination of other causes of fever such as malaria.

Schistosoma haematobium

In areas endemic for *S. haematobium*, the presence of haematuria (provided menstruating females are excluded) correlates well with the passage of schistosome eggs in the urine. With a dipstick-type test, provided it can detect both free haemoglobin and discrete red cells, the number of false-positives and false-negatives is very low. The false-positives are partly explained by glomerulonephritis and partly by the passage of dead eggs by patients whose worms are dead.

Radiological changes in the urinary tract may be very suggestive. Almost pathognomonic is the ring-like calcification of the bladder (Figure 17.4), which may also involve the ureters, prostate and seminal vesicles. Multiple, rounded filling defects produced by pseudopapillomas in the bladder are also very typical. Ultrasonography is clearly important in detecting obstructive uropathy. Otherwise, unaccountable pulmonary hypertension in an endemic area should also arouse suspicion of schistosomiasis.

Schistosoma mansoni and Schistosoma japonicum

The presence of colonic polyps in an endemic area incriminates schistosome infection as the most likely cause, as does the syndrome of portal hypertension with normal liver function tests. In recent years, ultrasonography of the liver has been used to detect the typical pipestem fibrosis and alteration to liver shape and size in order to grade liver pathology.

Neuroschistosomiasis

The most useful general clue, in cases with disease caused by ectopic worms or metastatic eggs, is the presence of eosinophilia. Unfortunately, eosinophilia is not invariably present, so immunodiagnostic tests may be particularly helpful. Diagnosis usually requires sophisticated brain imaging (Figure 17.5).

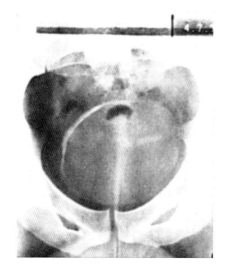

Figure 17.4 Calcified bladder in *Schistosoma haematobium* infection. Many such bladders are capable of entirely normal function, the calcification involving the eggs rather than the bladder tissues.

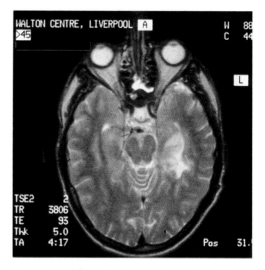

Figure 17.5 MRI scan demonstrating oedema around *S. haematobium* eggs in the left cerebral hemisphere. The clinical presentation was with motor seizures and haematuria (ova found in bladder).

Management

It is helpful to reach a definitive diagnosis with a direct test that confirms the presence of living worms before starting treatment. In practice therapy is increasingly accepted on the basis of indirect evidence such as the results of urine dipstick detection of haematuria in an endemic country or ELISA detection of antibody (where technology allows).

Drug treatment

All the available drugs (with the exception of artemisinin derivatives; discussed later) act on adult worm pairs only. After effectively eliminating the worms, the speed of resolution of the immunopathology induced by the eggs depends on how established the tissue damage has been.

Praziquantel (Biltricide)

This isoquinoline compound currently eclipses all other chemotherapy for schistosomiasis because of its ease of administration, lack of toxicity and price. It is effective against all human schistosomes. There has been some debate about the development of resistance in areas of intense transmission in West Africa, but the case for resistance remains unproven as yet. It is given in a dosage of 40 mg/kg as a single oral dose, which is sufficient for all species. Some argue that 30 mg/kg for two or three doses may be necessary for *S. mansoni* or *S. japonicum* infections. Side effects include giddiness and minor gastrointestinal disturbances. No serious toxicity has been reported, but unexplained abdominal pain and short-lived bloody diarrhoea are troublesome in heavy *S. mansoni* infections. The drug should be used with caution during pregnancy and breast-feeding.

Other drug options

Metriphonate (active against *S. haematobium* only) and oxamniquine (active against *S. mansoni* only) are occasionally still used in some countries.

Recent years have seen a rising interest in the use of the artemisinin derivatives in both treatment for and prophylaxis against schistosomiasis—particularly in China. This group of drugs appears to have effects against schistosomules as well as adult worms.

Management approaches for specific presentations

In the tropics, praziquantel is most frequently used to clear adult worms in patients presenting with symptoms caused by retained eggs in tissues or as part of mass chemotherapy (see later). The specific presentations peculiar to individuals from non-endemic areas who pick up infections during travel need to be mentioned.

Acute schistosomiasis

Praziquantel is often used in the management of this condition but the speed of its effect on symptoms is variable. On the whole, this is a self-limiting illness caused by an excess of egg antigen triggering aggressive immune responses. These will persist for a variable length of time even after the adult worms have been killed, and in severe cases, adjunctive corticosteroid therapy is occasionally advocated. It is wise to give a second dose of praziquantel 3 months after the first in order to clear worms that were only maturing during the initial illness.

Asymptomatic infection

Travellers who have one-off significant freshwater exposure (e.g. during water recreational activity such as snorkelling, windsurfing or scuba-diving) are often screened for schistosomal antibody even when they have no symptoms. It is common therefore for praziquantel treatment to be offered on the basis of a positive antibody test alone. On the whole this is a reasonable approach, but its overall effectiveness and cost-effectiveness in preventing later pathology has not been assessed and there are some pitfalls.

1 Screening before an adequate time (3 months) has elapsed since exposure.

2 Assuming that antibody tests can be used to monitor cure and that titres will fall to negative after treatment.

Neuroschistosomiasis

Praziquantel is used to kill the adult worms, but the offending circumoval granulomas in the nervous tissue will take a while to resolve and there is usually concern that the immunopathology will worsen on treatment. Adjunctive corticosteroid therapy is therefore the norm. In the case of cerebral involvement with epilepsy, it may take many months before anticonvulsant therapy can be withdrawn.

Monitoring treatment

It can be assumed that most light infections will be cured with a single praziquantel dose. However, when a direct diagnosis detecting viable eggs has been made, it is wise to check that egg production has ceased (in the absence of reinfection) at a 3-month follow-up.

Prevention and public health aspects

The schistosomiasis life cycle can be interrupted at various sites. Although some sites have proved more vulnerable than others, combined approaches, where possible, have most impact but are rarely implemented in a sustained fashion.
1 Contamination of water.
2 Intermediate host.
3 Human contact with infection.

Reducing contamination of water

The main methods used are:
1 Health education;
2 Provision of sanitation;
3 Prevention of access to transmission sites; and
4 Reduction of egg excretion by the definitive hosts (humans) by drug treatment.
Of all these measures, the one most immediately successful in most circumstances is mass chemotherapy (see later).

Attack on snails

Permanent results are possible if the habitats can be eliminated. It has been achieved in Japan and many parts of China by drainage and landfill. Temporary results are obtained with the application of poisonous chemicals (molluscicides such as niclosamide) to snail habitats. If used alone, this method is usually disappointing. The number of infected snails may not be reduced in proportion to the total snail reduction. Disadvantages include cost, the need to reapply chemicals for an indefinite period and undesirable effects such as killing fish. It is most effective in highly controlled environments, such as irrigated agricultural estates, and when used in combination with chemotherapy.

Reducing contact with infection

The necessity for contact can be reduced by the provision of a safe water supply for washing and drinking through chlorination or filtration which will clear water of cercariae. This will not prevent recreational or occupational contact. Attempts to fence off transmission sites are usually unsuccessful. Health education is important.

Mass chemotherapy

Mass chemotherapy of schistosomiasis is now receiving most support as the effective, modern approach to schistosomiasis control. It is recommended as part of a combined effort to implement the co-ordinated use of anthelmintic drugs in control interventions along with mass chemotherapy for lymphatic filariasis, onchocerciasis and soil-transmitted helminths. Dosages are dispensed according to gradations on ingenious height-poles which bypass the need for functional weight scales in small, peripheral treatment centres. The recommended treatment strategy is outlined in Table 17.1. As practical field experience is accumulating with this approach, consensus is developing around the following potential indicators for monitoring impact:
• presence of infection (by parasitological methods);

Table 17.1 Recommended treatment strategy for schistosomiasis mass chemotherapy

Category	Prevalence among school-aged children		Action to be taken
High risk community	• 50% by parasitological methods Or • 30% by questionnaire for visible haematuria	Treat all school-age children once a year	Also treat adults considered to be at risk (from special groups to entire communities living in endemic areas—e.g. fishermen and irrigation workers)
Moderate risk community	• 10% but <50% by parasitological methods Or <30% by questionnaire for visible haematuria	Treat all school-age children once every 2 years	Also treat adults considered to be at risk (special risk groups only—e.g. fishermen and irrigation workers)
Low risk community	<10% by parasitological methods	Treat all school-age children twice during their primary schooling	Praziquantel should be available in dispensaries and clinics for treatment of suspected cases

• intensity of infection (proportion of heavy-intensity infection);
• prevalence of macrohaematuria;
• prevalence of microhaematuria;
• prevalence of anaemia;
• prevalence of ultrasound-detectable lesions (urinary tract and liver).

Future developments

New diagnostics

As with all important tropical infections, there is clearly a need for a new diagnostic tool that is as robust and specific as direct microscopy for eggs, less dependent on laboratory skill and infrastructure, and more sensitive. However, as mass chemotherapy can be conducted without definitive diagnosis, the pressure to develop this tool has diminished and there are no obvious candidates for widespread use in developing countries.

New interventions

No new drugs look set to replace the current gold standard of single dose praziquantel.

Further reading

Carod-Artal FJ. Neurological complications of schistosoma infection. *Trans R Soc Trop Med Hyg* 2008; 102: 107–16. [Comprehensive review.]

Gryseels B, Polman K, Celrinx J, Kestens L. Human schistosomiasis. *Lancet* 2006; 368: 1106–1118. [Useful comprehensive review.]

Lloyd-Smith JO, Poss M, Grenfell BT. HIV-1/parasite coinfection and the emergence of new parasite strains. *Parasitology* 2008; 135: 795–806. [Review of interaction of HIV with several major tropical parasites including schistosomiasis.]

WHO website. http://www.who.int/schistosomiasis/en/index.html. [Includes useful background and country-specific information, including the downloadable manual for health professionals and programme managers 'Preventive chemotherapy in human helminthiasis, co-ordinated use of anthelminthic drugs in control interventions' ISBN 92 4 154710 3 (NLM classification: WC 800) ISBN 978 92 4 154710 9 World Health Organization, Geneva, 2006.]

Chapter 18

Leprosy

Leprosy is a chronic granulomatous disease caused by *Mycobacterium leprae*. The principal manifestations of disease are anaesthetic skin lesions and peripheral neuropathy with peripheral nerve thickening. The clinical form of the disease in any individual depends on the degree of cell-mediated immunity (CMI) expressed by that individual towards *M. leprae*. High levels of CMI with elimination of leprosy bacilli produce the tuberculoid form of disease, whereas absence of CMI results in lepromatous leprosy (LL). The medical complications of leprosy result from nerve damage, immunological reactions and bacillary infiltration. Nerve damage accompanying leprosy is a particularly serious complication because this will remain with the patient for the rest of his or her life and causes considerable morbidity. Currently available drug treatments are highly effective in clearing viable bacilli but do not prevent nerve damage. Leprosy has a long history as a deforming disease and leprosy patients all over the world are frequently stigmatized and ostracized. Words such as 'leper' should be avoided and using the term Hansen's disease may reduce stigmatization.

Leprosy must be considered in the differential diagnosis for any patient who has lived in the tropics and presents with chronic or bizarre acute skin lesions, peripheral neuropathy or apparent vasculitis.

Epidemiology

The infection is spread from human to human by droplets. There is a long clinical incubation period of 2–5 years for tuberculoid disease and 8–11 years for lepromatous disease. About 250 000 new cases per year are detected worldwide. The geographical distribution is patchy, with 62% of cases being detected in India, and Brazil, Congo, Mozambique and Nepal having the highest case rates. Age, sex and household contact are important determinants of disease. In the major leprosy endemic areas, the childhood case rate remains high, indicating ongoing transmission. HIV infection is not a risk factor for disease acquisition, and HIV-positive patients can develop all types of leprosy. Paradoxically HIV-positive patients with leprosy are a higher risk of developing Type 1 reactions and patients on ART may present with *de novo* leprosy as an IRIS.

Microbiology

M. leprae is an obligatory intracellular parasite which cannot be cultivated *in vitro*; although it can be grown in the armadillo and in footpads of nude mice. *M. leprae* has a doubling time of 12 days and is a remarkably hardy organism, remaining viable

Lecture Notes: Tropical Medicine, 6th edition.
By G.V. Gill and N.J. Beeching. Published 2009 by
Blackwell Publishing, ISBN: 978-1-4051-8048-1.

in the environment for up to 2 months. It has a highly resistant cell wall composed of lipids, carbohydrates and proteins. Phenolic glycolipid *M. leprae* is species specific. Numerous protein antigens have been identified as important immune targets using antibody and T cell screening. The *M. leprae* genome was completely sequenced in 2001. The organism has lost many genes and survives on only a few biochemical pathways. Only 40 genes are unique to *M. leprae*, and analysis of these genes will inform us about the unique biology of this organism.

Immune response in leprosy

The host immune response to *M. leprae* is crucial in determining either disease or immunity and the type of disease. The T cells and macrophages of the cell-mediated immune system have an important role in processing, recognition and response to *M. leprae* antigens. Antibodies to *M. leprae* antigens are produced but these do not appear to have any useful role in protection. Several stages in the immune response are recognized:

• phagocytosis of *M. leprae* by macrophages

• presentation of *M. leprae* antigens in association with human leucocyte antigen (HLA) class II molecules

• binding of antigen-specific T cells via the a/b T cell receptor

• activation of T cells and production of interleukin 2 (IL-2) and T cell proliferation

• IL-2 activates CD4, CD8, natural killer (NK) cells and macrophages, and

• interferon-γ (IFN-γ) is produced and activates bactericidal mechanisms within the macrophage.

Granuloma formation results from mycobacterial persistence with continued cytokine release. The leprosy granuloma has a core of macrophages, epithelioid cells and giant cells, with lymphocytes surrounding the core, and is dependent on tumour necrosis factor α (TNF-α) from activated macrophages and T cells.

The immunological and clinical effects vary across a spectrum between two 'poles' of presentations (Figure 18.1). In tuberculoid disease (TT), CMI is active and contains infection, so that few bacilli are found in tissues and CD4 cells and their cytokines (IL-2, IFN-γ) predominate (Th1 response). At the other pole of LL, the CMI

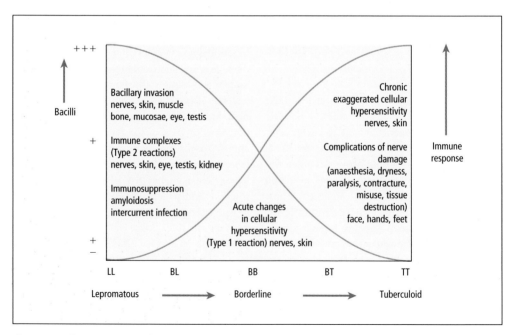

Figure 18.1 The immunological features of the different types of leprosy.

response is poor, there are many bacilli in the tissues and responses include both CD4 and CD8 cells. CD4 cells produce IL-4, IL-5, IL-6 and IL-10 (Th2 response); immunoglobulin G (IgG), IgM and IgA levels are also elevated. The unresponsiveness in LL disease is because of specific T cell anergy. It may be caused by T cell non-activation, suppression or clonal deletion and also involves defective macrophage function. Borderline states (borderline tuberculoid [BT]; borderline leprosy [BB]; borderline lepromatous leprosy [BL]) are intermediate between these poles.

There is no current immunological test that can determine whether a person has protective immunity against *M. leprae*.

Clinical features

The cardinal signs of leprosy are skin lesions, anaesthesia and thickened peripheral nerves.

Skin lesions

The most common skin lesions are macules or plaques; more rarely, papules and nodules are seen (Figures 18.2–18.5). In LL diffuse infiltration of the skin often occurs. Lesions may be found anywhere although rarely in the axillae, perineum or hairy scalp. The number of lesions indicates the ability of the CMI to limit the spread of bacilli. Tuberculoid patients have few hypopigmented lesions, while lepromatous patients have numerous sometimes confluent lesions. The few tuberculoid lesions are usually asymmetrical; more numerous lesions are likely to be distributed symmetrically.

Nerve damage

Only the peripheral nervous system is affected. Damage to peripheral nerve trunks is common and leads to motor weakness in the muscles supplied and to regional sensory loss (Figures 18.6 and 18.7). Sensory and autonomic fibres in skin lesions are also affected. The principal sites of peripheral nerve involvement are ulnar (elbow),

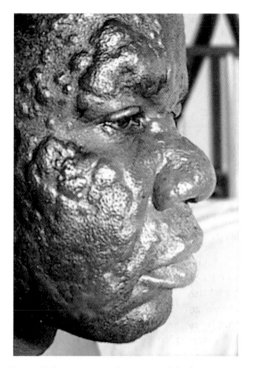

Figure 18.2 Lepromatous leprosy—nodular form.

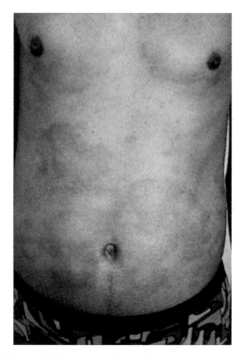

Figure 18.3 Skin lesions of borderline lepromatous leprosy.

173

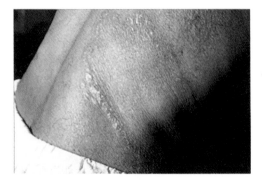

Figure 18.4 A patient from India with tuberculoid leprosy. The single lesion is anaesthetic, scaly, dry and has a raised edge.

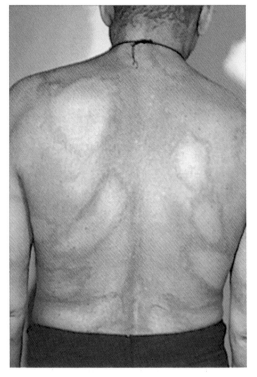

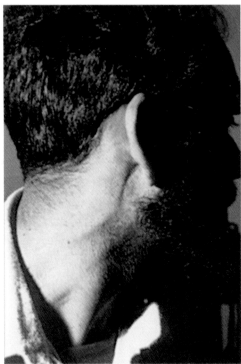

Figure 18.6 Visibly thickened posterior auricular nerve. The patient had a 'tuberculoid'-type lesion on the palm of his right hand and an associated thickening of the dorsal branch of the radial nerve.

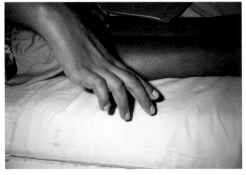

Figure 18.5 Borderline tuberculoid leprosy with numerous anaesthetic skin lesions.

Figure 18.7 An ulnar nerve lesion in a patient from South Africa with LL.

median (wrist), radial cutaneous (wrist), common peroneal (knee), posterior tibial and sural nerves (ankle) and the facial nerve (zygomatic arch). All these nerves should be examined for enlargement and tenderness. Nerve function impairment occurs before, during and after treatment. In field cohort studies, 16–56% of newly diagnosed patients had functional nerve impairment.

Table 18.1 Main clinical characteristics of polar leprosy

	Tuberculoid	Lepromatous
Skin and nerves		
Number and distribution	One or a few sites, asymmetrical	Widely disseminated
Skin lesions		
Definition		
Clarity of margin	Good	Poor
Elevation of margin	Common	Never
Colour		
Dark skin	Marked hypopigmentation	Slight hypopigmentation
Light skin	Coppery or red	Slight erythema
Surface	Dry, scaly	Smooth, shiny
Central healing	Common	None
Sweat and hair growth	Impaired early	Impaired late
Loss of sensation	Early and marked	Late
Nerve enlargement and damage	Early and marked	Late
Bacilli (bacterial index)	Absent (0)	Many (5 or 6+)
Natural outcome	Healing	Progression

Leprosy classification

Classification of the stage of disease helps to predict the future likelihood and types of reaction that a patient may experience and also guides the content and duration of specific chemotherapy. Polar forms of disease are stable but borderline disease is unstable. BT/BL disease is associated with severe large nerve damage caused by Type 1 'reversal' reactions and neuritic reactions, and LL/BL patients suffer with erythema nodosum leprosum (ENL) (Type 2) reactions. Multibacillary disease requires longer treatment with more drugs to prevent relapse or the development of drug resistance.

The Ridley–Jopling classification uses clinical and microbiological features of the patient, which mirror the immunological state (Table 18.1).
- Skin lesions
  Number
  Distribution and symmetry
  Definition and clarity
  Anaesthesia
  Loss of sweating and hair growth
- Peripheral nerve involvement
- Mucosal and systemic involvement
- Bacillary load

A simpler WHO field classification merely divides patients into those with few lesions (paucibacillary) or those with more (multibacillary) if skin smears are not available (see Management section, p. 178).

Tuberculoid leprosy

Infection is localized and asymmetrical. The skin lesions are few, hypopigmented and have sharp borders. Anaesthesia is usually present in the lesion and is often accompanied by loss of sweating, indicating local autonomic nerve damage. The cutaneous nerve on the proximal side of the lesion is frequently thickened. If peripheral nerve trunk involvement is present, usually only one nerve trunk is enlarged. No *M. leprae* are found in the skin. True tuberculoid leprosy has a good prognosis; many infections resolve without treatment and peripheral nerve trunk damage is limited.

Borderline tuberculoid

The skin lesions are similar to TT leprosy but are larger and more numerous. The margins are less well-defined and there may be satellite lesions. Damage to peripheral nerves is widespread and severe, usually with several thickened nerve trunks. BT patients are at risk of severe reversal (Type 1) reactions with rapid deterioration in nerve function with consequent deformities.

Borderline leprosy

BB disease is the most unstable part of the spectrum and patients usually downgrade towards LL if they are not treated or upgrade towards tuberculoid leprosy as part of a reversal reaction. There are numerous skin lesions, which may be macules, papules or plaques and vary in size, shape and distribution. The edges of the lesions may have streaming irregular borders. Annular lesions with a broad irregular edge and a sharply defined punched-out centre are characteristic of BB disease. Nerve damage is common with involvement of several peripheral nerve trunks.

Borderline lepromatous leprosy

Borderline lepromatous leprosy is characterized by widespread, small but variable macules all over the body. With disease progression, the macules become infiltrated. Peripheral nerve involvement is widespread and often severe. Patients with BL leprosy are at risk of both reversal and ENL (Type 2) reactions.

Lepromatous leprosy

The patient with untreated polar LL may be carrying 10^{11} leprosy bacilli and the characteristic signs of LL are caused by the widespread dissemination of organisms throughout the body. The onset of disease is frequently insidious, the earliest lesions being ill-defined, widely distributed hypopigmented macules. Gradually, the skin becomes infiltrated and thickened and nodules develop. Thickening of facial skin gives rise to the characteristic leonine facies. Hair is lost, especially the lateral third of the eyebrows (madarosis) (Figure 18.8). Dermal nerves are destroyed and there is sensory loss (light touch, pain and temperature) which begins at the hands and feet. Sweating is lost and this can cause profound discomfort in a tropical climate as compensatory

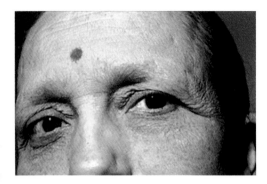

Figure 18.8 Lateral eyebrow loss or 'madarosis' in a patient with LL.

sweating occurs in the remaining intact areas. Damage to peripheral nerves is symmetrical and occurs late in disease.

Nasal symptoms (stuffy nose, nose bleeds, loss of sense of smell) can often be elicited early in the disease, and 80% of newly diagnosed lepromatous cases have invasion of the nasal mucosa. Bone involvement is common, with osteoporosis and fractures. Testicular atrophy results from diffuse infiltration and the acute orchitis that occurs with ENL reactions. The consequent loss of testosterone leads to azoospermia and gynaecomastia.

Other forms of leprosy

These include pure neuritic, histoid and Lucio's leprosy, and will not be considered further here.

The eye in leprosy

Blinding complications include lagophthalmos, decreased corneal sensation, acute iritis, chronic iritis and cataract. Patients at risk include those with BL and/or LL disease, those with facial patches, patients experiencing reactions and those with disease of long duration (Table 18.2).

Diagnosis

The diagnosis of leprosy is essentially a clinical one made on finding one or more of the cardinal signs of leprosy (typical skin lesions and peripheral nerve thickening) and supported by finding

Table 18.2 Key features of eye disease in leprosy

Conjunctivitis
Infectious/allergic aetiology
Redness throughout and inside eyelids
Treat with tetracycline ointment

Acute iritis
Conjunctiva reddest next to cornea
Eye painful
Sensitive to light
Poor pupil reactivity

Corneal ulcer
Roughness
Discharge and redness
Treat with tetracycline ointment

Chronic iritis
Pupil constricted and irregular
Sluggish reaction
Treat with atropine eye drops

acid-fast bacilli on slit skin smears. The whole body should be inspected in a good light otherwise lesions may be missed, particularly on the buttocks. Skin lesions should be tested for anaesthesia to light touch, pinprick and temperature. The peripheral nerves should be palpated systematically, examining for thickening and tenderness. Wherever possible the diagnosis should be supported by a skin biopsy, which is essential for accurate classification. The presence of neural inflammation in the skin biopsy will help to distinguish leprosy from other granulomatous conditions. Serology is not usually helpful diagnostically because antibodies to the species-specific glycolipid PGL-1 are present in 90% of untreated lepromatous patients but only 40–50% of paucibacillary patients and 5–10% of healthy controls. PCR for detecting *M. leprae* DNA is not used as a routine diagnostic test.

Slit skin smears

The bacterial load is assessed by making a small incision through the epidermis, scraping dermal material and smearing it evenly onto a glass slide. At least six sites should be sampled (earlobes, eyebrows, edges of active lesions). The smears are then stained and acid-fast bacilli are counted. Scoring is performed on a logarithmic scale per high-power field (the bacterial index [BI]). A score of 1+ indicates 1–10 bacilli in 100 fields and 6+ indicates >1000 per field. Smears are useful for confirming the diagnosis and should be carried out annually to monitor response to treatment.

Differential diagnosis

A wide variety of dermatological conditions might be considered in the differential diagnosis of manifestations of leprosy, which include erythematous macules, hypopigmented macules, papules and nodules. Neurological problems include both mononeuropathies and polyneuropathies. Diabetes is a common cause of peripheral neuropathy and may coexist with leprosy but does not cause nerve thickening.

Management

Educating a leprosy patient about their disease is the key to successful management. Key issues to be discussed include the low infectivity, the importance of treatment adherence and/or compliance, warnings about reactions, the care of anaesthetic hands and feet and support with social issues.

Chemotherapy

The effectiveness of dapsone against *M. leprae* was discovered in the late 1940s and it was used widely as a single agent. This led to the widespread development of dapsone resistance and in 1982 the WHO proposed a multidrug regimen for the treatment of leprosy. The first-line antileprotic drugs are rifampicin, dapsone and clofazimine.

Rifampicin

Rifampicin is a potent bactericidal for *M. leprae*. Four days after a single 600 mg dose, bacilli from a previously untreated lepromatous patient are no longer viable. It acts by inhibiting DNA-dependent RNA polymerase, thereby interfering with bacterial RNA synthesis. Rifampicin is well absorbed orally. Hepatotoxicity is rarely a problem.

Because *M. leprae* resistance to rifampicin can develop as a one-step process, rifampicin should always be given in combination with other anti-leprotic drugs.

Dapsone

Dapsone (DDS; 4,4-diaminodiphenylsulphone) acts by blocking folic acid synthesis. It is only weakly bactericidal. Oral absorption is good and it has a long half-life, averaging 28 h. Haemolytic anaemia is the most common side effect of dapsone treatment and patients with G6PD deficiency are particularly at risk. The 'DDS syndrome', which is occasionally seen in leprosy, starts 6 weeks after commencing DDS and manifests as exfoliative dermatitis associated with lymphadenopathy, hepatosplenomegaly, fever and hepatitis. Agranulocytosis, hepatitis and cholestatic jaundice occur rarely with DDS therapy.

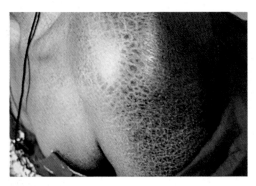

Figure 18.9 Icthyotic skin changes in a patient on clofazimine treatment.

Clofazimine

Clofazimine is a dye that has a weakly bactericidal action. It also has an anti-inflammatory effect and helps prevent ENL. The major side effect is skin discoloration, ranging from red to purple-black, the degree of discoloration depending on the dose and the amount of leprous infiltration. The pigmentation usually clears up within 6–12 months of stopping clofazimine, although traces of discoloration may remain for up to 4 years. Clofazimine also produces a characteristic icthyosis on the shins and forearms (Figure 18.9). Gastrointestinal side effects, ranging from mild cramps to diarrhoea and weight loss, may occur as a result of clofazimine crystal deposition in the wall of the small bowel.

Multidrug therapy

This has been used to treat over 14 million people since 1982. Relapse rates are low, ranging from 0% in China and Ethiopia to 2.04 per 100 person-years in India. Patients with high initial bacterial loads are at greater risk of relapse (8 per 100 person-years). So far there has been no reported drug resistance. Toxicity is limited, response is rapid and the duration of therapy is greatly shortened compared to historical treatment regimens. Multidrug therapy (MDT) is provided free of cost to all patients through the WHO and funded by Novartis. The recommended regimens are summarized in Table 18.3 and include both monthly directly observed therapy and daily

Table 18.3 Modified multidrug therapy regimens recommended by WHO

Type of leprosy	Drug treatment		Duration of treatment
	Monthly supervised and	Daily self-administered	
Paucibacillary (PB)	Rifampicin 600 mg	Dapsone 100 mg	6 months
Multibacillary (MB)	Rifampicin 600 mg	Clofazimine 50 mg	24 months
	Clofazimine 300 mg	Dapsone 100 mg	

Children
PB: Rifampicin 450 mg monthly and dapsone 50 mg daily.
MB: Rifampicin 450 mg and clofazimine 150 mg monthly, clofazimine 50 mg alternate days and dapsone 50 mg daily.

Table 18.4 WHO classification for field use when slit skin smears are not available

Paucibacillary	Up to 5 skin lesions
Multibacillary	≥6 skin lesions

self-administered therapy. The WHO now recommends treatment of multibacillary (Table 18.4) patients for 12 months only, although there were no controlled trial data to guide this decision. Ofloxacin 400 mg and minocycline 100 mg are useful second-line drugs that can be used to replace components of WHO-MDT if patients experience adverse effects or drug interactions.

Reactions and nerve damage

These include Type 1 (reversal) reactions, Type 2 (ENL) reactions and acute neuritis.

Type 1 (reversal) reactions

These are caused by delayed hypersensitivity towards *M. leprae* antigens in skin and nerve (Figure 18.10). Those at risk include all borderline (BT, BB and BL) patients and women in the post-partum. The peak time for reactions is during the first 2 months of treatment. Type 1 reactions occur in 30% of BL patients. Clinical manifestations include erythema, swelling and tenderness of skin lesions, and pain and tenderness of peripheral nerves with loss of sensory and motor function. Rapid severe nerve damage may occur with Type 1 reactions, so patients must be warned about symptoms and advised to return for treatment if they develop new weakness or numbness. Nearly all reactions, and especially those with nerve inflammation, must be treated with 40 mg/day prednisolone, reducing by 5 mg/day every month. Physiotherapy will be needed for affected hand, foot and eye muscles.

Erythema nodosum leprosum reaction

This is also known as a Type 2 reaction (Figure 18.11) and is caused by immune complex deposition, T cell dysregulation and overproduction of TNF. It affects up to 50% of LL and 10% of

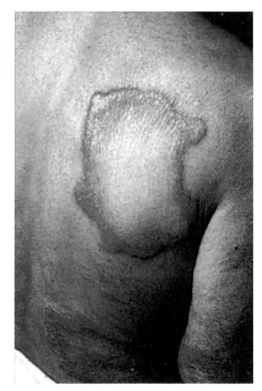

Figure 18.10 A reversal reaction in leprosy. The previously flat lesions suddenly become hot, painful and raised.

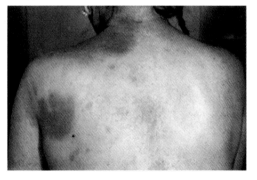

Figure 18.11 Erythema nodosum leprosum in an Asian patient who presented with fever, leucocytosis and painful red skin swellings.

BL patients. There is systemic illness with malaise, fever and raised white cell count and erythrocyte sedimentation rate. Manifestations include widespread erythema nodosum, neuritis, iritis, arthritis, orchitis, lymphadenopathy and renal disease. ENL usually starts in the first year of chemotherapy and may relapse intermittently over several years. It is often difficult to treat. Most episodes of ENL require treatment with high-dose prednisolone (60–80 mg/day) or thalidomide. Thalidomide is very effective in relieving the symptoms and signs of ENL, gives better long-term control of the reaction and avoids the adverse effects of long-term steroid treatment. Increasing the dosage of clofazimine up to 300 mg daily for 3 months may also reduce inflammatory responses. Iritis should be treated with 1% atropine and 1% steroid eye drops. Antileprosy drugs should be continued, and the patient should be reassured that the reaction will settle.

Neuritis

Neuritis refers to acute and chronic nerve inflammation that may occur without evidence of either a Type 1 or Type 2 reaction. Nerve damage may also occur as silent neuropathy which is defined as 'the development of functional deficit of a major nerve without a manifest neuritis'. Nerve function should be checked carefully during treatment so that silent neuropathy can be detected. Treatment is with 40 mg/day prednisolone as for reversal reactions, reducing slowly over a period of months. Over 60% of patients who present with nerve damage at diagnosis are at risk of developing further nerve damage during and after treatment especially during the first 12 months of treatment.

Prevention of disability

Nerve damage produces anaesthesia, dryness and muscle weakness. These three factors lead to misuse of the affected limb with resultant ulceration, infection and, ultimately, severe deformity (Figure 18.12). Keys to prevention include regular monitoring of nerve function and recording of problems secondary to nerve dysfunction. Patients who need self-care should be identified and their understanding and implementation of this should be monitored (Table 18.5). All

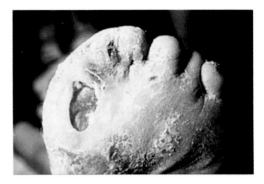

Figure 18.12 Perforating neuropathic plantar foot ulcer in a patient with LL and extensive lower limb denervation.

Table 18.5 General care of hands and feet

Self-care training
Inspect for injury
Understand why injuries happen
Soak feet and oil
Remove callus
Exercise hands and feet
Treat injuries promptly
Hands
Problems with heat/pressure/sharp objects
Feet
Plantar ulcers occur at pressure sites
Either walk less or use protective shoe insoles
Footwear
Check shoe fittings
Provide insoles
Arch supports, metatarsal pads
Orthopaedic footwear
Management of plantar ulcers
Clean wound
Bed rest, walking plaster
Check footwear
Find out why it happened

patients need general training and social support; some may need surgical referral.

Reconstructive surgery

Reconstructive surgery has a role in both improving function and appearance. Lagophthalmos can be ameliorated by tarsorrhaphy or temporalis muscle transfer. Appropriate tendon transfers can reduce the effects of ulnar and median nerve paralysis and improve drop foot and claw toes. Cosmetic surgery—in particular eyebrow replacement, nasal reconstruction and reduction of gynaecomastia—is important in the rehabilitation of severely deformed patients.

Women and leprosy

Women with leprosy are in double jeopardy. Not only may they develop postpartum nerve damage, but they are at particular risk of social ostracism with rejection by spouses and family. There is little good evidence that pregnancy causes new disease or relapse. However, there is a clear temporal association between parturition and the development of Type 1 reactions and neuritis when CMI returns to prepregnancy levels. ENL in pregnancy is associated with early loss of nerve function compared with non-pregnant individuals. Rifampicin, dapsone and clofazimine are safe during pregnancy, but ideally pregnancies should be planned for when leprosy is well controlled. Women may breast-feed while on multidrug therapy but should be warned that low levels of clofazimine are excreted in the breast milk and may cause some skin discoloration in the infant.

Leprosy in childhood

All types of leprosy are seen in childhood, usually after the age of 5 years. Children are at the same risk as adults of developing nerve damage and reactions, and often present with established nerve damage. Reactions should be treated with prednisolone 0.5 mg/kg/day. The WHO has produced separate multidrug therapy paucibacillary (PB) and multibacillary (MB) blister packs for treating children.

Control and prevention

Vaccines

The substantial cross-reactivity between BCG and *M. leprae* has been exploited in attempts to develop a vaccine against leprosy. Trials of BCG as a vaccine against leprosy showed it to confer variable protection, ranging from 80% in Uganda to 20% in Burma. A case-control study in Venezuela showed BCG vaccination to give 56% protection to the household contacts of leprosy patients. Combining BCG and killed *M. leprae* has been tried, but in both a large population-based trial in Malawi and an immunoprophylactic trial in Venezuela there was no advantage for BCG plus *M. leprae* over BCG alone.

Leprosy provision in general health services

For much of the twentieth century, leprosy patients were detected and treated within vertical programmes dedicated to leprosy. Although these were effective, they also became inefficient as the numbers of leprosy patients declined. The management of leprosy patients is now being integrated into a range of health services including combined leprosy and tuberculosis programmes, dermatology programmes and full integration with general health services. The current WHO strategy emphasizes the importance of quality services that are accessible, patient-centred, provide free treatment with MDT, do appropriate prevention of disability and refer patients on for the management of complications. There are now huge training needs to train people to recognize leprosy. The development of referral services is also a critical need if an integrated approach is to work well.

Further reading

Britton WJ, Lockwood DNJ. Leprosy. *Lancet* 2004; 363: 1209–1219. [Up-to-date overview of leprosy.]

Kahawita IP, Walker SL, Lockwood DNJ. Leprosy type 1 reactions and erythema nodosum leprosum. *An Bras Dermatol* 2008; 83: 75–82. [Good overview of leprosy reactions and their management. Free download.]

LEPRA, Fairfax House, Causton Road, Colchester CO1 1PU, UK. [International leprosy charity, can provide posters, pamphlets, etc.]

Lockwood DNJ, Suneetha S. Leprosy: too complex a disease for a simple elimination paradigm. *Bull World Health Organ* 2005; 83: 230–235.

Report of the International Leprosy Association Technical Forum. Evidence-based assessment of leprosy management issues. *Lepr Rev* 2002; 73 (Suppl). [Covers everything from epidemiology through diagnosis and treatment to prevention of disability.]

Srinivasan H. *Prevention of Disabilities in Patients with Leprosy: A Practical Guide*. Geneva: World Health Organization, 1993.

World Health Organization. Global Strategy for further reducing the leprosy burden and sustaining leprosy control activities 2006–2010.

www.ilep.org.uk. ILEP (International Federation of anti-leprosy associations). Website with teaching materials and links.

www.lepra.org.uk. *Leprosy Review*. [The premier leprosy journal, free internet access.]

Part 3

Other Tropical Diseases

Chapter 19

Amoebiasis

Introduction and epidemiology

Entamoeba histolytica is an intestinal protozoan parasite with the ability to invade and cause lysis of cells. *E. histolytica* occurs worldwide, particularly in situations of poor hygiene and sanitation. Thus, infections are commonly found among people living in developing countries and immigrants or travellers from such countries. In addition, people with learning difficulties in residential institutions, men who have sex with men and people who are immunosuppressed are also at increased risk.

The most common clinical presentation is dysentery. Extra-intestinal infections also occur, notably amoebic liver abscess (ALA). It has been shown experimentally that the majority of infections are asymptomatic, and only about 20% of people who swallow cysts develop symptoms of dysentery. It is estimated that there are 40–50 million cases of symptomatic amoebiasis per year, resulting in 40 000–110 000 deaths.

In the past, the prevalence of infection in developing countries has been estimated to exceed 90% in some communities. This is probably an overestimate as cysts of *E. histolytica* are microscopically identical to cysts of the non-pathogenic *Entamoeba dispar*. *E. dispar* is about three times

as common as *E. histolytica* in developing countries and about 10 times as common in industrialized countries. Other non-pathogenic protozoa found in the human intestine include *E. moshkovskii* (which also produces cysts identical to those of *E. histolytica/E. dispar*), *E. coli*, *E. hartmanni* and *Endolimax nana*.

Other amoebae sometimes associated with disease in humans include *E. gingivalis* (periodontal disease), *E. polecki* and *Dientamoeba fragilis* (diarrhoea), *Acanthamoeba* species and *Balamuthia mandrillaris* (acanthamoebic keratitis/granulomatous amoebic encephalitis) and *Naegleria fowleri* (primary amoebic meningoencephalitis).

Parasite and life cycle

E. histolytica is principally an infection of humans, although some monkeys also harbour the parasite. The four-nucleated cyst is ingested in food or water contaminated by human faeces. The cyst is digested in the gut releasing eight amoebic trophozoites. These live in the colon, normally on the surface of the mucosa, feeding on bacteria and other food residues. The amoebic trophozoite is variable in size, highly motile by means of its pseudopodia and characteristic flowing motion and, when invasive, usually contains ingested red cells.

The amoebae multiply in the gut by simple binary fission. As they move around the colon from right to left, the colonic contents become

Lecture Notes: Tropical Medicine, 6th edition.
By G.V. Gill and N.J. Beeching. Published 2009 by
Blackwell Publishing, ISBN: 978-1-4051-8048-1.

more solid and the actively motile amoebae stop feeding, empty their food vacuoles, become rounded and secrete a cyst wall.

The cysts are spherical, measuring 10–15 μm, and when mature contain four nuclei, and sometimes a glycogen mass and a refractile chromidial bar. Amoebic cysts are passed in the formed stool of people with, usually asymptomatic, amoebiasis. The cysts can survive for prolonged periods in normal environmental conditions, for example, for more than 12 days in cool faeces and for several weeks in water. They are killed by drying at temperatures above 50°C, freezing below −5°C and standard treatment of water supplies.

Under normal circumstances, amoebic trophozoites are said to be non-infective; however, an epidemic of amoebic dysentery was caused by the introduction of trophozoites via an incorrectly functioning enema machine used by chiropractors in the United States and resulted in several deaths. Person–person transfer and inoculation of trophozoites into skin abrasions or mucous membranes can also occur resulting in cutaneous amoebiasis.

Pathogenesis

E. histolytica binds to host intestinal cells by means of a galactose-binding lectin on its surface. Following attachment, the amoeba uses pore-forming molecules called amoebapores and, possibly, phospholipidases, to disrupt the target cell, triggering a process of apoptosis or 'cell suicide'. The amoeba then phagocytoses the dead cell and in due course, the process leads to the development of mucosal ulcers with undermined edges commonly described as 'flask-shaped' ulcers. However, this 'bind–lyse–eat' model for invasive amoebiasis may be oversimplistic. Invasion also appears to depend on cytoskeleton motility, the secretion of proteases that degrade the extracellular matrix and antibody. The host inflammatory response, including the production of cytokines and inflammatory mediators, accompanied by an influx of neutrophils, is also important in the pathogenesis of invasive amoebiasis.

Clinical studies show some of evidence of mucosal immunity to recurrent infections;

however, protective immunity does not appear to follow an amoebic liver abscess. Acquired immunity to recurrent infection with *E. histolytica* has been shown to be linked to a mucosal immune response against a major virulence factor of the parasite, a Gal/GalNAc lectin responsible for adherence and killing of the host tissue. Small peptides derived from the galactose-binding adhesin administered by the parenteral or oral route have been shown to protect gerbils against experimental amoebic liver abscess. Therefore, the prospects for a vaccine are brightening.

Clinical features

The incubation period may range from a few days to many years. Amoebiasis is one of the several 'tropical' diseases that can have a prolonged latent period and may be present more than a decade following exposure.

Intestinal amoebiasis

The clinical spectrum ranges from asymptomatic infections (the majority) to fulminant amoebic colitis. The onset of invasive disease may be precipitated by another gastrointestinal infection or other illness, debility or immunosuppression. Symptoms are usually insidious with abdominal discomfort and loose stools sometimes containing mucus and blood. Patients with mild disease are relatively well with a history of a few loose stools. Investigations may reveal scanty trophozoites in faeces and a few ulcers on endoscopy. Patients with more extensive disease usually remain afebrile and ambulant despite producing 5–15 bloody stools per day containing numerous trophozoites. They are likely to have obvious rectal ulceration on endoscopy. Debilitated or immunosuppressed patients are more likely to present with rapid onset of abdominal pain, vomiting, dysuria, tenesmus and frequent bloody stools. They are likely to be febrile, dehydrated, toxic and anaemic. Abdominal tenderness may be marked and there may be evidence of peritonitis. Endoscopy is contraindicated. The most extreme presentation is that of extensive fulminating necrotizing colitis, which occurs in a minority of, usually immuno-compromised, patients and is often fatal.

Complications of intestinal amoebiasis include the following:
- *Peritonitis*—abrupt/insidious onset; may occur after the patient has commenced treatment.
- *Haemorrhage*—resulting in anaemia or shock.
- *Stricture*—especially of the colon and rectum.
- *Post-dysenteric ulcerative colitis*—mimicking classical ulcerative colitis; usually resolves slowly without specific treatment; rarely progresses to massive necrosis and toxic megacolon.
- *Skin ulceration*—usually perianal and anogenital regions, but may occur elsewhere, for example in surgical wounds and ileostomy/colostomy sites.
- *Amoeboma*—chronic inflammatory mass, single or multiple, most commonly developing in the ileocaecal region presenting as an acute/subacute obstruction or causing an intussusception.
- *Amoebic abscess*—most commonly in the liver (see later).

The differential diagnosis of amoebic colitis includes the following:

1 Other causes of dysentery or bloody stools such as *Shigella*, typhoid, other *Salmonella*, enteroinvasive and enterohaemorrhagic *Escherichia coli*, schistosomiasis (especially *Schistosoma mansoni* and *S. japonicum*), *Balantidium coli*, *Trichuris trichiura*, tuberculosis, carcinoma, inflammatory bowel disease, ischaemic colitis, arteriovenous malformation and diverticulitis.

2 Any other cause of acute or chronic abdominal pain.

The differential diagnosis of an amoeboma includes tuberculosis, carcinoma, actinomycosis, an 'antibioma' or appendix mass.

Amoebic liver abscess

Trophozoites of *E. histolytica* invade the liver via the portal vein and set about destroying hepatocytes, resulting initially in the formation of microabscesses that subsequently coalesce to form multiple abscesses (25–35% of patients) or, more commonly, a single abscess (65–75% of patients) by the time the diagnosis is made. The surrounding tissue becomes oedematous with a chronic

inflammatory infiltrate. Secondary bacterial infection may occur but is unusual.

Right lobe abscesses are four times more common than those on the left. Amoebic liver abscess is about 10 times more common in males than in females. All age groups may be affected, from neonates to the elderly, but ALA is most common in males aged between 20 and 40 years. Fewer than 50% have a history of dysentery within 1 month prior to presentation and many have no history of dysentery at all. A patient may present with an ALA many years after exposure, the transition from latent infection to clinical disease often being precipitated by immunosuppression or debility.

Clinical features

Patients who present in the early precoalescence stage of the development of an amoebic liver abscess may complain of low-grade fever and (usually) right upper quadrant discomfort and tenderness. This stage is sometimes referred to as 'amoebic hepatitis', a term that is perhaps misleading as it is unusual for such patients to have raised transaminases or bilirubin.

Most patients with ALA present when the abscess or abscesses are more 'mature' and the clinical symptoms and signs are more florid. The history is usually one of gradually increasing, but sometimes acute, pain in the right upper quadrant of the abdomen. In some cases, there is referred pain to the shoulder. Symptoms such as fever, sweats and rigors are common. In some cases, the pain is localized to the lower chest wall and may be pleuritic in nature. The patient may also complain of cough and breathlessness and have evidence of a pleural effusion, leading to a mistaken diagnosis of pneumonia. Weight loss, wasting and anaemia occur more frequently in chronic presentations and such patients may be afebrile. Most patients have tender hepatomegaly, sometimes with inflammation and oedema of the overlying tissue. There may be tenderness in the intercostal spaces (Durban's sign). Signs of a pleural effusion may be evident and the apex beat displaced, especially if the left lobe is affected. Chest

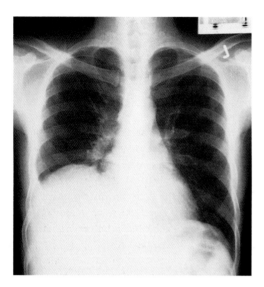

Figure 19.1 Chest X-ray of a patient with a large amoebic liver abscess, showing a grossly elevated right hemidiaphragm.

X-ray frequently reveals a raised hemidiaphragm or a pleural effusion (Figure 19.1). Jaundice is uncommon and less than half of the patients with an established ALA have a raised bilirubin and transaminases, although most have a raised alkaline phosphatase. A neutrophil leucocytosis is present in around 80% of cases.

In patients with a suspicious history but without obvious tender hepatomegaly, it may be possible to elicit tenderness resulting from a deep-seated abscess by means of a gentle 'thump' over the lower rib cage. This should be regarded as something of a last resort in a situation where more sophisticated diagnostic techniques are unavailable, and caution is advised if you do decide to thump your patient: (i) because your patient may thump you back (liver abscesses are usually extremely tender) and (ii) worse still, the abscess may rupture.

Complications of ALA include

• rupture through the skin or into the peritoneum, lung, pleura or pericardium (a particular risk with left lobe abscesses possibly resulting in cardiac tamponade);
• haematogenous seeding causing abscesses in any organ or tissue, for example brain, muscle, kidney or spleen.

The differential diagnosis of an ALA includes pyogenic abscess, hepatocellular carcinoma, liver secondaries, hydatid cyst, hepatitis, tuberculosis, syphilitic gumma and lung pathology.

Investigations

Microscopy

The presence of cysts only on stool microscopy is of little diagnostic value because of the problem in distinguishing between *E. histolytica* and *E. dispar*. A diagnosis of amoebic dysentery depends on finding trophozoites of *E. histolytica* containing ingested red blood cells in a fresh stool sample. Ideally, the stool sample should be examined within 15 min of being produced or should be maintained at body temperature until examined. This is advised because the trophozoites lose their motility and tend to round up as the specimen cools, thus becoming more difficult to identify. Trophozoites of *E. histolytica* may also be seen in scrapings or biopsies of ulcers identified endoscopically. Non-pathogenic amoebae do not contain ingested red blood cells. In contrast to patients with bacillary dysentery, leucocytes are usually scanty in the faeces of patients with amoebic dysentery. It is rare for trophozoites of *E. histolytica* to be identified in the faeces of patients with ALA and less than half have cysts.

On aspiration, the pus from an ALA ranges in colour from pink to brown, darkening on exposure to air and is sometimes described as resembling 'anchovy sauce' (in appearance, not odour). Characteristic trophozoites of *E. histolytica* can be identified in the pus or, more reliably, in scrapings from the wall of an ALA. Antigen detection is more sensitive. Cysts of *E. histolytica* are never found in abscesses. Leucocytes are scanty in pus obtained from an amoebic liver abscess unless there is secondary infection.

Antigen detection and polymerase chain reaction

Microscopy remains the principal method of investigation in settings with limited resources.

However, stool antigen detection is more sensitive and specific and is being increasingly adopted in more affluent countries. This reliably differentiates between *E. histolytica* and *E. dispar*, but a positive test does not guarantee that *E. histolytica* is responsible for the patient's symptoms. Antigen can also be detected in pus from an ALA. Sensitive PCR techniques have recently been developed for detection of *E. histolytica* in faeces and in ALA, and may be useful in epidemiological studies and in determining the virulence characteristics of different isolates.

Serology

A variety of serological tests have been developed for the diagnosis of invasive amoebiasis. Of these, indirect haemagglutination assay appears to be the most sensitive, particularly in the diagnosis of ALA. However, antibodies may persist for years following a significant infection, and 10–35% of people living in developing countries have positive serology. Therefore, caution should be exercised in interpreting the results of serological tests.

Endoscopy

Colonoscopy is helpful in investigating patients with suspected intestinal amoebiasis in whom stool microscopy or antigen tests are negative or inconclusive. Bowel preparation with enemas or cathartics is not advised because this may interfere with the identification of the parasite. The endoscopic appearance of amoebic colitis resembles that of inflammatory bowel disease, and there have been numerous examples of misdiagnosis and consequently disastrous mismanagement. Discrete patchy ulceration with a granular friable mucosa may be seen in acute cases. Larger ulcers with loosely adherent yellowish or grey 'pseudomembranes' tend to occur in more chronic disease. *E. histolytica* may invade areas of the bowel affected by other pathology, such as a carcinoma, leading to diagnostic confusion. Aspirates, scrapings or superficial biopsies from the ulcer edge should reveal motile erythrophagocytic trophozoites of *E. histolytica* if examined immediately

and should also be positive when tested for antigen. The parasites are readily identified by their magenta colour in biopsy specimens using a periodic acid–Schiff stain.

Imaging

Barium enema may demonstrate areas of ulceration, stricture or a filling defect from an amoeboma; however, none of these appearances are specific for amoebiasis, and there is a risk of perforation in patients with severe disease. Ultrasound, CT and magnetic resonance imaging (MRI) are very useful in identifying a liver abscess but cannot reliably differentiate an ALA from a pyogenic abscess. An abscess may not be evident if the patient presents in the early 'precoalescence' stage of disease, and it is worth repeating the scan after a few days if there is a high index of suspicion.

Management

Invasive amoebiasis

Treatment with one of the following tissue amoebicides is usually effective:
- *Metronidazole*—Adults 800 mg three times daily orally for 5–10 days; children 35–50 mg/kg/day in three divided doses for 5–10 days.
- *Tinidazole*—A single oral dose of 2 g is better tolerated but more expensive. This dose should be continued for 3–6 days in case of more severe infections; children 50–60 mg/kg/day for 3–5 days.
- *Oral chloroquine* 600 mg base daily for 2 days followed by 300 mg base daily for 2–3 weeks is also effective in the treatment of ALA; children 10 mg/kg/day (maximum 300 mg/day base) in 2–4 divided doses for 2–3 weeks.

Eradication of cysts

One of the following luminal amoebicides is usually recommended:
- *Diloxanide furoate*—Adults 500 mg orally three times daily for 10 days; children 20 mg/kg/day in three divided doses for 10 days.
- *Paromomycin*—Adults and children 25–35 mg/kg/day in three divided doses for 7 days.

- *Iodoquinol*—Adults 650 mg three times daily for 20 days; children 30–40 mg/kg/day (maximum 2 g) in three divided doses for 20 days.
- *Quinfamide* given in three doses of 100 mg each in a single day. This regimen has been used in both adults and children; however, full prescribing information is not yet available.
- *Tetracycline* may also be used as a luminal amoebicide.

Some practical points

A 5-day course of metronidazole is usually sufficient for the treatment of amoebic dysentery and most other forms of invasive amoebiasis. In affluent settings, it is usual to follow on with a course of a luminal amoebicide. If a luminal amoebicide is unavailable, patients with severe infections should be given a 10-day course of metronidazole. Patients treated with tinidazole or chloroquine should also receive a luminal amoebicide.

Parenteral metronidazole is indicated for patients who are severely ill with the addition of gentamicin and a third-generation cephalosporin (if available) or ampicillin to cover secondary sepsis from bowel pathogens. Attention should also be paid to the management of fluid and electrolyte disturbances, anaemia, ileus and other complications.

Surgery is recommended in cases of acute colonic perforation in the absence of diffuse colitis and in cases of ruptured amoebic appendicitis. Surgery should be avoided in patients with severe amoebic colitis because the bowel is very friable and difficult to repair or anastomose. However, patients presenting with toxic megacolon or an abdominal abscess should be managed surgically.

Amoebomas usually respond rapidly to medical treatment and failure to do so should raise suspicion of coincidental pathology, such as a carcinoma. Surgery may be indicated in cases of obstruction or intussusception.

Most patients with an uncomplicated ALA will respond to a 5-day course of metronidazole. However, it may be advisable to extend this to 10 days, particularly if a luminal amoebicide is not available. The best guide to the efficacy of treatment is the patient's clinical response. Unless indicated

on clinical grounds, there is little point in repeating scans as these are likely to remain abnormal for several months despite successful treatment.

Indications for aspiration and drainage of an ALA include failure to respond to medical treatment, impending rupture, suspected secondary bacterial infection and diagnostic uncertainty.

Management of asymptomatic individuals passing cysts depends on the clinical context and the availability of resources for diagnosis and treatment. Ideally, one should differentiate between *E. histolytica* and *E. dispar* using a stool antigen test and prescribe a luminal amoebicide for those with *E. histolytica*. This is unlikely to be possible or practical in a resource-poor setting. In these circumstances, there is little point in attempting to identify and treat such individuals, particularly as the majority have *E. dispar* and all are likely to become reinfected. It is very important to eliminate *E. histolytica* from the gut of asymptomatic patients prior to immunosuppressive treatment and such patients should receive either a 5-day course of metronidazole (or single dose of tinidazole) followed by a luminal amoebicide, or a 10-day course of metronidazole.

Prevention and public health aspects

Improved hygiene, sanitation and access to safe drinking water are the main issues in preventing infection with *E. histolytica*. 'Boil it, cook it, peel it or leave it' is the message for travellers.

Interactions with immunosuppression

Topical and/or systemic steroids given for misdiagnosed inflammatory bowel disease can exacerbate amoebic colitis and lead to extension into the perineum or into the abdominal wall. Amoebic liver abscess and colitis had been reported to be more frequent in HIV positive Taiwanese men, but this association is found only in men who have sex with men and probably reflects increased epidemiological risk of acquiring amoebic infections, rather than a true interaction with HIV.

Recent developments

Nitazoxanide, a thiazolide compound, has been shown to be well tolerated and effective in the treatment of a wide range of gastrointestinal infections in adults and children including *E. histolytica* (effective as both a tissue and luminal amoebicide), *Giardia intestinalis* (*G. lamblia*), *Blastocystis hominis, Isospora belli, Cyclospora cayetanensis, Dicrocoelium dendriticum, Cryptosporidium parvum, Trichomonas vaginalis, Balantidium coli, Ascaris lumbricoides, Strongyloides stercoralis, T. trichiura, Enterobius vermicularis, Taenia saginata, Hymenolepis nana, Fasciola hepatica, Clostridium difficile, Helicobacter pylori,* rotavirus and norovirus. In immunocompetent patients, a 3-day course of oral nitazoxanide is usually recommended in the following doses:

- adults and children over 12 years, 500 mg b.d.
- children aged 4–11 years, 200 mg b.d.
- children aged 1–3 years, 100 mg b.d.

Further reading

Aslam S, Musher DM. Nitazoxanide: clinical studies of a broad-spectrum anti-infective agent. *Future Microbiol* 2007; 2: 583–590. [Recent summary about this increasingly versatile drug.]

Haque R, Huston CD, Hughes M, Houpt E, Petri WA. Amebiasis. *N Engl J Med* 2003; 348: 1565–1573. [Beautifully illustrated state-of-the-art review.]

Hung CC, Ji DD, Sun HY. Increased risk for *Entamoeba histolytica* infection and invasive amoebiasis in HIV seropositive men who have sex with men in Taiwan. *PLOS Negl Trop Dis* 2008; 2(2): e175. [Nicely illustrated article from the only group who previously linked amoebiasis with HIV.]

Petri WA. *Entamoeba histolytica*: clinical update and vaccine prospects. *Curr Infect Dis Rep* 2002; 4: 124–129. [Summarizes recent findings on *E. histolytica* infection in children, differentiation of *E. histolytica* from *E. dispar*, outcome of *E. histolytica*/HIV coinfection in pregnant women in Tanzania, acquired immunity to *E. histolytica* and prospects in vaccine development.]

Stanley S. Amoebiasis. *Lancet* 2003; 361: 1025–1034. [Comprehensive overview of pathogenesis, clinical and diagnostic features, and treatment.]

Chapter 20

Bacillary dysentery

The term 'dysentery' is generally used to describe diarrhoea with visible blood and mucus. The term 'bacillary dysentery' is used interchangeably with 'shigellosis' although numerous other bacteria also cause bloody diarrhoea, including several that are bacilli. Shigellosis occurs worldwide and is associated with poverty, crowding and lack of hygiene and sanitation.

Microbiology and epidemiology

Shigellae are non-motile Gram-negative rod-shaped bacteria belonging to the family Enterobacteriaceae. According to current criteria for classification on the basis of DNA, Shigellae belong to the genus *Escherichia coli*. However, for historic and clinical reasons, *Shigella* has retained its identity as a separate genus.

Four groups or species are described, all but one of which include several serotypes and subtypes.
1 Group A: *Shigella dysenteriae* (serotypes 1–15) tends to cause epidemics (especially *S. dysenteriae* type 1).
2 Group B: *S. flexneri* (serotypes 1–6, with 15 subtypes) commonly causes endemic dysentery in developing countries.

3 Group C: *S. boydii* (serotypes 1–18) is common on the Indian subcontinent.
4 Group D: *S. sonnei* (one serotype) is an important cause of dysentery in the industrialized world.

Studies in animals and epidemiological evidence in humans indicate that *Shigella* infections elicit serotype-specific immunity. Humans are the only important reservoir of infection. People who have asymptomatic infections are important carriers. Transmission is faecal–oral via flies, food, water and person–person contact including various sexual practices. Shigellae are notably resistant to gastric acid and a very small ingested dose, as few as 10 bacilli, may cause clinical disease. It is estimated that over 160 million clinical infections occur each year, resulting in more than one million deaths. Children aged less than 5 years account for 70% of cases and 60% of deaths. Dietary supplementation with both zinc and vitamin A have been shown to reduce the incidence and severity of diarrhoeal diseases, including dysentery.

Clinical features

Shigellosis principally affects the colon and, sometimes, the terminal ileum. Clinical manifestations are brought about by a combination of enteroinvasion and toxin production. Organisms invade and multiply in the mucosa causing cell death, inflammation, ulceration, haemorrhage

Lecture Notes: Tropical Medicine, 6th edition.
By G.V. Gill and N.J. Beeching. Published 2009 by Blackwell Publishing, ISBN: 978-1-4051-8048-1.

and formation of microabscesses. Shiga toxin, an exotoxin produced by certain strains of *S. dysenteriae* type 1, consists of an enterotoxin causing secretory diarrhoea, a cytotoxin causing cell necrosis and a neurotoxin that may cause CNS complications in children. Shiga toxin may also be involved in the pathogenesis of haemolytic uraemic syndrome (HUS).

The incubation period usually ranges from 1 to 8 days with a median of 5 days. The clinical spectrum of shigellosis may range from asymptomatic to fulminant with fatal attacks. Many clinical episodes are mild and self-limiting, with watery diarrhoea without blood or mucus, which resolve spontaneously after a few days.

Sh. sonnei infections are usually milder, but may be severe in infants. *Sh. dysenteriae* and *Sh. flexneri* tend to cause more severe disease with an abrupt onset of bloody, mucoid stools, cramps and tenesmus often accompanied by fever and, sometimes, dysuria and confusion. Fever, confusion, meningism and convulsions often precede the onset of diarrhoea in young children.

Sh. dysenteriae type 1 may cause a fulminating gangrenous infection with an abrupt onset of fever, chills, rigors, vomiting and toxaemia. The patient can pass 20–60 bloody stools per day, often containing mucus and pus, and sometimes even sloughs of mucosa. Perforation is relatively rare, but severe dehydration, blood loss and sepsis can lead to acute renal failure. HUS occurs in 13% of cases of *Sh. dysenteriae* type 1, usually 1–5 days after the onset of the dysentery. Rarely, a choleraic form may occur with an abrupt onset of profuse watery diarrhoea that later becomes bloody and is associated with a high mortality.

Other complications and sequelae of shigellosis include toxic megacolon, post-dysenteric colitis, strictures, protein-losing enteropathy, granular proctitis, piles, parotitis and rectal prolapse in children. Peripheral neuropathy can also occur, particularly in children. Post-dysenteric Reiter's syndrome and symmetrical arthritis are also well-recognized sequelae.

For the differential diagnosis of bacillary dysentery, see Chapter 1, p. 7, and 19, p. 187.

Investigation

The typical stool of shigellosis is often described as like 'redcurrant jelly'. Microscopically, red blood cells and pus cells are usually numerous whereas bacilli are scanty. Stool culture, even if the sample is fresh, is often difficult, and rectal swabs are more likely to be positive, particularly if directly inoculated onto appropriate culture media at the bedside.

Management

Most cases can be managed supportively with oral rehydration solution. In more severe cases, intravenous fluids such as normal saline (with or without potassium, depending on renal function) or Ringer's lactate solution will be required. Blood transfusion may be indicated, and patients with HUS may require dialysis.

The WHO recommends that all cases of bloody diarrhoea should be treated promptly with an effective antibiotic. The choice depends on local sensitivity. Multidrug resistance is now very common and widespread, especially with *Sh. dysenteriae* type 1. Empirical treatment with ciprofloxacin, or another fluoroquinolone, is currently recommended as first-line therapy. Second-line choices include pivmecillinam, ceftriaxone or azithromycin. The possibility of secondary septicaemia from gut anaerobes and other enteropathogens should be considered in severely ill patients.

The use of antibiotics in children with dysentery caused by *E. coli* 0157:H7, which produces a Shiga-like toxin, is associated with an increased risk of development of HUS. However, at the time of writing, this association has not been demonstrated among patients with shigellosis. Daily zinc supplements are recommended for 10–14 days in children aged less than 5 years. Vitamin A also reduces the severity of episodes of diarrhoea, including dysentery.

Prevention and public health aspects

Prevention of shigellosis is very much a matter of basic hygiene and sanitation. Hand washing, preferably using soap, is very important especially in relation to food preparation and consumption. Food and utensils should be protected from flies. At community level, provision of an adequate quantity of water is more important than the quality of water, although quality is also important, as is sanitary disposal of faeces. Epidemic shigellosis can be devastating in refugee and displaced populations. In unstable situations associated with poor hygiene and sanitation, attack rates may be greater than 30%. Severe malnutrition and extremes of age are associated with more severe disease and fatal outcome. Laboratory confirmation and antibiotic sensitivity testing is a priority. Early access to oral rehydration fluids and antibiotic treatment should be coupled with hygiene promotion and other appropriate public health measures.

The need for an effective vaccine has become more urgent with the emergence of multidrug-resistant strains of *Shigella*. Several promising candidate vaccines are currently under development but it is likely to be some time before an effective vaccine becomes widely available.

Further reading

World Health Organization (2005). Guidelines for the control of shigellosis, including epidemics due to *Shigella dysenteriae* 1. http://www.who.int/vaccine_research/documents/Guidelines_Shigellosis.pdf

Chapter 21

Cholera

Cholera is a bacterial infection of humans caused by *Vibrio cholerae* 01 (of classical or El Tor biotypes) and *V. cholerae* 0139, which characteristically cause severe diarrhoea and may lead to death—in those severely affected—from water and electrolyte depletion. Spread is directly from person to person by the faecal–oral route or indirectly by infected food or water. It can spread to any part of the world and may become endemic where standards of environmental sanitation and personal hygiene are low.

Humans are the only animal reservoir of infection. However, *V. cholerae* can survive for several months in aquatic environments and transmission may be maintained from such sources. The El Tor biotype has now largely displaced classical cholera as the major pathogen of public health importance with 0139 responsible for infection in some areas of South Asia.

Microbiology and pathogenesis

V. cholerae, a Gram-negative comma-shaped bacillus of the family Vibrionaceae comprises over 100 serogroups, distinguished by the composition of the oligosaccharide antigen of the cell wall. Only serogroups 01 and 0139 cause the clinical disease cholera. The classification of *V. cholerae* is important in understanding the global epidemiology of the disease, and it is shown in Figure 21.1. The classical biotype is now found only in limited areas of Bangladesh. Most current outbreaks of cholera are caused by *V. cholerae* 01 El Tor biotype, serotype Ogawa or Inaba.

The infective dose of cholera is relatively high (10^2–10^6) and infectivity is increased in achlorhydria and chronic gastritis. In the ileum, vibrios adhere to ganglioside receptors of the epithelial cells. The principal pathogenic factor is the polypeptide cholera toxin released by the vibrios. Cholera toxin comprises two subunits, A and B. The B subunit attaches to the epithelial cells and 'allows' entry of the A subunit into the cells. The A subunit 'switches on' cyclic AMP, resulting in the efflux of water, bicarbonate and electrolytes and the clinical dehydration and electrolyte imbalance that characterizes cholera.

In 2000 the full genome of *V. cholerae* was characterized, and the location of the genes coding for the A (*ctx*A) and B (*ctx*B) toxin subunits was determined. A further regulatory gene, *Tox*R, has been shown to be influenced by environmental factors and may be linked to the seasonal pattern of cholera. An understanding of the pathogenic mechanism and the toxin genes has enabled the development of improved cholera vaccines.

Lecture Notes: Tropical Medicine, 6th edition.
By G.V. Gill and N.J. Beeching. Published 2009 by
Blackwell Publishing, ISBN: 978-1-4051-8048-1.

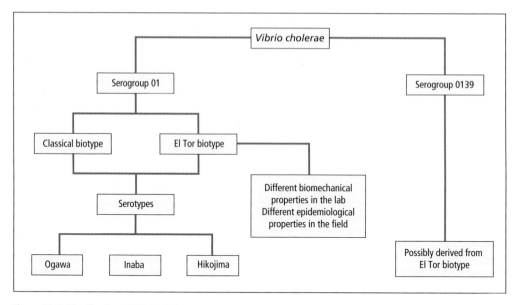

Figure 21.1 Classification of *Vibrio cholera.*

Epidemiology

Pandemics of cholera have been described for several centuries. The current pandemic began in 1961 in Indonesia and spread relentlessly through south and east Asia, the Middle East, in the 1970s into Africa and finally in 1990 to Latin America. The pandemic strain is *V. cholerae* 01 El Tor. In 1993 a new serotype, *V. cholerae* 0139, was reported in southern India and has been responsible for outbreaks in Bangladesh and Thailand.

Cholera is transmitted by the faecal–oral route and occurs where sanitation and water supplies are inadequate, particularly in the poorer areas of the developing world, and in refugee and complex emergencies. Vibrios can survive for long periods in aquatic environments and so provide a reservoir of infection when public health infrastructure is compromised. The El Tor biotype has an improved environmental survival compared to classical and a higher number of asymptomatic carriers:case ratio, which has contributed to its displacement of the classical biotype. Large-scale epidemics have occurred in the last decade among Rwandan refugees in the Democratic Republic of Congo, in southern Sudan, Angola and Somalia and Zimbabwe. Smaller outbreaks have occurred in hospitals with limited facilities for isolation and infection control.

Diagnosis

In outbreaks of cholera, diagnosis is usually made on clinical grounds following the WHO suspected case definition: '(i) in an area where cholera is not endemic, severe dehydration or death from watery diarrhoea in a patient aged 5 years or more; (ii) in an area where there is a cholera epidemic, acute watery diarrhoea with or without vomiting in a patient aged 5 years or more'. Laboratory investigation is required to confirm the diagnosis and to determine the serogroup and serotype for epidemiological purposes. Cholera vibrios can survive for several days in alkaline peptone water or Cary Blair medium for transport to a laboratory distant from the epidemic. Specimens are cultured at 37°C on thiosulphate citrate bile salt sucrose (TCBS) agar. *V. cholerae* produces characteristic yellow, oxidase positive, colonies that can be tested for agglutination with 01 or 0139 anti sera. Recently, immunodiagnostic dipsticks have been developed for the rapid diagnosis of cholera in field conditions.

Treatment

Initial rehydration

Rehydration is the mainstay of cholera treatment. In severe cases with hypovolaemic shock, the restoration of blood volume is urgently needed, and this can be achieved rapidly only by intravenous infusion (see also p. 9). Because peripheral veins are collapsed in such patients, the initial resuscitative infusion may have to be given via the femoral or subclavian vein in adults or the internal jugular vein or intraosseous route in children.

Fluid in the initial stages is run in as quickly as possible; an initial rate of 4 L/h for the first few litres is the norm in adults. The best guide to success is the return of a palpable arterial pulse. As soon as the systolic blood pressure reaches 90 mmHg, renal function usually returns. Tubular necrosis only usually develops if resuscitation is delayed.

In all patients with hypovolaemic shock, the initial fluid deficit will be at least 10% of the body weight. It is a safe rule of thumb to give one-third of the total estimated deficit in the first 20–30 min.

The type of fluid is less important than an adequate quantity. However, because patients usually have a metabolic acidosis as a result of bicarbonate loss, a deficiency of potassium and a loss of water greater than of salts, a slightly hypotonic alkaline fluid enriched with potassium is the most physiological choice.

The single fluid that meets all these needs, and is suitable for both adults and children, is Ringer's lactate solution. This contains calcium 2 mmol, chloride 111 mmol, lactate 27 mmol, potassium 5 mmol and sodium 131 mmol/L. It is suitable for both initial rehydration and maintenance therapy. Simpler solutions can be used with almost as good results, certainly in adults.

As soon as the blood volume has been restored and the pulse has returned, the drip can be moved to a more convenient site as peripheral veins reappear.

Maintenance hydration

When the patient has been resuscitated, careful charting of fluid intake and output must be started. The urine output must also be charted accurately, and intravenous fluid input should equal the combined volume of stool and urine, and 500 mL added for insensible losses. Once the patient is rehydrated and able to take fluids by mouth, oral rehydration should begin, although diarrhoea may be continuing.

Oral rehydration with glucose–electrolyte solution is used for maintenance hydration in severe cases following resuscitation and for all milder cases from the beginning. It is cheaper than intravenous therapy, requires no special apparatus or skills and is free from the dangers of fluid overload. Its success depends on the fact that the active transport of electrolytes into the mucosal cells is glucose dependant. If glucose is not available, sucrose can be used with almost as good results, as it is rapidly split into glucose and fructose by intestinal enzymes. The WHO-recommended solution comprises 1 L of 'clean' water, dextrose (glucose) 20 g, potassium chloride 1.5 g, sodium bicarbonate 2.5 g and sodium chloride 3.5 g. Oral rehydration should initially be given frequently and in small amounts and can be successfully done by family members rather than health workers.

Antimicrobial agents in cholera management

Tetracycline, doxycycline and furazolidone have all been shown to reduce the volume and duration of diarrhoea, particularly in those with severe disease. The normal adult regimens are tetracycline 500 mg 6 hourly for 3 days, furazolidone 400 mg/day for 3 days or a single dose of doxycycline 300 mg. Resistance, particularly to tetracycline, is frequently reported and indiscriminate use of antibiotics for mild cases should be discouraged.

Control of cholera and prevention

Control involves effective case detection and management of cases, improvements in public health to reduce spread and the possible use of cholera vaccine. Symptomatic cases are a major source of infection to household contacts, both directly and by contaminating food and water, and in crowded refugee camps can lead to explosive epidemics. Isolation facilities for symptomatic cases will vary with the location. In hospitalized patients, single rooms and toilet facilities and standard barrier precautions are necessary, and the use of chlorine-based disinfectants after discharge. Where epidemics occur in refugee camps or crowded urban slums, locally appropriate strategies will be needed to isolate or cohort patients to reduce the risk of transmission. Facilities will be required for effective case treatment with adequate supplies of intravenous replacement fluids for severe cases and supplies of oral rehydration solution.

The challenges involved in managing large numbers of cases in the most difficult of situations have been well reported from the 1990s Rwanda refugee outbreak, where case fatality rates were reduced from over 30% to less than 5% by appropriate rehydration centres.

During outbreaks emergency public health measures will be necessary to improve sanitation, control polluted water supplies and improve hygiene at the household level by safe water storage, provision of soap and appropriate education and information.

Longer term control depends mainly on improving standards of environmental sanitation and water supply, which should be a sustained objective of international health programmes.

The role of vaccination in cholera prevention and control has become an important issue with the availability of oral cholera vaccines. The principal of these vaccines is based on an understanding of the pathogenesis and genetics of *V. cholerae*. The objective of the vaccine is to produce gut mucosal antibodies to the B subunit of cholera toxin. These antibodies then prevent the B subunit adhering to the mucosal cells, thus preventing the entry of the A subunit (see Microbiology and pathogenesis section). Antibodies to the *V. cholerae* cell wall are also required. Oral vaccines have been developed by two strategies. In the Whole Cell B subunit vaccine (WC-B vaccine), a synthesized or recombinant B subunit polypeptide is combined

with a suspension of four strains of killed *V. cholerae* 01: El Tor and Classical Ogawa and Inaba. In the genetically engineered vaccine (103HgR), living *V. cholerae* El Tor has the *ctx*A gene deleted producing a living strain that is deficient in the A subunit. The first type has been licensed for use in United Kingdom for travellers to cholera endemic areas, particularly those who may be working with refugees or going to remote areas.

There have been various studies to determine whether the mass use of the oral vaccine could play a role for populations in cholera endemic areas or as a control measure in large epidemics. At present there are no specific recommendations, but recent WHO documentation suggests possible strategies. Current WHO recommendations do not support the use of antimicrobials as prophylaxis against cholera in endemic or epidemic situations.

Cholera continues to be a major public health problem among poorer communities in endemic areas, and among refugees and displaced communities in complex emergencies. While new vaccines and new diagnostics may have a role to play, political and public health initiatives are essential for control.

Further reading

Gordon M. Cholera. In: Parry EPO, Godfrey R, Mabey D, Gill GV, eds. *Principles of Medicine in Africa*, 3rd edn. Cambridge: Cambridge University Press, 2004: 591–595. [Good overview.]

Hill DR, Ford L, Lalloo D. Oral cholera vaccines – use in clinical practice. *Lancet Infect Dis* 2006; 6: 361–373. [Comprehensive but succinct overview of trials of cholera vaccines in endemic settings and for travellers. Critical review of controversy over use for preventing other traveller's diarrhoea.]

Role of cholera vaccination in emergencies: www.who.int/cholera/publications/cholera_vaccines_emergencies_2005.pdf

Updated information on cholera outbreaks: www.who.int/csr/don/archive/disease/cholera/en

WHO Guidelines on prevention and control: www.who.int/topics/cholera/control/en

Chapter 22

Giardiasis and other intestinal protozoal infections

Giardiasis

Epidemiology

Giardiasis occurs worldwide, particularly in areas of poor hygiene and sanitation. Humans are the main reservoir of infection, although beavers have been implicated in outbreaks in North America. It is uncertain whether several species that occur in various domestic pets and other animals actually cause disease in humans. Most infections are acquired through drinking water contaminated with *Giardia* cysts. These are relatively resistant to chlorination and large community outbreaks have occurred from drinking chlorinated but unfiltered water. Cysts may also be ingested on food, particularly salads, and by direct faeco–oral spread, for example among preschool children in day-care centres or in other situations of poor hygiene and sanitation. Cysts can survive outside the body for several weeks under favourable conditions.

Parasite and life cycle

Giardia lamblia (also known as *G. intestinalis* or *G. duodenalis*) is a flagellate protozoon that inhabits the upper small bowel. The trophozoite stage

of the parasite is a flattened pear-shaped creature about 15 μm long, 9 μm wide and 3 μm thick. It is concave on its ventral surface where it attaches itself, by its sucking disc, to the intestinal mucosa but does not invade. It has four pairs of flagella for locomotion and multiplies in the gut by binary fission. Large areas of the mucosal surface may be colonized in heavy infections.

Trophozoite adherence disrupts the intestinal brush border and interferes with enzyme activity. Attachment also stimulates an inflammatory cytokine response resulting in secretion of fluid and electrolytes and damage to enterocytes. Trophozoites usually encyst as they pass distally along the intestine. The cyst is oval, 8–12 μm long by 6–8 μm wide, and contains four small nuclei and a central refractile axoneme. The cysts are infective as soon as passed. When swallowed by a new host, they excyst in the upper gastrointestinal tract and liberate trophozoites.

Occasionally, *Giardia* may colonize the biliary tract and—in patients with achlohydria—the stomach, usually in association with *Helicobacter pylori*.

Clinical features

The median incubation period is 7–10 days but ranges from 3 days to several months. Susceptibility to infection and disease depends on parasite and host factors. Clinical symptoms may develop after ingesting as few as 10 cysts. Most

Lecture Notes: Tropical Medicine, 6th edition.
By G.V. Gill and N.J. Beeching. Published 2009 by Blackwell Publishing, ISBN: 978-1-4051-8048-1.

infections are asymptomatic. Clinical symptoms are more likely to develop and tend to be more severe in initial infections and tend to be more difficult to treat in persons with impaired immunity (e.g. HIV and B cell deficiencies).

Symptoms are often abrupt with diarrhoea, abdominal cramps, bloating and flatulence. Often there is associated malaise, nausea and belching accompanied by a taste of rotten eggs. The diarrhoea can be variable in character, ranging from watery to greasy but does not contain blood. Most patients have been symptomatic for several days before seeking medical help and may have significant weight loss by the time they present. Untreated, the clinical course is variable. Many patients, often after periods of fluctuating symptoms, eventually become asymptomatic. Others continue to have persisting diarrhoea, associated with malabsorption, malnutrition and failure to thrive. In some patients, chronic diarrhoea may be partly related to lactose intolerance, which may persist despite eradication of the *Giardia*.

Differential diagnosis

The differential diagnosis includes a wide range of causes of acute and chronic non-bloody diarrhoea and other causes of malabsorption, including:
- parasitic (fasciolopsiasis, capillariasis, strongyloidiasis, isosporiasis, cryptosporidiosis)
- tropical sprue
- hypolactasia
- chronic calcific pancreatitis
- malnutrition
- intestinal tuberculosis
- alpha-chain disease
- coeliac disease
- small bowel lymphoma.

Investigations

The standard method of diagnosis is stool microscopy for the characteristic cysts. Passage of cysts can be intermittent, and it may be necessary to examine repeated samples. Motile trophozoites are sometimes seen in saline preparations. Concentration and special staining techniques increase the sensitivity of stool microscopy and it should be possible to diagnose 50–70% of infections on examination of a single stool sample and more than 90% of infections if three samples are examined.

Various techniques are now available for the rapid detection of *Giardia* antigen in stool samples, for example using ELISA and direct fluorescence antibody techniques. These are more sensitive and less time consuming than stool microscopy, although occasionally it is necessary to test more than one stool sample. A panel EIA has been developed for the detection of *G. lamblia*, *Entamoeba histolytica* and *Cryptosporidium parvum* with sensitivities and specificities of over 95% for identification of these organisms. However, antigen testing should not replace stool microscopy because other pathogens may be present and may, in fact, be responsible for the patient's symptoms.

Other methods of diagnosis include duodenal fluid aspiration and microscopy for trophozoites. Duodenal fluid can also be sampled using the 'string test' in which the patient swallows a length of string, one end of which is entwined in a gelatin capsule. The capsule dissolves and the string passes into the duodenum. Having taped the proximal end to the patient's cheek, the string is left *in situ* overnight or with the patient fasting for 4–6 h. The string is then withdrawn; the duodenal fluid is squeezed from the distal end onto a microscope slide and examined for *Giardia* trophozoites. This technique is also useful in diagnosing strongyloidiasis (Chapter 52).

Small bowel biopsy may be helpful in patients in whom an alternative or concurrent diagnosis is being considered, for example patients with HIV/AIDS, common variable immunodeficiency or suspected tropical sprue. The typical picture in giardiasis is of villous flattening, deepening of crypts and an increased inflammatory infiltrate in the lamina propria. *Giardia* trophozoites may also be seen in the intervillous spaces.

Management

Most patients respond to oral metronidazole 400 mg three times daily for 5 days or 2 g/day for 3 days. Paediatric regimens are 15 mg/kg/day in three divided doses or 40 mg/kg/day for 3 days. Tinidazole is effective as a single oral dose of 2 g for adults and 50 mg/kg (maximum 2 g) for children. Albendazole 400 mg/day for 5 days is also effective. Nitazoxanide is also effective and has proved useful in treating patients who are HIV positive, who fail to respond to standard treatment. Other drugs that are sometimes used include quinacrine, furazolidone and paromomycin. Paromomycin is not absorbed and thus is safe to use throughout pregnancy, though it is inferior to metronidazole, which may be used in the second and third trimesters.

Failure to eradicate the organism following a standard course of treatment may be because of poor compliance, reinfection or, possibly, antimicrobial resistance or underlying immunodeficiency. Persisting symptoms despite eradication of the parasite raises the possibility of continuing lactose intolerance or that *Giardia* was a coincidental finding and the patient's symptoms are attributable to another aetiology.

Prevention and public health

Prevention is all about improving hygiene, sanitation and access to safe water. Cysts of *Giardia* are resistant to standard chlorination of water, therefore flocculation, sedimentation and filtration are of greater importance. Cysts are killed if water is boiled. Micropore filters, with or without iodine resins, are available for personal use and may be handy for travellers.

Other intestinal protozoa of importance

C. parvum

Parasite and life cycle

Cryptosporidium spp. are coccidian protozoans with a worldwide distribution found in mammals, reptiles, fish and birds. Two major, distinct species have been identified in waterborne epidemics: (i) *C. hominis*, which is predominantly an infection of humans and (ii) *C. parvum,* which infects a broader range of animals. Transmission is faeco–oral and

infection most commonly occurs when the oocyst is ingested via contaminated water or food, or following person–person contact. The oocyst releases four sporozoites into the lumen of the small bowel, which invade the epithelial cells where they undergo further stages in a life cycle that, in many ways, resembles that of malaria. *Cryptosporidium* may also invade the colon and biliary tree. *Cryptosporidium* has the ability to produce thin-walled oocysts that maintain its life cycle within the host ('internal autoinfection') or thick-walled oocysts that are excreted in faeces. The latter are highly resistant to chlorination and small enough to pass through conventional filters. *Cryptosporidium* is notorious in causing epidemics of diarrhoea even among communities in developed countries with access to treated water supplies.

Clinical features

The incubation period for *Cryptosporidium* has not been clearly established but usually ranges from 1 to 12 days, with an average of 7 days. *Cryptosporidium* is important in four clinical settings:

1 childhood diarrhoea in developing countries
2 travellers' diarrhoea
3 protracted diarrhoea in immunocompromised patients
4 waterborne outbreaks in developed and developing countries.

Clinical features frequently include watery diarrhoea, abdominal cramps, bloating, weight loss, fever and malaise. Episodes are usually self-limiting but may become chronic or fulminant, particularly in immunocompromised patients, for example with HIV/AIDS, and associated biliary tract disease may also occur in this population.

Isospora belli

I. belli is a protozoan parasite with a worldwide distribution, usually acquired from faecally contaminated water or food. Disease may occur following ingestion of the mature oocyst and pathology is similar to *Cryptosporidium*. Clinical presentation is usually with watery diarrhoea—sometimes with blood and pus cells—abdominal pain and malabsorption. Infections are usually self-limiting but may become chronic or relapsing in immuno-compromised patients.

Cyclospora cayetanensis

Cyclospora is usually acquired from faecally con-taminated water, fruit or herbs. Clinically simi-lar to *Cryptosporidium* and *Isospora*, symptoms include prolonged watery diarrhoea, cramps, fever and fatigue.

Balantidium coli

The largest and probably least common protozoan pathogen of humans, *B. coli*, can cause a spectrum of disease similar to that of amoebiasis, including severe, life-threatening colitis. The pig is the most important animal reservoir for human disease. Monkeys and other mammals may also be infected.

Blastocystis hominis

Although, like many of the other protozoa, *B. hominis* can infect humans without causing diarrhoea, it is now evident that it can cause acute and chronic diarrhoea, particularly in indi-viduals who are immunocompromised.

Microsporidia

Various species of the order Microsporidia are pathogenic in humans and are increasingly recog-nized to be important, particularly in HIV-infected individuals. The most common is *Enterocytozoon bieneusi*, which occurs in 7–50% of HIV-infected persons with chronic diarrhoea. Microsporidia species may invade the biliary tree and liver and may also affect other organ systems, particularly the CNS, including the eye, respiratory and geni-tourinary systems.

Investigations

The diagnosis of cryptosporidiosis is usually made by demonstrating acid-fast oocysts in faeces

or luminal aspirates using a modified Kinyoun acid-fast stain. *Cryptosporidium* oocysts appear as round pinkish-red bodies measuring 4–6 μm. A sensitive and specific panel EIA test has recently been developed.

Isospora oocysts are larger and oval measuring 10×30 μm. They may be visible in an unstained saline preparation and appear red with the modi-fied acid-fast stain. Unusually for a protozoal infection, *Isospora* may cause an eosinophilia.

Cyclospora oocysts are round and measure 8–10 μm. They may be seen in unstained faecal preparations and stain (variably) red with the modified acid-fast stain. They do not stain with iodine. They can be detected as blue fluorescent dots when examined in ultraviolet light.

Modified trichome stains, calcofluor or chem-ofluorescent stains can be used in expert hands for the diagnosis of *E. bieneusi* and other micro-sporidia in faeces, and electron microscopy is used in reference laboratories to confirm the iden-tity of the organism. None of these modalities are routinely available in the tropics and underdiag-nosis is the norm.

Management

Most patients with normal immunity recover from these infections spontaneously. HIV-related cryptosporidiosis and other protozoal infections described earlier usually improve following the initiation of antiretroviral treatment.

Treatment of symptomatic patients with crypt-osporidiosis poses problems as few of the avail-able antimicrobials have proven and consistent efficacy. In the past, paromomycin was the agent most commonly recommended for the treatment of *Cryptosporidium* associated with HIV. Trials using azithromycin have also yielded promising results.

Recently, Nitazoxanide has been shown to be effective against a wide range of intestinal patho-gens, including *B. hominis*, *I. belli*, *C. cayetanen-sis*, *C. parvum*, *E. bieneusi*, *B. coli* (see Chapter 19, p. 190).

Nitazoxanide is now emerging as the drug of first choice for treatment of HIV-related cryptosporidiosis and, because of its broad spectrum of activity, may also have a role in the 'blind' treatment of persistent diarrhoea in circumstances where diagnostic facilities are limited or absent.

Isospora and *Cyclospora* respond to oral trimethoprim-sulfamethoxazole 160–800 mg four times daily for 7–10 days. HIV-positive patients should then receive a maintenance dose three times weekly or a weekly dose of Fansidar. Pyrimethamine can be used if the patient is allergic to sulphonamides. Ciprofloxacin is also effective against *Cyclospora*.

B. coli usually responds to tetracycline 500 mg four times daily for 10 days. Bacitracin, ampicillin, metronidazole and paromomycin are alternatives. Surgery may be required in fulminant colitis.

B. hominis also responds to metronidazole and trimethoprim-sulfamethoxazole.

Albendazole may produce clinical improvement in patients with *E. bieneusi*, despite persistence of the parasite in stool samples and small bowel biopsies following treatment. It is more effective for treating the less common gut microsporidian *Encephalitozoon intestinalis*. Improvement may also occur with the introduction of antiretroviral treatment.

Further reading

Aslam S, Musher DM. Nitazoxanide: clinical studies of a broad-spectrum anti-infective agent. *Future Microbiol* 2007; 2: 583–590. [Recent summary about this increasingly versatile drug.]

Didier ES, Weiss LM. Microsporidiosis: current status. *Curr Opin Infect Dis* 2006; 19: 485–492. [Recent review describing the epidemiological and clinical features of this important group of emerging pathogens.]

Farthing MJ. Treatment options for the eradication of intestinal protozoa. *Nat Clin Pract Gastroenterol Hepatol* 2006; 3: 436–445. [Excellent review covering recent developments in the management of intestinal protozoal infections.]

Gardner TB, Hill DR. Treatment of giardiasis. *Clin Microbiol Rev* 2001; 14: 114–128. [Useful summary including recommendations for treatment during pregnancy.]

Chapter 23

Intestinal cestode infections (tapeworms) including cysticercosis

Tapeworms

Tapeworms are flat segmented hermaphrodites measuring from 10 mm to 20 m. The head (scolex) attaches to the intestinal mucosa by means of suckers or hooklets. All, with the exception of *Hymenolepis nana*, require a secondary intermediate host in which the larvae develop into cysts, usually in muscle. Human infection follows consumption of cysts in undercooked meat or fish. Larval cestode infections can also occur in humans following the ingestion of the egg, the most important being cysticercosis.

Parasites and life cycles

Taenia saginata, the beef tapeworm, is a cosmopolitan infection in which humans harbour the adult worm and cattle harbour the larval stage. Its main importance is in economic losses caused by condemnation of beef carcasses. Human infection is of social importance only. Ethiopia has the highest infection rate in the world. People acquire infection by eating undercooked meat containing cysticerci, the larval stages of the parasite encysted in the muscles of infected herbivores. The cysts evaginate in the intestine, and the head

of the worm attaches itself to the mucosa of the upper third of the small intestine by its suckers. Segments called proglottids grow from the head, and new segments are added until the worm contains a chain of 1000–2000 segments.

Proglottids at the tail end of the worm develop fertilized eggs in the uterus and are called gravid segments. When mature, the gravid segments break off the chain (strobila) and leave the anus in the stool or by their own movements. Proglottids sometimes rupture in the intestine, and free eggs are also passed in the stool. The eggs that reach pasture, mainly after disintegration of the mature proglottids, are infective to cattle (and several other herbivores) when swallowed. They hatch in the bovine gut to become oncospheres and enter the circulation where they are carried to the muscles and encyst as cysticerci. The meat is described as 'measly', and the cysticerci are easily visible to the naked eye.

T. saginata cysts can occur in other domestic bovines, and a closely related Asian species has been shown to infect pigs, ungulates and monkeys. *T. solium*, the pork tapeworm, is a much less common infection than *T. saginata* but far more important because of its ability to cause severe disease in humans. Humans are the definitive host; pigs are the normal intermediate host. It is found all over the world where people eat cysts in raw or undercooked pork. For this reason, intestinal infection with *T. solium* is rare in Muslims,

Lecture Notes: Tropical Medicine, 6th edition.
By G.V. Gill and N.J. Beeching. Published 2009 by Blackwell Publishing, ISBN: 978-1-4051-8048-1.

Orthodox Jews and vegetarians. *T. solium* cysts also occur in dogs and cats.

Ingestion of eggs of *T. solium* can give rise to human cysticercosis, a major cause of epilepsy and other neurological disease in some parts of the world such as Central America and India. Human cysticercosis can occur regardless of religious or dietary affiliation. Human cysticercosis does not occur following the ingestion of eggs of *T. saginata*.

Beef and pork tapeworm maturation takes up to 12 weeks. A fully grown tapeworm may be 5–10 m long, live up to 25 years and produce about 50 000 eggs/day.

A third species of human *Taenia*, *T. asiatica*, which is also transmitted in pigs, has recently been described in Asia. Prevalence rates of up to 20% have been documented among villagers in Indonesia.

Clinical features of taeniasis

Intestinal infections are usually asymptomatic. The host may only realize that a tapeworm is on board when a proglottid segment appears in faeces or is felt as it passes through the anus. Symptoms may include loss of appetite, nausea or vague abdominal pain. Rarely, complications arise when a proglottid migrates to an unusual site, such as the appendix or pancreatic and bile ducts. Patients who are vomiting profusely for whatever reason may be further distressed by the appearance of several metres of tapeworm in the vomit.

Investigations

The eggs of *T. saginata* are indistinguishable from those of *T. solium* on routine microscopy. To make a specific diagnosis, a mature proglottid is pressed between two microscope slides and the number of lateral branches of the uterus counted. *T. saginata* has 15–20 main branches on each side while *T. solium* has 13 or fewer; but this criterion is not as reliable as once thought. The scolex, measuring about 1 mm, may be found among the smallest immature segments with the aid of

a magnifying glass. The presence of hooks distinguishes the scolex of *T. solium* from that of *T. saginata*, which has no hooks. Coproantigen detection tests and PCR are also available.

Serology is sometimes used for epidemiological surveys and may be useful in the diagnosis of cysticercosis. DNA probes have also been developed to differentiate between *T. saginata* and *T. solium*.

Cysticercosis

Tissue cysts of *T. solium* are usually 1–2 cm in size and can be found in many tissues, especially subcutaneous, muscle and brain. During the initial phase of invasion and development, there may be pain and swelling accompanied by eosinophilia. Subsequently, skin nodules can sometimes be felt as movable, small, painless nodules, especially on the arms or chest. Muscle cysts eventually calcify and can be seen as calcified streaks that follow the planes of the fibres of skeletal muscle on X-ray of the forearms, psoas or thigh muscles.

The most important effect of cysticercosis is in the brain. Initially there may be a diffuse encephalitic picture. More usually the patient presents with single or repeated seizure. Neurocysticercosis is the most important cause of epilepsy in many parts of Africa, South America and India. A small proportion of cases present with features of hydrocephalus. CT and MRI are needed to delineate the number, location and 'activity' of cysts in the brain. About 15–25% of patients with neurocysticercosis have a tapeworm at presentation or have a past history of tapeworm infection.

There is still controversy about the benefits and drawbacks of active antiparasitic treatment, but expert consensus is that treatment will benefit some patients with neurocysticercosis. Active parenchymal neurocysticercosis may be treated with albendazole 15 mg/kg/day or 800 mg/day in divided doses for 10–28 days or as second choice, praziquantel 50–100 mg/kg/day divided in three doses for 14 days. Cimetidine 400 mg three times daily may be used to increase the levels of both albendazole and praziquantel. Dexamethasone

6–12 mg/day in divided doses should be given before and during antiparasitic treatment to reduce the effects of inflammation around damaged cysts. Dexamethasone increases levels of albendazole and decreases levels of praziquantel. Steroids are also needed (in neurosurgical doses) for short-term management of occasional flare-ups of inflammation, and cerebral oedema that occur as cysts degenerate as part of their natural history. Inactive parenchymal cysts do not require treatment with antiparasitic agents. Seizures usually respond to first-line anticonvulsant drugs. Surgical intervention, for example shunting, may be required for obstructive hydrocephalus and intracranial hypertension. Extraparenchymal cysts, depending on number, size and location, may require treatment with combinations of antiparasitic drugs, steroids and, possibly, surgery (see Chapter 59).

Other intestinal cestode infections

Diphyllobothriasis

Diphyllobothrium latum is the most common of more than a dozen species of fish tapeworm affecting humans. Human infection follows ingestion of undercooked or raw fish or roe. Infection usually involves a single worm and most are asymptomatic or associated with vague non-specific abdominal symptoms. Megaloblastic anaemia can occur in severe cases.

Hymenolepiasis and dipylidiasis

H. nana, the dwarf tapeworm, occurs worldwide, mainly among children. Infections are usually asymptomatic, but abdominal pain, nausea, vomiting, pruritis ani and diarrhoea—sometimes containing blood—have been described in heavy infections. Headache, dizziness, sleep and behavioural disturbances are relatively frequent, and convulsions have also been reported. Autoinfection is common.

H. diminuta, the rat tapeworm, may affect humans following ingestion of the intermediate host, commonly a weevil, flea or cockroach. Infections are usually asymptomatic and short lived.

Dipylidium caninum may infect humans, usually young infants, following accidental ingestion of a flea, the intermediate host. Infections are usually asymptomatic; however, symptoms may include abdominal pain, diarrhoea, pruritis ani and urticaria.

Management of intestinal cestode infections

A single oral dose of praziquantel (10 mg/kg) is the drug of choice for all the aforementioned intestinal cestode infections. *H. nana* requires 25 mg/kg as a single dose. Caution is advised in populations in which cysticercosis is common, because of the risk of precipitating or aggravating neurological symptoms.

Niclosamide, as a single oral dose (500 mg if <11 kg; 1 g if 11–34 kg; 1.5 g if >34 kg; 2 g for adults) is also effective. Tablets should be well chewed and swallowed with plenty of water. The routine use of purgatives and antiemetics in patients with *T. solium* prior to cestocidal treatment, in order to prevent retrograde peristalsis of eggs and possible risk of cysticercosis, is not justified on the basis of clinical evidence.

Albendazole, which is used in the treatment of cysticercosis and hydatid cyst, is also effective in treating intestinal taeniasis. Nitazoxanide has also been shown to be effective in infections with *T. saginata* and *H. nana*.

Prevention and public health aspects

Control measures for taeniasis are aimed at environmental sanitation, meat inspection and adequate cooking or freezing of meat. Effective vaccines are available to prevent *T. saginata* and *T. solium* infection in livestock.

Further reading

Craig P, Akira I. Intestinal Cestodes. *Curr Opin Infect Dis* 2007; 20: 524–532. [Excellent recent review summarizing the biology, clinical aspects, diagnosis, treatment and epidemiology of intestinal cestodes.]

García HH, Gonzalez AE, Evans CAE *et al. Taenia solium* cysticercosis. *Lancet* 2003; 361: 547–556. [Comprehensive review with superb illustrations and references; clear discussion of areas of controversy.]

Nash TE, Singh G, White AC *et al.* Treatment of neurocysticercosis: current status and future research needs. *Neurology* 2006; 67: 1120–1127. [Authoritative and detailed review addressing an often controversial and difficult clinical problem.]

Chapter 24

Soil-transmitted helminths

The term 'soil-transmitted helminths' applies to a group of parasites whose life cycle usually depends on a period of development outside the human host, typically in moist, warm soil. The most important of these globally are the roundworms (*Ascaris lumbricoides*), whipworms (*Trichuris trichiura*) and hookworms (*Necator americanus* and *Ancylostoma duodenale*). In some species, infection occurs following the ingestion of eggs that have been passed in the faeces, and that only become infectious after a period of time undergoing further development, usually in soil, for example, *A. lumbricoides*.

Penetration of the skin is the method of infection used by the hookworms, *Anc. duodenale* and *N. americanus*. Under favourable environmental conditions, larvae hatch from eggs deposited in the soil. The larvae lie in wait in the surface layers of the soil until they come into contact with the skin of their unsuspecting host. *Strongyloides stercoralis* employs a similar *modus operandi*, but instead of eggs, larvae are passed in faeces which either can cause autoreinfection by direct penetration of the perianal skin, or go on to establish an independent life cycle in the soil awaiting the appearance of a new host.

The prevalence and distribution of soil-transmitted helminth infections is a product of lifestyle and life cycle. Soil-transmitted helminths do not multiply within the host. Their ability to evade the host immune response and avoid causing acute and fatal disease enables them to achieve a state of balanced parasitism that optimizes transmission. The down-regulatory immune responses induced in the host may have a fortuitous role in reducing host susceptibility to atopy and may explain why children living in regions that are highly endemic for these infections appear to be less likely to develop diseases associated with allergy, a theory known as the 'hygiene hypothesis'. Furthermore, infection with *A. lumbricoides* has been shown to dampen the immune response to a recombinant cholera toxin, whereas albendazole treatment of children with ascariasis enhances the vibriocidal antibody response to the live attenuated oral cholera vaccine CVD 103-HgR.

There is also some evidence indicating that these infections may increase host susceptibility to malaria, tuberculosis and HIV. However, studies from Thailand indicate that intestinal helminth infections, particularly with *A. lumbricoides*, appear to be protective against cerebral malaria, even though such infections are also associated with an increased risk of infection with *Plasmodium falciparum*.

Lecture Notes: Tropical Medicine, 6th edition.
By G.V. Gill and N.J. Beeching. Published 2009 by Blackwell Publishing, ISBN: 978-1-4051-8048-1.

About two billion people worldwide are infected with soil-transmitted helminths, often with several different species simultaneously, resulting in significant morbidity in about 300 million. The greatest burden of disease occurs among children, particularly in areas of poor hygiene and sanitation, and has a significant effect on the physical and intellectual development. The WHO is currently promoting the periodic mass chemotherapy of schoolchildren and women of childbearing age in an attempt to reduce the burden of disease in vulnerable populations. Reinfection is common; however, regular re-treatment should reduce associated morbidity. There is concern that this mass-treatment approach may hasten the development of resistance to mainstay antihelminthics such as albendazole and mebendazole.

Future developments are likely to include strategies involving combination treatment with existing antihelmintics and the wider use of newer drugs with antihelmintic properties, for example nitazoxanide and tribendimidine. A promising hookworm vaccine that has been shown to be effective in animal models is currently being developed for use in humans. Prevention of infection, disease and transmission of soil-transmitted helminths in a single step by vaccination is an attractive, if ambitious, goal for the future.

cny update in journals?

Ascariasis

Epidemiology

A. lumbricoides affects over 600 million people worldwide with a peak prevalence and intensity of infection among children aged 3–8 years. Infection is found wherever conditions of environmental hygiene are poor.

Parasite and life cycle

Ascaris eggs, contaminating vegetables, soil or dust, are swallowed, and liberate larvae as they pass through the stomach and small intestine. The larvae penetrate the intestinal mucosa, enter the bloodstream and lymphatics and reach the lungs 4–16 days after infection. The larvae penetrate the alveoli, moult and migrate via the respiratory tract to the oesophagus and on to the small intestine, where they develop into adults, mate and start producing eggs 9–11 weeks after infection. Adults are large, cream-coloured worms; males are 15–30cm long, and females 20–40cm. They live in the small intestine and obtain nourishment from the intestinal contents. They do not suck blood or damage the mucosa significantly. Females produce up to 200000 eggs per day. These are excreted in faeces, and their ova mature into infective embryos within 1–4 weeks and may remain viable in soil for years.

The morphologically similar *Ascaris* of pigs, *A. suum*, also infects humans.

Clinical features

Ascaris pneumonitis

Fever, cough, dyspnoea, wheeze and urticaria may occur in a proportion of those infected during the migration of larvae through the lungs. Chest pain, cyanosis and haemoptysis occur in more severe cases. Ascaris pneumonitis accompanied by eosinophilia is known as Löffler's syndrome. Symptoms usually resolve spontaneously within 10 days. Pneumonitis is more common in children and tends to be more severe on reinfection.

Clinical features resulting from adult worms

Intestinal worms are rarely noticed unless passed in the stool. Lactose intolerance and malabsorption of vitamin A and other micronutrients may sometimes occur. Worms may form a bolus in heavy infections causing intestinal obstruction, volvulus or perforation and peritonitis. Intestinal obstruction is more common in children, whereas obstruction of biliary ducts is more likely in adults. Obstruction of ducts or diverticula may cause biliary colic, cholangitis, liver abscess, pancreatitis or appendicitis, or wandering worms can make an unwelcome appearance in an endotracheal tube during anaesthesia. They have also been known to obstruct nasogastric tubes and even enter the paranasal sinuses. Even if these nomadic nematodes do not cause an obvious pyogenic peritonitis, they may continue to lay eggs, giving rise to a granulomatous peritonitis. Pneumothorax and pericarditis have also been reported.

Investigations

Ascaris pneumonitis is diagnosed on clinical grounds; the presence or absence of eggs in the stools is irrelevant. Larvae and/or eosinophils may be found in the sputum. Chest X-ray findings range from discrete densities to diffuse interstitial—or more confluent—infiltrates. Stool microscopy for eggs is usually adequate for diagnosing established infection, although stools may be negative if all the worms are male. Worms may also be found by means of barium studies, ultrasonography and endoscopy.

Management

- Albendazole 400 mg as single oral dose clears most infections. Heavy infections may need repeated doses for 2 or 3 days. The recommended dose in children aged 1–2 years is 200 mg.
- Mebendazole 100 mg orally twice daily for 3 days is effective. Its use in children younger than 2 years is not recommended by the manufacturer. Ectopic migration of *Ascaris* has been reported following the use of mebendazole. A single dose of 500 mg may also be effective.
- Piperazine 75 mg/kg (to a maximum of 3.5 g for adults and children >12 years and a maximum of 2.5 g for children aged 2–12 years). Side effects are relatively common and can be serious. Therefore, piperazine should only be used if safer alternatives are unavailable.
- Pyrantel pamoate (11 mg/kg up to a maximum of 1 g) can be given as a single dose. Pyrantel and piperazine have antagonistic effects and should never be prescribed concurrently.
- Levamisole 2.5 mg/kg as a single dose may also be effective.
- Nitazoxanide is also effective.

Ascaris pneumonitis is managed symptomatically with bronchodilators and steroids if indicated. Symptoms may be exacerbated by larval death, therefore the use of antihelmintics is questionable.

Intestinal obstruction is usually managed conservatively with nasogastric aspiration, intravenous fluids and antispasmodics, followed by an antihelmintic when the obstruction has subsided. Laparotomy may be necessary if this fails or if the patient is seriously ill. It may be possible to manipulate the worms through the ileocaecal valve without having to open the bowel. Surgical or endoscopic removal of single worms blocking bile or pancreatic ducts may be necessary for patients who fail to respond to antihelmintic treatment and those with persisting pain or raised serum amylase.

Prevention and public health aspects

Improved hygiene and sanitation, access to clean water and health education are particularly important. In some communities, human excrement ('night soil') is used to fertilize vegetables and poses an obvious risk. Periodic mass chemotherapy of vulnerable schoolchildren and women of childbearing age is currently being promoted by the WHO.

Hookworm

Epidemiology

Anc. duodenale and *N. americanus* are widely distributed in the tropics and subtropics, affecting approximately 900 million people worldwide. *N. americanus* predominates in the Americas, Australia, sub-Saharan Africa, South Asia and the Pacific islands, whereas *Anc. duodenale* is more prevalent in the Middle East, northern Africa, southern Europe, northern India and northern China. In Africa and Asia, 30–54% of moderate and severe anaemia in pregnancy is attributable to infection with hookworm. Hookworm infections commonly cause significant anaemia in all age groups, particularly if dietary iron intake is limited.

Parasites and life cycle

Hookworms are slender tubes about 1 cm long. They have a mouth and an oesophagus at the front, connected by the gut to the anus at the rear. *Ancylostoma* is larger than *Necator*. The female body is largely occupied by eggs. The teeth in *Anc. duodenale* and the cutting plates in *N. americanus* are used to pierce the intestinal mucosa. The mouth and pharynx are used to attach the worms to the mucosa by suction.

Hookworm eggs passed in the faeces hatch in warm, moist conditions, liberating rhabditiform larvae. These develop into filariform larvae, which inhabit the surface layer of soil. Filariform larvae penetrate human skin via fissures or hair follicles and are carried in the lymphatics and venous circulation to the lungs. Here they enter the alveoli, migrate to the pharynx and then to the small intestine, where they mature into adults. Adult hookworms attach themselves to the upper half of the small intestine and feed on blood. An adult *Anc. duodenale* may consume between 0.15 and 0.26 mL/day. *N. americanus* consumes a relatively modest 0.03 mL/day. Blood loss also occurs at the site of attachment. Loss of plasma proteins may result in hypoproteinaemia. The journey to the intestine takes about a week. Adults are fully grown (approximately 1 cm) in 2–3 weeks and sexually mature in 3–5 weeks, after which eggs begin to appear in the faeces.

Rarely, infection with *Anc. duodenale* may occur following the ingestion of larvae on contaminated vegetables. Infantile hookworm disease has been described in China and attributed to transmammary transmission, laying infants on contaminated soil or using nappies made of cloth bags stuffed with infected soil.

Clinical features

Most infections are asymptomatic. Problems arise when dietary iron intake is poor or demands are high, resulting in a gradually worsening iron-deficient anaemia, sometimes associated with hypoalbuminaemia and oedema. Eventually this may lead to cardiac failure. Pregnant women,

women with menorrhagia and children are at the greatest risk of developing anaemia.

Other symptoms are uncommon and tend to be associated with the early stages of initial infection. 'Ground itch' may occur at the site of larval penetration and, if severe, may be associated with the development of vesicles or pustules. The serpiginous rash of cutaneous larva migrans may be seen in human hookworm infections, although this is more commonly associated with infection with dog or cat hookworm. Larval migration through the lungs may cause a pneumonitis. Occasionally, within a few weeks of a heavy infection, there may be abdominal discomfort, flatulence, anorexia, nausea, vomiting and diarrhoea, sometimes containing blood and mucus. Life-threatening gastrointestinal haemorrhage has been reported as a rare complication in young children with severe primary infections.

'Wakana syndrome' (nausea, vomiting, pharyngeal irritation, cough, dyspnoea and hoarseness) may follow oral ingestion of *Anc. duodenale* larvae.

Investigations

Eosinophilia is common. Characteristic eggs can be identified by standard faecal microscopy. Concentration methods may be necessary for light infections. Culture techniques similar to those used for *Strongyloides* may also be used. Eggs may hatch in stool samples that are left for a few days before examination, liberating larvae that may be mistaken for those of *S. stercoralis*, although they are morphologically distinct. Mixed infections of hookworm and *Strongyloides* may also occur.

Humans may be infected with largely non-pathogenic worms whose eggs resemble those of hookworm. The most important is *Ternidens diminutus*, a common parasite in monkeys, baboons and humans in southern Africa. The worms inhabit the large bowel, where they may cause cystic nodules. Because they suck blood, they can cause anaemia in heavy infections. Their eggs closely resemble those of the hookworm, but are larger.

Trichostrongylus worms of many species are natural parasites of herbivores in many parts of the world, and humans can become infected by ingesting the infective larvae on raw vegetables or salads. The adult worms are attached to the small intestine, but cause only slight damage and insignificant blood loss. The eggs of *Trichostrongylus* spp. have more pointed ends than the eggs of true hookworms.

Management

- Albendazole 400 mg as a single dose is usually effective.
- Mebendazole 100 mg twice daily for 3 days is commonly prescribed.
- Pyrantel pamoate 11 mg/kg (maximum 1 g) for 3 days is also effective.
- Levamisole 2.5 mg/kg as a single dose repeated after 7 days may also be used.

Treatment for iron-deficiency anaemia may be required, preferably with oral iron. Transfusion is rarely necessary.

Prevention and public health aspects

Improved standards of hygiene and sanitation and the wearing of shoes reduce the likelihood of infection. Periodic mass chemotherapy of vulnerable schoolchildren and women of childbearing age is currently being promoted by the WHO.

Interestingly, lower incidence, prevalence and intensity of infection have been noted among children who have received BCG.

Trichuriasis

Epidemiology

T. trichiura, the whipworm, has a global distribution, most prevalent in warm, humid climates, and infects about 900 million people worldwide.

Parasite and life cycle

Infection occurs when eggs contaminating soil, food or fomites are swallowed. Larvae are liberated in the caecum, penetrate the crypts of Lieberkühn and migrate within the mucosa. Mature adult worms are 2–5 cm long, the thinner anterior half of the body being normally partly buried in the mucosa of the large bowel of the host (caecum, colon and rectum). They feed on tissue juices, not blood. Female worms release several thousand eggs per day. After about 2 weeks' development in warm, moist soil, the eggs are embryonated and infective.

Interestingly, *T. suis*, the swine whipworm, which does not develop to maturity in humans, has been used in the management of pro-inflammatory autoimmune diseases such as Crohns disease because of its ability to secrete, so far undefined, molecules that create an anti-inflammatory local environment.

Clinical features

Most infections are asymptomatic. Heavy infestations may cause severe gastrointestinal symptoms resembling inflammatory bowel disease. Bleeding from the friable mucosa may result in iron-deficiency anaemia in children on poor diets. Chronic infection is associated with growth retardation. Severe trichuris dysentery syndrome frequently leads to rectal prolapse.

Investigations

The diagnosis is obvious in children presenting with rectal prolapse when adult worms can be seen attached to the mucosa of prolapsed bowel. In other circumstances, the characteristic eggs may be identified in the stool. Concentration techniques can be used for light infections; however, if eggs cannot be found on direct examination, the infection is unlikely to be of clinical significance. Trichuriasis may cause a significant eosinophilia.

Management

A single oral dose of mebendazole 500 mg is more effective than albendazole 400 mg. Severe infections require either mebendazole 100 mg twice daily for 3 days, or albendazole 400 mg daily for 3 days. Single dose combination treatment using albendazole 400 mg plus ivermectin 200 µg/kg is also highly effective. More recently, nitazoxanide has also been shown to be effective.

Prevention

Prevention consists of simple standard methods of improved hygiene and sanitation. Periodic mass chemotherapy of vulnerable schoolchildren and women of childbearing age is currently being promoted by the WHO.

Toxocariasis

info on parasites?!

Epidemiology

Young children are at the greatest risk of infection with *Toxocara canis* and *T. cati*, parasitic round-worms of dogs and cats. Seroprevalence may exceed 80% among children in poorer communities. Sandpits in public parks fouled by dog faeces are particularly notorious as sources of infection.

Parasite and life cycle

Infection in humans occurs following the ingestion of eggs in sand or soil contaminated by dog or cat faeces. The larva from the ingested egg is released in the intestine, which then goes on a prolonged safari through the tissues, lasting 1–2 years. Worms seldom develop beyond the larval stage, so do not reach maturity in the intestine. Thus, eggs are not excreted in human faeces.

Clinical features, investigations and management

Clinical disease is relatively uncommon and depends on the intensity of infection and the organs involved. There are two distinct clinical syndromes: visceral and ocular.

Visceral larva migrans

Visceral larva migrans (VLM) is caused by migrating larvae. Pneumonitis, fever, abdominal pain, myalgia, lymphadenopathy, hepatosplenomegaly, sleep and behavioural disturbances and focal or generalized convulsions can occur. Investigations commonly reveal eosinophilia, anaemia, hyper-gammaglobulinaemia and elevated titres of blood group isohaemagglutinins. Serological diagnosis may be established using an ELISA.

The treatment of choice for VLM is albendazole 10 mg/kg/day for 5 days. Alternatives include mebendazole 100 mg twice daily for 5 days, tiabendazole 50 mg/kg/day in three divided doses for at least 5 days or diethylcarbamazine 3 mg/kg thrice daily for 21 days. Symptomatic treatment with bronchodilators, steroids or antihistamines may also be indicated.

Ocular larva migrans

Ocular larva migrans (OLM) may occur in lighter infections. A larva invades the eye producing a granulomatous reaction, usually in the retina, resulting in visual disturbance or blindness in the affected eye. This may present as strabismus or go unnoticed. The diagnosis is sometimes made by chance on routine opthalmoscopy. The appearance is usually of choroidoretinitis with a mass lesion, which may be mistaken for a retinoblastoma. Serology is usually positive. Antibody detection in vitreous fluid is more sensitive and specific. Patients with eye involvement seldom have eosinophilia or other evidence of generalized VLM.

Topical or systemic steroids are indicated in the management of acute OLM. There is no consistent evidence of benefit from the additional use of antihelmintics. Destruction of the larva is possible using laser photocoagulation. Steroids may also be useful in exacerbations of chronic OLM. Surgery is often required for adhesions.

The terms 'covert' or 'occult' toxocariasis are sometimes used in situations where serology is positive, eosinophilia is absent or low and symptoms are absent or relatively mild and more chronic than those described in VLM. Treatment is not usually indicated for asymptomatic infections.

Prevention and public health measures

In most urban environments, children have to compete with increasing numbers of domestic pets for diminishing open spaces where they can play safely. Pet owners are advised to regularly deworm their dogs and cats and keep them away from children's play areas. In many towns and cities, protected play areas are provided for children in public parks. There are also designated areas for pet owners to exercise their animals, and pet owners are legally required to clean up if their animals defecate in a public area. Even so, when playing football in most public parks, you are as likely to be fouled by dog faeces as by a member of the opposing team.

Further reading

Awasti S, Bundy DAP, Savioli L. Helminthic infections. *Br Med J* 2003; 327: 431–433. [Concise review of rationale for global control, and role of helminths in causing cognitive impairment in children.]

Bethony J, Brooker S, Albonico M, *et al*. Soil-transmitted helminth infections: ascariasis, trichuriasis, and hookworm. *Lancet* 2006; 367: 1521–1532. [Excellent comprehensive review focusing on three of the most important helminth infections in humans.]

Information on WHO's programme for reducing the global burden of soil-transmitted helminth infections can be accessed via http://www.who.int/intestinal_worms/en/index.html.

World Health Organization. Guidelines for the evaluation of soil-transmitted helminthiasis and schistosomiasis at community level. WHO/CTD/SIP/98.1 http://www.who.int/ctd/intpara/98–1.pdf. [This manual has been compiled to assist health planners at national, regional or district levels in the organization, management and evaluation of surveys on soil-transmitted helminthiasis and schistosomiasis for the development and implementation of control activities.]

Chapter 25

Viral hepatitis

The differential diagnosis of jaundice in the tropics includes a variety of causes that are seen less often in developed countries (Table 25.1). Schistosomiasis does not usually cause jaundice, but schistosomal liver damage frequently coexists with chronic viral hepatitis. Many of the infectious causes of jaundice are common in childhood and are less likely in the differential diagnosis of a jaundiced adult in the tropics (e.g. glandular fever group, hepatitis A). The history should always include careful questioning about the past and present use of alcohol, 'western' drugs and traditional herbal remedies, many of which can be hepatotoxic. Non-alcoholic fatty liver disease is becoming increasingly important as a cause of 'cryptogenic' cirrhosis in the tropics. This chapter focuses on the effects and prevention of hepatitis A, B, C, D and E in a tropical context.

General clinicoepidemiological features

The acute syndromes produced by hepatitis A, B, D or E are indistinguishable clinically except that acute hepatitis B patients are a little more likely to experience generalized arthralgia and

Lecture Notes: Tropical Medicine, 6th edition.
By G.V. Gill and N.J. Beeching. Published 2009 by Blackwell Publishing, ISBN: 978-1-4051-8048-1.

rashes than patients with the other viruses, and acute hepatitis C rarely causes symptoms severe enough to seek medical treatment. In all cases, a prodrome of malaise, nausea and vomiting, fever and often diarrhoea leads to a phase of jaundice with dark urine and pale faeces. This is often followed by a cholestatic phase, especially in older adults in whom the recovery period can take several months.

No drugs have been shown to alter the course of acute hepatitis caused by these viruses. This includes the ayurvedic remedy 'Liv-52', popular in the Indian subcontinent, vitamin injections and steroids. Full supportive therapy may be required for patients with severe liver failure, which is characterized by an altered (and falling) level of consciousness, metabolic flap of outstretched hands, ascites, peripheral oedema and a rising international normalized ratio (INR) or prothrombin ratio. Such patients have a high mortality and should be transferred early to a specialist centre if possible.

The water- and food-borne viruses, hepatitis A and E, have no significant chronic sequelae or carriage state, whereas the parenterally and sexually transmitted viruses, hepatitis B, C and D, can cause long-term problems in those patients who go on to become chronic carriers. The effects are worse in patients with dual infection (e.g. hepatitis B plus C) and especially with concurrent alcohol abuse, and in the tropics schistosomal

Table 25.1 Some causes of jaundice in the tropics

Prehepatic	Hepatic	Posthepatic
Haemolysis (e.g. favism with G6PD deficiency)	Viral hepatitis	Pigment gallstones
	Q fever	Hydatid in biliary tree
Haemoglobinopathies	Drugs	Ectopic ascariasis
Sepsis	Traditional medicines	Opisthorchis/Clonorchis infection
Malaria	Leptospirosis	Gall bladder cancer (associated with typhoid carriage)
	Yellow fever	
	Toxins, for example, acute aflatoxin poisoning	Cholangiocarcinoma (associated with Opisthorchis/Clonorchis)

hepatic fibrosis commonly coexists with chronic viral hepatitis.

Hepatitis A

Hepatitis A virus (HAV) is a single-stranded RNA virus, which is primarily spread by the faeco-oral route. It is so common in the tropics that almost all individuals in a developing country will have the infection by the age of 10 years, although most will not realize this because young children rarely have significant symptoms. Adults are more likely to become jaundiced, and those over 40 years have a small risk of dying from fulminant hepatitis.

The incubation period is 2–6 weeks, and most patients already have detectable anti-HAV IgM antibodies in their blood by the time they develop symptoms. Over time, the IgM antibody is lost and is replaced by a long-lasting anti-HAV IgG response, with solid immunity (i.e. second infections are very rare). Patients excrete virus from before the onset of jaundice and are infectious to others who do not wash their hands after contact.

Hepatitis A is mainly a problem for travellers to the developing world. Paradoxically, the older a 'western' person is, the more likely they are to have had hepatitis A in childhood before sanitation was improved. However, the minority of older adults who have no immunity may have substantial morbidity or mortality if they acquire HAV during a visit to the tropics.

There are no significant clinical interactions with HIV, except that individuals with very low CD4 counts are less likely to seroconvert after hepatitis A immunization.

Prevention is very effectively provided by active immunization with hepatitis A vaccine, followed by a booster 6–12 months later to produce life-long immunity. Anti-HAV IgG levels are not measured routinely to monitor vaccine response. Passive immunity can be provided by intramuscular gamma globulin made from sera of individuals known or presumed to be immune; however, this is rarely used in the modern era.

Some tropical countries such as Singapore have experienced such an improvement in standard of living that children are no longer exposed to HAV in childhood, but are becoming symptomatically affected at a later age. In such a setting, active immunization of the population might become appropriate, but, in general, HAV vaccines have little role in the tropics except for travellers.

Hepatitis B

Hepatitis B virus (HBV) is a major cause of death worldwide, with 1–2 million deaths per year mainly because of the sequelae of chronic liver disease and hepatocellular carcinoma (HCC). The DNA virus replicates in the hepatocytes which then express antigens such as HBsAg (surface antigen) on their surface, provoking both cell-mediated and humoral responses. These cause liver cell destruction associated with a rise in transaminases and clinical hepatitis, followed by loss of the circulating antigens HBsAg and HBeAg, and a rise in antibodies anti-HBs, anti-HBc and anti-HBe (Figure 25.1). Thus, the marker for current hepatitis B infection is HBsAg (and HBV DNA) in blood. A positive anti-HBc antibody test represents exposure to HBV at any time, and a positive anti-HBs antibody alone is a marker for past immunization. In some cases, immunity is insufficient to clear all the infected hepatocytes and the patient becomes a carrier, defined as having detectable hepatitis B (HBsAg) for over 6 months. Carriers with high HBV DNA levels usually have positive HBeAg tests, and 'HBeAg seroconversion' with loss of HBeAg and rise in anti-HBe antibody is a surrogate for reduced HBV DNA levels (Figure 25.2). The presence of chronic liver disease (e.g. chronic active hepatitis) can only be determined by clinical examination, by checking liver function tests and by liver biopsy, in addition to serological tests. In future, imaging modalities tests such as the 'Fibroscan' may be accepted as a surrogate for liver biopsy. Point-of-care tests are increasingly used in the tropics to detect HBsAg, but there are concerns that their sensitivity and specificity require further validation in African settings, particularly in HIV-coinfected patients.

Chronic carriage is currently conceptualized as going through four phases over a lifetime, associated with rises and falls in HBV DNA levels which are related to the risk of developing HCC. During the first 'immune-tolerant' phase, there are high HBV DNA levels and little immune reaction damaging infected hepatocytes, and hence normal liver function tests. During the second phase, which typically occurs in early adulthood, there is increased recruitment of cell-mediated immunity, with active hepatitis which may lead to partial clearance of HBV, characterized by loss of HBeAg, appearance of anti-HBe antibody and reduced HBV DNA levels. However, there is wide variation in the age at which this phase commences, and it may persist rather than leading to HBeAg seroconversion. A third prolonged phase follows with low-grade chronic hepatitis, and this can occasionally lead to complete clearance of hepatitis B, with loss of HBsAg and circulating HBV DNA. Finally, in some patients, a fourth phase develops with rising HBV DNA levels, associated with emergence of 'precore mutant' HBeAg, increased activity in the liver and a new rise in transaminases. The patient is now more infectious and at increased risk of developing HCC. This phase

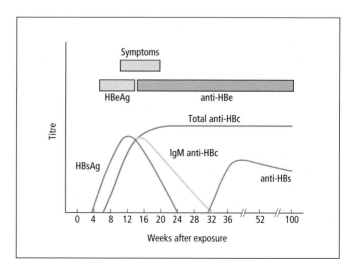

Figure 25.1 Acute hepatitis B virus (HBV) infection, followed by recovery.

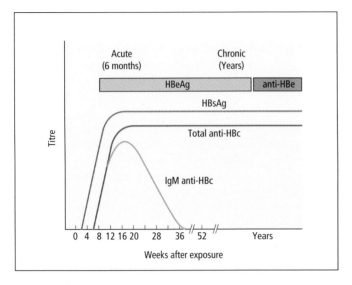

Figure 25.2 Progression of acute to chronic hepatitis B virus (HBV) infection (two patterns). Presence of HBeAg is used as a surrogate for high HBV DNA levels.

may not be detected unless liver function is monitored, together with HBV DNA levels (rarely available in the tropics), as the precore mutant is not detectable by the ELISA tests used to monitor HBeAg levels.

Conditions that favour infection progressing to carriage include the neonatal state, chronic illness, such as renal failure, and immunosuppression because of HIV or chemotherapy. Immunosuppressed individuals may have high levels of virus but no illness, because the destruction of liver cells relies on having a strong immune response. If this is improved (e.g. by successful antiretroviral therapy or by stopping chemotherapy), patients with chronic carriage may paradoxically develop severe hepatitis.

Infants infected at the time of birth have a 90% chance of becoming carriers, this risk falling to 10% after infection at 1 year of life and to less than 5% for adults. In the Far East, Polynesia and West Africa, 30–50% of carriers are infected from their mothers at birth and most of the rest are infected by uncertain means in early childhood. This tends to cluster in families with a carrier mother. In such populations, carriage rates in adults are high (≥8%) and carriers tend to have

high levels of circulating virus. In other parts of the tropics, most infections are acquired in childhood or infancy, and intermediate HBsAg prevalence rates between 2% and 7% are seen in adults (Figure 25.3; Table 25.2).

In industrialized countries, sexual transmission and shared drug-injecting paraphernalia are the major routes of transmission in adulthood. Sexual transmission is important in the tropics, but the major threat in this setting is nosocomial and/or iatrogenic hepatitis caused by the reuse of needles and infusion sets. Other factors contributing to the spread of HBV in the tropics include traditional practices such as scarification or circumcision using non-sterile instruments, tattooing, acupuncture and barbering practices. Bedbugs (but not mosquitoes) have a small role in transmission in some settings, but control of bedbugs has little effect on reducing transmission.

Treatment for chronic HBV is only appropriate for those with high HBV DNA levels. Endpoints are easier to define for HBeAg positive carriers, for whom the aim is to convert them to anti-HBe antibody positivity. A small minority subsequently lose HBsAg as well, after a delay of several years. For patients with precore mutant HBeAg, the only

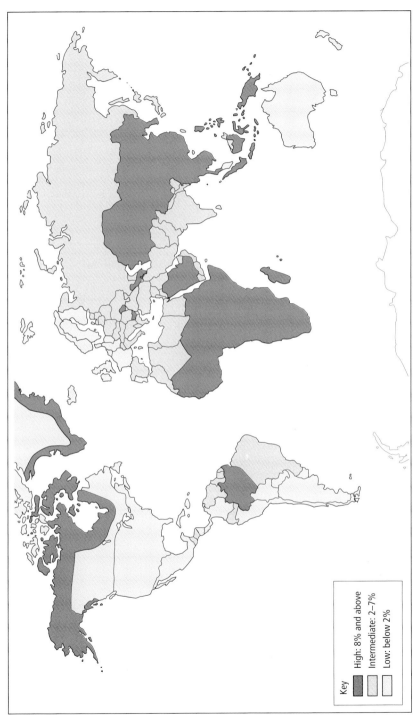

Figure 25.3 Patterns of HBsAg endemicity as defined by WHO.

Key

High: 8% and above

Intermediate: 2–7%

Low: below 2%

Table 25.2 Patterns of hepatitis B prevalence (WHO definitions)

Prevalence	Adults with HBsAg (%)	Anti-HBc (%)	Incidence of infection Infant	Child	Adult	Location
High	8–20	70–95	+++	++++	++	China, South East Asia, Polynesia, West Africa
Intermediate	2–7	20–60	++	+++	++	South West Asia, eastern Europe, East and Central Africa, South and Central America
Low	<2	2–6	+	−	+	North, West and Central Europe, North America, Australia

measurable endpoint is reduction in HBV DNA levels (or subsequent loss of HBsAg). Two approaches are currently favoured, using injectable interferons or oral nucleoside analogues. Pegylated interferon given as a weekly subcutaneous injection for 12 months will induce HBeAg seroconversion in about 30% of carefully selected patients. This option is better than high-dose interferon α (IFN-α) injections given three times a week. Both types of interferon are very expensive, carry significant side effects and require regular injections. On the plus side, there is no emergence of resistant virus if treatment fails, and if it succeeds, the effect is usually durable and further treatment is not required. The second approach is the prescription of oral nucleoside reverse transcriptase inhibitors as long-term suppressive therapy. Lamivudine was the first drug to be used, and other agents include adefovir, tenofovir and entecavir. This is a rapidly changing area, which is hampered by predictable emergence of drug-resistant virus when patients take monotherapy. Although cheaper in the medium term than interferons, with similar or slightly lower success in inducing HBeAg seroconversion, it carries significant risk of emergence of untreatable virus in those that do not respond. Further trials of double and triple therapy regimens and of new agents are in progress. All are limited by cost and side effects, and require specialist supervision.

Treatment of HIV-coinfected patients is even more complex, as lamivudine-resistant HBV emerges very fast in HIV-positive patients who receive ART such as Triomune, a common triple

regimen in sub-Saharan Africa, containing lamivudine without a second antiretroviral that also has anti-HBV activity. In resource-rich settings, a typical ART regimen for such patients would include tenofovir and lamivudine or emtricitabine, but this is not readily available in much of sub-Saharan Africa, where 10–20% of HIV-positive patients have HBV coinfection. Patients with coinfection will often experience immune reconstitution-related flares of hepatic activity after starting any form of ART, and there are theoretical concerns that these could be severe if effective anti-HBV treatment is stopped at this point, leading to a rapid rise of HBV DNA concurrent with improved cell-mediated immune activity. Conversely, coinfected patients who do not require ART for their HIV but require HBV treatment should not receive drugs such as lamivudine alone, as this may prejudice their future HIV treatment by encouraging emergence of drug-resistant HIV. Overall, HBV is thought to upregulate HIV and vice versa, and it is likely but not established that each promotes perinatal transmission of the other virus. The significance of possible effects of HBV on the natural history of HIV and on the response of HIV to ART remain controversial and need further study.

Hepatitis B immunization

Very effective vaccines against hepatitis B have been available for over three decades, containing HBsAg. This may be harvested from the plasma of chronic HBV carriers, and cheap vaccines from this source were routinely used in the tropics until recently, but are now being replaced by recombinant vaccines with support from the GAVI Alliance. The vaccine is effective in neonates, and three doses of vaccine produce a long-lasting response in 80–90% of children and young adults. Vaccine schedules 'approved' for western licensing are usually 0, 1 and 6 months, or 0, 1, 2 and 12 months (booster fourth dose), or 0, 7 and 21 days followed by a late booster at 12 months. However, many other strategies are in use and it can be given alongside other Extended Programme on Immunization (EPI) scheduled vaccines in infancy. In western practice, it is usual to confirm seroconversion only in people at continued risk of infection, such as health care workers or partners or children of carriers. Seroconversion is defined as a rise in anti-HBs antibody >10 units/L, 4–6 weeks after the third dose of vaccine. With or without such confirmation, a final booster vaccination 5 years later should provide life-long protection.

Factors that reduce the efficacy of active immunization include male gender, age >40 years, smoking tobacco and immunosuppression for any reason. The vaccine must be given into muscle (deltoid or thigh), and inappropriate administration into adipose tissue (e.g. buttocks) is ineffective. Active vaccination can be given at the same time as passive immunization with hyperimmune hepatitis B immunoglobulin (HBIg), a strategy that is used in some countries for extra, early protection of infants born to HBeAg-positive (high-grade) carrier mothers. Immunization of infants within 48h of birth prevents almost all such transmissions, which is usually perinatal rather than intrauterine.

Large community-based studies in different parts of the tropics and in Italy have shown that infant or childhood vaccination programmes reduce the rate of infection by 90% or more. Most of the few who do become infected have subclinical disease, and very few become carriers. The protective effects in reducing community rates of infection, hepatitis B carriage and hepatocellular carcinoma persist for at least 15–20 years after

such programmes, without further boosters being administered.

Over 150 countries have adopted policies of universal immunization against HBV. This depends on adequate supplies of affordable vaccine, which in turn requires an intact cold chain to maintain vaccine potency. In most tropical settings, the majority of infections occur in infancy or early childhood, and universal infant immunization is therefore the most appropriate strategy. Subsequent boosters are not needed in tropical settings. In western settings, in which infections predominantly occur in infants and children of carrier mothers or in adolescence and early adulthood, selective immunization of children of identified carriers may be employed. However, it is more difficult to then arrange for universal or selective adolescent or adult immunization, and most countries have opted for universal immunization in early childhood.

Hepatitis D

Hepatitis D virus (HDV, formerly delta hepatitis) resembles some plant viruses in that it is incomplete. The outer coat is derived from hepatitis B surface antigen, which means that the virus can only infect individuals who have acute hepatitis B or who are chronic HBV carriers. The virus is transmitted by the same routes as HBV, and two epidemiological and clinical patterns are seen, so called 'coinfection' and 'superinfection'. Patients who are infected by hepatitis B and D viruses at the same time (coinfection) have clinical acute hepatitis that is no more severe than hepatitis B alone, and are no more or less likely to progress to chronic liver carriage and disease. More importantly, chronic HBV carriers who acquire acute hepatitis D (superinfection) are likely to develop fulminant hepatitis with a high mortality rate. In western and tropical settings, where intravenous drug misuse is a problem, the clue to the arrival and spread of the virus is an epidemic of severe liver disease with high mortality in drug users. In tropical settings, similar epidemics are seen in previously asymptomatic HBV carriers of all ages. Such epidemics are regularly reported in South America, examples being epidemics of 'L'abrea' or 'Santa Marta' fever. The epidemiological clue is the high proportion of affected patients who develop severe or fatal disease, and would be confirmed by the detection of both HBV antigens and anti-HDV antibody responses. However, the latter serological tests are rarely available in a tropical setting.

As HDV only affects patients with concurrent acute or chronic HBV, it is prevented by immunization against hepatitis B and by other control measures used to prevent nosocomial or sexual transmission of hepatitis B.

Hepatitis C

Hepatitis C virus (HCV) is an RNA virus that is predominantly spread by blood–blood contact, and reuse of syringes and infusion equipment is responsible for high rates of hepatitis C endemicity in many parts of the tropics. Other factors encouraging blood–blood contact are also likely to be important in a tropical setting, as for HBV. Sexual and perinatal transmission of HCV is relatively inefficient but accounts for low background prevalence rates. However, the risk of sexual and perinatal transmission rises to about 10% if the 'donor' is also HIV positive. The prevalence of anti-HCV antibodies in Egypt and parts of Yemen is extraordinarily high, affecting over one-third of adults aged >40 years. This is because of past well-intentioned mass treatments of populations with tartar emetic for endemic schistosomiasis. The same syringes were used sequentially for many people, resulting in the largest described iatrogenic epidemic of a blood-borne virus in the world.

Hepatitis C rarely causes symptomatic acute hepatitis, but 70–80% of those infected will become chronic carriers, and there is a prolonged 'window' of antibody seronegativity of 2–3 months (ranging up to 6 months) after initial infection. Molecular methods (PCR) are now routinely used in western settings to detect early infection and to confirm the presence of viraemia in patients who are anti-HCV antibody positive. Like HIV, HCV has different genotypic groups and a very high rate of viral turnover, leading to

frequent mutations of viral quasispecies, so immunity is not solid and patients can be reinfected by HCV after successful treatment.

Chronic HCV is defined by the presence of viraemia for more than 6 months, associated with abnormal hepatic histology (on liver biopsy) and/or abnormal liver function tests. Normal liver function tests do not exclude abnormal histology, so liver biopsy is often part of the full workup of patients. The natural history is still poorly understood, and patients who have had single or few exposures to small amounts of virus seem less likely to progress. Overall, the '20' rule applies: 20% of patients initially infected will clear the virus (but still remain antibody positive). Of the remaining 80%, 20% will develop significant liver disease over 20 years. Of those with cirrhosis, up to 20% might develop HCC over a further 20 years. The most important determinant for the development of serious liver disease and HCC is concurrent alcohol abuse, and the most important aspect of clinical management is to persuade chronic carriers to reduce or discontinue their alcohol intake.

Other factors that favour more rapid progression (and also resistance to treatment) include older age, obesity, male gender, infection with genotypes other than genotypes 2 or 3 and the presence of stainable iron in liver biopsies. In counselling patients, it is important to emphasize that most will not develop clinically apparent liver disease, and that the main risk to partners and families is sharing of needles and other sharps such as razors, nail scissors and toothbrushes. In trop-ical settings, concurrent infection with hepatitis B and/or schistosomiasis is common and worsens the prognosis, as does HIV infection. A minority of HIV-positive individuals develop fulminant or rapidly progressive HCV for unknown reasons.

Treatment is expensive but increasingly effective. The current optimum regimens include weekly injections of pegylated (PEG) IFN-α, together with daily oral ribavirin for 6–12 months, producing viral remission in over 50% of cases. Genotypes 2 and 3 will be cured in 75% of cases by treatment for 6 months, compared to about 40% of other genotypes treated for a year. Treatment can be discontinued if not effective (PCR test negativity or substantial drop in HCV RNA levels) early in the course of treatment. Similar results are obtained in HIV-coinfected patients. There are no immediate prospects for vaccination, and the only means of control is to educate health care workers and others not to reuse any kind of injection or infusion equipment. Intravenous drug misusers (most are anti-HCV antibody positive within 3 years of starting injecting) should not share any kind of injecting equipment, including water and spoons or cookers used to dissolve drugs. Monogamous couples may choose not to start to use condoms (as the risks are small), but HCV carriers should otherwise be encouraged to use condoms with new partners. There is no evidence against breast-feeding.

Hepatitis E

Hepatitis E virus (HEV) is another virus spread by the faeco-oral route, usually by the contamination of water supplies, with a similar incubation period and clinical outcome to HAV infection. The key difference from HAV is that immunity after natural infection is not solid, so that older children and adults can suffer repeated symptomatic infections. Large epidemics that affect people of all ages have been described in the Indian subcontinent and central Asia for over 50 years, whereas epidemics of HAV primarily affect children. It is also well recognized in Mexico and North Africa (Figure 25.4) but increasingly diagnosed in other areas in Africa. HEV is less common in western countries unless there is a history of travel to the tropics or of contact with a recent traveller, but it is increasingly recognized as a cause of subclinical infection and as a cause of 'cryptogenic' acute hepatitis. Some of this is zoonotic in origin, with links to pig farming and butchering, and to the consumption of under-cooked deer or badger meat.

HEV is endemic in the Indian subcontinent, where it accounts for the majority of symptomatic acute viral hepatitis admissions to hospital of both adults and children. Like HAV, there are usually no chronic sequelae, although progressive chronic infection has recently been described in transplant patients, and further clinical–epidemiological studies are essential worldwide.

The second major difference from other forms of viral hepatitis is the high incidence of fulminant hepatitis in pregnant women, with a mortality of 30–50%, particularly in the later stages of pregnancy. Perinatal transmission also occurs with a high mortality in infants who are infected.

Diagnosis is by detection of anti-HEV IgM followed by anti-HEV IgG antibodies. However, assays are not well standardized and titres of both antibodies decline rapidly (within 1–2 years), so detection of antibodies late after infection is problematic. Passive immunization with pooled immunoglobulin from donors living in endemic areas is not effective. A very effective vaccine has been produced and tested in Nepal. Unfortunately, the protective immunity declines within a year or two, and the vaccine may find use in military settings but is not likely to be available for other travellers in its current formulation.

Hepatocellular carcinoma (hepatoma)

This aggressive tumour is common in the tropics, and is multifactorial in aetiology. Any patient with chronic active hepatitis is at risk, especially if cirrhosis has developed. Both chronic HBV and HCV are important causes, particularly if patients abuse alcohol. In many parts of the tropics, aflatoxins ingested in food are epidemiologically important as primary or cofactor causes, although it is usually impossible to determine this in individual patients.

Patients usually present at a late stage with several months of weight loss, a painful hard irregular mass in an enlarged liver, often with ascites which may be bloodstained. Other signs of chronic liver disease may be obvious, and a 'bruit' or arteriovenous hum can be heard on auscultation over the liver. This is almost pathognomonic of hepatoma, although a 'bruit' can occasionally be heard over the liver in acute alcoholic hepatitis. Ultrasound shows diffuse infiltration of the

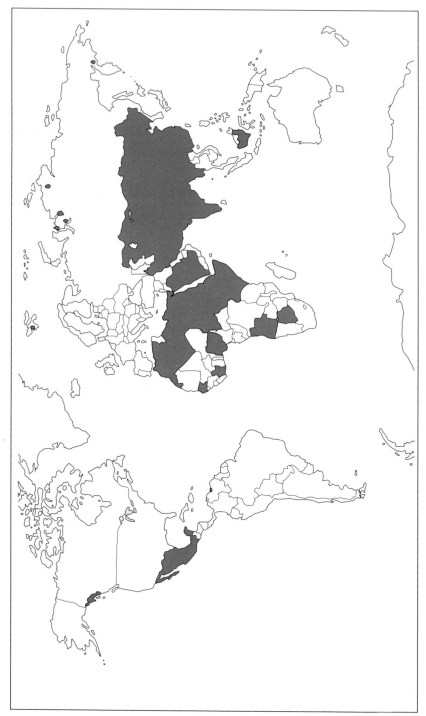

Figure 25.4 Countries with recognized hepatitis E outbreaks (after WHO).

liver by one or more tumours, often with central necrosis, which may resemble metastases from other sites. The other main differential diagnosis is acute amoebic liver abscess, which has a more acute presentation, typical ultrasound appearances, peripheral neutrophil leucocytosis and positive amoebic antibody tests. Most HCC patients have very elevated levels of alpha-fetoprotein in the serum, although this is absent in a minority. By the time that patients present with symptoms, the prognosis is very poor. Surgical removal, embolization and chemoembolization can all be attempted, and liver transplantation may be possible in some cases. In most resource-poor settings, the only therapeutic option is palliation.

Prevention is by measures to control HBV and HCV infections, and countries that have initiated mass infant HBV immunization programmes have experienced marked fall in HCC incidence. Control of alcohol abuse is also important, especially in those with chronic HBV or HCV carriage.

Further reading and other resources

Centers for Disease Control—National Center for Infectious Diseases. Viral hepatitis www.cdc.gov/ncidod/diseases/hepatitis/ index.htm. [Western-orientated patient information sheets, detailed statements of best practice and large downloadable teaching slide sets. First source for hepatitis C.]

Fattovich G, Bortolotti F, Donato F. Natural history of chronic hepatitis B: special emphasis on disease progression and prognostic factors. *J Hepatol* 2008; 48: 335–352. [Review of current thoughts on staging and progression of hepatitis B.]

Frank C, Mohamed MK, Strickland GT *et al*. The role of parenteral antischistosomal therapy in the spread of hepatitis C virus in Egypt. *Lancet* 2000; 355: 887–891. [Describes the largest single iatrogenic blood-borne virus epidemic in the world.]

GAVI Alliance. www.gavialliance.org/. [Formerly the Global Alliance for Vaccines and Immunization, this alliance of public health institutions, industry and donors underpins development and provision of vaccines to many resource-poor settings.]

Viral Hepatitis Prevention Board. www.vhpb.org. [Pressure group with industry funding. Large numbers of useful PowerPoint presentations and region-specific reports particularly related to epidemiology and prevention of hepatitis A and B.]

WHO website. www.who.int/csr/disease/hepatitis/resources/en/. [Excellent essays, illustrations, maps about all aspects, with extensive electronic links to online resources and full scientific referencing for those who want more information. First port of call for hepatitis A, B, D and E.]

Chapter 26

Liver and intestinal flukes

Food-borne trematodes include liver, lung and intestinal flukes. One-fifth of the world's population is at risk from these infections, which are endemic in at least 100 countries, half of which are among the poorest in the world. Forty million people are infected and there are at least 10 000 deaths per year. Praziquantel is the drug of choice for most food-borne trematode infections. However, a notable exception is *Fasciola hepatica*, for which triclabendazole is the drug of choice.

Liver flukes

Epidemiology

F. hepatica and *F. gigantica* occur in sheep- and cattle-rearing areas worldwide, notably in the South American Andes, especially Bolivia and Peru.

Parasites and life cycles

In common with other flukes, the life cycles of *F. hepatica* and *F. gigantica* involve certain species of freshwater snail that are infected by miracidia liberated from eggs passed in herbivore (or human) faeces. The snails act as intermediate amplifying hosts, eventually liberating free-swimming cercariae which encyst as metacercariae on water plants.

Lecture Notes: Tropical Medicine, 6th edition.
By G.V. Gill and N.J. Beeching. Published 2009 by Blackwell Publishing, ISBN: 978-1-4051-8048-1.

Human infection occurs when the metacercarial cysts on raw water vegetables (e.g. watercress) are eaten, or are swallowed with contaminated water. These excyst in the duodenum, releasing larvae which then penetrate the intestinal wall and migrate via the peritoneal cavity to the liver. Having penetrated the liver capsule, they make their way to the bile ducts, where they mature into adults. Maturation in the human host takes 3–4 months. Adult flukes can survive for up to 10 years.

Clinical features

Acute symptoms, including fever, malaise, abdominal pain, weight loss, urticaria and respiratory symptoms, caused by migrating flukes may develop 6–12 weeks after infection. Tender hepatomegaly may be evident. Liver enzymes are sometimes mildly elevated. Ectopic flukes can cause granuloma or abscess formation in various organs and migrating erythematous cutaneous nodules, a form of cutaneous larva migrans, may also be seen. Mature flukes in the bile ducts may initially cause fever, anorexia and abdominal pain.

Symptoms usually subside spontaneously once the adult flukes have made themselves at home. Blood loss into the bile resulting in anaemia occurs in heavy infections. Chronic symptoms include recurrent cholangitis or intermittent biliary obstruction in a minority of patients and fatigue which can persist for more than 10 years.

Investigations

Eosinophilia is common. Ultrasound is usually normal. CT scan of the liver may reveal numerous hypodense lesions, and peripheral branched hypodense hepatic lesions, best seen on CT using contrast, are relatively specific for fascioliasis. Serology may be helpful in diagnosing *F. hepatica* infections towards the end of the acute phase when eggs are still unlikely to be present in faeces. Blood spots can be collected on filter paper for later serological testing in large-scale surveys. Serology is less reliable for *F. gigantica*. In established infections, eggs may be present in faeces or in bile aspirate. Concentration techniques may be required. Fasciola excretory–secretory (FES) antigen detection in faeces is useful both in prepatent and patent infections with *F. hepatica*.

Management

In contrast to other fluke infections, praziquantel is unreliable in the treatment of fascioliasis.

Triclabendazole, a new benzimidazole with few side effects, has become the drug of choice for treating *F. hepatica*. A single dose of 10 mg/kg taken with food is usually effective. This may be repeated after 12 h in severe infections. Biliary colic, associated with the expulsion of dead or damaged parasites, commonly occurs 3–7 days after treatment and responds well to antispasmodic therapy. Unfortunately, cases resistant to triclabendazole have been reported in Ireland, UK and Australia.

Bithionol, 30–50 mg/kg/day in three divided doses on alternate days for 10–15 days, was the preferred treatment previously. Side effects include mild gastrointestinal upset and pruritus.

Recently, nitazoxanide, 500 mg every 12 h for 7 days, has proven to be an effective treatment for adults with *F. hepatica*.

Prevention and public health aspects

Avoid eating potentially contaminated watercress and other water plants. Treatment of herbivores and snail control measures may sometimes be feasible. A promising vaccine is currently under development for use in sheep.

Oriental liver flukes

Epidemiology

Opisthorchis sinensis (also known as *Clonorchis sinensis*) and *O. viverrini* affect about 20 million people in China and South East Asia. *O. felineus*, a related species, occurs in eastern Europe and Russia. Animal hosts include domestic dogs and cats. This has important implications for control programmes.

Parasites and life cycles

Eggs passed in human or animal faeces on contact with freshwater release miracidia that infect and multiply in certain species of freshwater snail which act as intermediate amplifying hosts. The snails eventually liberate free-swimming cercariae that, as metacercariae, encyst on susceptible species of freshwater fish.

Human infection occurs when metacercariae are consumed in raw or undercooked fish, or after ingesting metacercariae contaminating cooking surfaces and utensils. Metacercariae excyst in the small bowel, migrate along the common bile duct and colonize the biliary tree where they mature into adults within about 4 weeks. All adult oriental flukes are hermaphrodite creatures of similar appearance, lanceolate in shape, translucent and brownish in colour. In common with other flukes, they possess two suckers. *O. sinensis* is about 10–25 mm long by 3–5 mm wide. The other species are about half as big.

Clinical features

Most infections are asymptomatic. Heavy initial infections may present with an illness similar to Katayama fever. Patients with established infections may have vague right upper quadrant abdominal pain that typically occurs in the late afternoon and lasts a few hours. Patients may actually complain of feeling something moving about the liver. Other symptoms include lassitude, anorexia, flatulence, diarrhoea and fever. Hepatomegaly may be evident on examination, and heavily infected patients may also be jaundiced. Some patients appear malnourished and are deficient in fat-soluble vitamins.

Recurrent bouts of ascending cholangitis, jaundice and pancreatitis can occur. Biliary cirrhosis and, rarely, cholangiocarcinoma may develop in chronic infections. Cholangiocarcinoma associated with *O. viverrini* is the most common form of liver cancer in north-eastern Thailand, where an estimated 70% of the population are infected with the parasite. In Hong Kong, 15% of all primary liver cancers were found to be cholangiocarcinomas associated with *C. sinensis*. Genetic factors, dietary nitrosamines and aflatoxins have been implicated in the development of this malignancy.

Investigations

Diagnosis is established by identifying characteristic eggs in faeces or in biliary aspirate. Concentration techniques may be required. A number of serological tests are available with a variable range of sensitivity and specificity. A coproantigen test is now available for *O. viverrini*. Ultrasound may reveal gallstones and abnormalities of the biliary tree. Endoscopic retrograde cholangiopancreatography (ERCP) is also useful.

Management

Praziquantel is effective, either 40 mg/kg in a single dose or 25 mg/kg three times in 24 h after meals. A 3-day course should be used for heavy infections.

Prevention and public health aspects

Health education, improving sanitation and annual treatment with praziquantel can dramatically reduce the prevalence of infection and, on the face of it, infection with oriental liver flukes should be easy to prevent by avoiding raw fish. However, food habits are very difficult to change, even with vigorous health education. It seems that once you have tasted well-prepared raw fish, the cooked item never tastes as good.

Intestinal flukes

Fasciolopsis buski, the most important intestinal fluke in humans, is widely distributed from India to South East Asia, particularly in pig-rearing communities. Metacercariae attached to edible water plants, such as the water caltrop, are ingested and after excystation attach to the mucosa of the duodenum and jejunum and develop into adults causing inflammation and ulceration.

Most infections are asymptomatic. Symptoms are more likely to occur in heavy infections, and tend to be most severe in children. These include epigastric pain, vomiting and diarrhoea, initially alternating with constipation but later becoming persistent. Wasting, oedema and ascites may also occur in severe cases. Characteristic eggs, and sometimes adult flukes, can be identified in faeces, and adult flukes sometimes also appear in vomit. Echinostome species, principally found in Asia, can also infect humans causing symptoms similar to *F. buski*. Heterophyids, a group of smaller intestinal flukes affecting humans, cause milder gastrointestinal symptoms than *F. buski*. However, ectopic eggs may be deposited in other organs, for example the CNS, presenting as a space-occupying lesion, and the heart, causing myocarditis or valve damage. Praziquantel is usually effective in the treatment of intestinal flukes.

Further reading

Garcia HH, Moro PL, Schantz PM. Zoonotic helminth infections of humans: echinococcosis, cysticercosis and fascioliasis. *Curr Opin Infect Dis* 2007; 20: 489–494. [Recent review of these important zoonotic infections.]

Gillespie SH, Pearson RD, eds. *Principles and Practice of Clinical Parasitology*. John Wiley and Sons, 2001. Chapters 17 and 24. [This excellent volume on clinical parasitology includes two useful chapters on food-borne trematode infections.]

Chapter 27

Hydatid disease

Hydatid disease results from the larval stage of a small tapeworm of dogs and other canines developing in humans. The infection is a zoonosis, normally maintained in dogs and sheep or cattle in close association with humans (*Echinococcus granulosus*), or in a wild cycle such as in wild canines and rodents (*E. multilocularis*). Most human infections are with *E. granulosus* and are associated with the rearing of sheep and cattle in climatic conditions varying from tropical to subarctic regions. The third, and rarest species of importance in man, is *E. vogeli* which has been reported mainly in southern regions of South America.

Echinococcus granulosus (hydatid cyst disease)

Life cycle

Infected dogs harbour the 3–6 mm adult tapeworms in their small intestine. The worms possess only three proglottids, the end one being mature. The eggs are liberated either before or after the proglottid escapes in the faeces, and contaminate pasture. When ingested by the normal herbivorous intermediate host, the oncospheres liberated in the gut enter the circulation and are trapped in the capillaries of various viscera, where they develop into cysts. A cyst is composed of a sphere of germinal epithelium containing protruding invaginations (brood capsules) and fluid. From the inner surface of the brood capsules, protoscolices develop, invaginated in much the same way as the cysticerci of *Taenia* spp. The whole structure is a hydatid cyst, and it becomes surrounded by fibrous capsule derived from the host tissue. The cyst may develop large daughter cysts in its cavity, each containing more brood capsules. The cyst continues growing for years. Brood capsules that break free from the cyst wall, and individual scolices in the cyst cavity, are called hydatid sand.

Dogs become infected by eating the contents of hydatid cysts in infected carcasses. Sheep or other herbivores become infected by swallowing the *Taenia*-like eggs passed in dog faeces. The strain of *E. granulosus* in the UK that commonly infects horses and has the foxhound as its definitive host is probably not pathogenic for humans. There are several other biological complexes in nature that probably do not pose the risk of human infection.

Clinical features

About 70% of cysts develop in the liver, usually the right lobe, 20% in the lungs and the rest in rarer sites. Cysts may be single or multiple. Symptoms

Lecture Notes: Tropical Medicine, 6th edition.
By G.V. Gill and N.J. Beeching. Published 2009 by
Blackwell Publishing, ISBN: 978-1-4051-8048-1.

are caused by a mass effect produced by the growing cyst, secondary bacterial infection of the cyst or because of leakage of fluid from the cyst. Hepatic cysts are initially asymptomatic until they become large. A non-tender mass may be evident on examination. If secondary bacterial infection occurs, the cyst may mimic a liver abscess. Spillage or leakage of the cyst fluid, during surgery or following rupture, can precipitate hypersensitivity reactions ranging from urticaria, pruritus and fever to fatal anaphylaxis. Secondary cysts may develop following spillage and seeding in the peritoneal cavity. Leakage from a cyst into the biliary tree may cause colic, urticaria and obstructive jaundice, sometimes complicated by secondary bacterial infection.

Most lung cysts are asymptomatic, found incidentally on a chest X-ray (Figure 27.1). Symptomatic patients may complain of fever, dyspnoea, chest pain and cough, occasionally with haemoptysis. Secondary infection may result in development of a lung abscess. Pneumothorax, empyema or a hypersensitivity reaction may occur following rupture into the lung. Seeding of pulmonary cysts is uncommon. Rupture of a cyst into a bronchus may cause the patient to cough up clear salty tasting liquid, sometimes followed by the soft white outer membrane of the cyst. A collapsed cyst may have a characteristic 'water lily' appearance on chest X-ray.

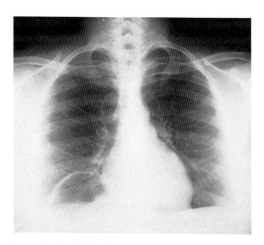

Figure 27.1 A hydatid cyst at the base of the right lung, found in an African patient 'incidentally'.

Hydatid cysts occur at a variety of other sites including spleen, bone (causing pain and pathological fracture), brain (causing convulsions or a mass effect) and eye (causing proptosis and chemosis).

Investigations

Imaging

Ultrasound is useful for abdominal cysts. X-ray, CT or MRI may be useful for detecting cysts elsewhere.

Serology

The specific IgG ELISA antigen B-rich fraction (AgB) is the most sensitive serological test. Others include an enzyme-linked immunotransfer blot (EITB) assay and the double diffusion test for arc 5 (DD5). Current serological tests lack sensitivity for extrahepatic cysts. The DD5 may give false-positive results in patients with cysticercosis.

Others

Urine antigen detection tests are promising. Eosinophilia may follow leakage or rupture of a cyst.

Treatment

In the past, surgical removal was the preferred method of managing accessible cysts. Small cysts can be removed intact. Larger cysts should be carefully aspirated and the aspirate replaced with an equivalent volume of a scolicide, such as hypertonic saline, reaspirated after 5–10 min and the procedure repeated. Following re-aspiration, the cyst cavity is opened, the membranes are removed and the cavity closed. Great care should be taken to avoid spillage of cyst fluid.

Percutaneous aspiration of cysts under ultrasound control is now used increasingly as an alternative to surgery. Following initial aspiration, hypertonic saline is injected into the cyst and reaspirated after 20 min. The procedure is summarized by the acronym PAIR (Puncture, Aspiration, Injection, Re-aspiration).

Indications for PAIR are:
- Non-echoic lesion >5 cm in diameter
- Cysts with daughter cysts and/or with detachment of membranes
- Multiple cysts if accessible to puncture
- Infected cysts

PAIR is also recommended for:
- Pregnant women
- Patients who fail to respond to chemotherapy alone
- Patients in whom surgery is contraindicated
- Patients who refuse surgery
- Patients who relapse after surgery

Contraindications to PAIR are:
- Non-cooperative patients, children <3 years
- Inaccessible or risky location of the cyst (e.g. spine, brain, heart)
- Inactive or calcified lesion
- Cysts communicating with the biliary tree
- Cysts opening into the abdominal cavity, bronchi and urinary tract.

Patients undergoing surgery or PAIR should receive albendazole—either alone or in combination with praziquantel—for 1–3 months prior to, and covering, the procedure. PAIR should be followed by an 8-week course of albendazole. Laparoscopic treatment of hydatid cysts of the liver and spleen is also effective. Anthelmintic treatment may reduce the need for surgery in patients with uncomplicated pulmonary cysts.

Albendazole is useful for patients with inoperable, widespread or numerous cysts and in patients who are unfit for surgery. The course usually recommended is 400 mg twice daily for adults (5–7.5 mg/kg twice daily for children) for 28 days. This is followed by 14 days' rest and then repeated for 3–12 cycles depending on response, although many experts now just give continuous therapy without the 14 days rest periods. Albendazole absorption is enhanced if taken with fatty meals. Albendazole plus praziquantel has been shown to have greater protoscolicidal activity in animal studies and *in vitro* compared with either drug alone. Combined therapy has

been used successfully in managing inoperable spinal, pelvic, abdominal, thoracic and hepatic hydatidosis and as an adjunct to surgery.

Prevention and control

Large-scale programmes involving public health education and strict dog-control measures have led to elimination of hydatid disease in certain regions (Iceland, Cyprus, Australia, Tasmania, New Zealand). Similar programmes have met with less success elsewhere. Recent advances include the development of a promising new recombinant vaccine (EG95) against ovine echinococcus and a vaccine against the dog tapeworm stage.

Alarmingly for Liverpool DTM&H students who enjoy weekend country rambles in Snowdonia, the prevalence of infected dogs in Wales is currently approaching 10%, having more than doubled in the past decade following policy changes in favour of health education instead of regular dosing of dogs with praziquantel. Remember: "boil it, cook it, peel it or leave it" (and don't stroke it or pet it)!

Echinococcus multilocularis (alveolar hydatid disease)

Life cycle

Humans become infected by swallowing the eggs passed by foxes and other Canidae, possibly mainly from contaminated wild ground fruits such as bilberries and their close relatives, lingonberries and cloudberries, widely eaten in northern Europe. Recent surveys in central Europe have extended the known geographical occurrence of *E. multilocularis* in foxes from four countries at the end of the 1980s to at least eleven countries in 1999. Factors with the potential of enhancing the infection risk for humans in the future include increasing fox populations and parasite prevalences, progressing invasion of cities by foxes, the establishment of urban cycles of the parasite and the spillover of the *E. multilocularis* infection from wild carnivores to domestic dogs and cats. Infection is spreading in North America and Japan. An intense focus of infection has been described in Gansu province, China. Various rodents are the intermediate hosts.

Clinical features

Unlike *E. granulosus*, the cyst produces daughter cysts by external and not internal budding, so it tends to invade progressively into surrounding tissues like a malignant tumour and is not contained in a well-defined fibrous capsule. It may be 30 years before a patient becomes symptomatic. The primary site of tissue invasion is usually the liver, mimicking hepatic carcinoma or cirrhosis. Metastatic lesions may occur in other tissues (lung, brain, bone) and are evident in over 10% of patients. Patients usually present with right upper quadrant pain, hepatomegaly and a palpable mass. Complications arise in around 2% of patients, either because of local invasion or as a result of metastatic lesions involving brain, lung or mediastinum. Untreated, 90% of patients die within 10 years of presentation.

Investigations

Ultrasound, CT, MRI and serology are useful in establishing the diagnosis. Histology provides confirmation.

Treatment

Surgical excision is preferred for the primary lesion. Pre- and postoperative treatment with albendazole is recommended. Albendazole 10 mg/kg in cycles of 28 days followed by 14 days' rest is recommended postoperatively and for inoperable patients. Treatment cycles are usually continued for more than 1 year. The optimal duration of treatment remains uncertain. Mebendazole 40–50 mg/kg/day has also been used extensively, sometimes for up to 10 years. Serology may remain positive for several years following successful treatment. A 90% 10-year survival rate is possible with early diagnosis and appropriate treatment.

Further reading

Eckert J, Conraths FJ, Tackmann K. Echinococcosis: an emerging or re-emerging zoonosis? *Int J Parasitol* 2000; 12–13: 1283–1294. [An excellent recent review of the epidemiology and control of human echinococcal infections.]

Garcia HH, Moro PL, Schantz PM. Zoonotic helminth infections of humans: echinococcosis, cysticercosis and fascioliasis. *Curr Opin Infect Dis* 2007; 20: 489–494. [Recent review of these important zoonotic infections.]

PAIR: Puncture, Aspiration, Injection, Re-Aspiration. An option for the treatment of cystic Echinococcosis. WHO/CDS/CSR/APH/2001.6 http://www.who.int/emc-documents/zoonoses/whocdscsraph20016.html. [Practical guidelines and useful images.]

Chapter 28

Pneumonia

Pneumonia is an acute inflammatory disease of lung parenchyma occurring in response to microbial invasion of the distal bronchial tree and alveoli. It is a leading cause of morbidity and mortality in all parts of the world. The incorporation of a chapter on pneumonia in a tropical medicine text underlines the importance of this condition in the developing world—the WHO World Health Report 2000 placed lower respiratory tract infections as the leading global cause of ill health. This chapter also serves to highlight the role of specific pathogens, and the difficulties of management when only limited investigational and therapeutic resources are available.

Microbiology

Streptococcus pneumoniae is the most important—by virtue of both frequency and severity—aetiological agent of pneumonia throughout the world and particularly so in the tropics (Table 28.1). Preceding viral upper respiratory tract infections may be important precipitants, although the role of viruses as a primary cause of pneumonia in adults is unclear. Likewise, the contribution of the 'atypical' pneumonia group of bacteria is uncertain, and the infrequency of reporting may

Lecture Notes: Tropical Medicine, 6th edition.
By G.V. Gill and N.J. Beeching. Published 2009 by Blackwell Publishing, ISBN: 978-1-4051-8048-1.

simply reflect inadequate surveillance and study. Most importantly, patients with *Mycobacterium tuberculosis* frequently present with an acute pneumonic illness and can also present with a dual infection with *S. pneumoniae*. In adults, *M. tuberculosis* may be identified in as many as 10% of cases of severe acute pneumonia admitted to hospitals in sub-Saharan Africa. Acute presentations of pulmonary tuberculosis in children are also well recognized.

Epidemiology

Pneumonia affects individuals of all ages and the risk of disease exists throughout the year with seasonal variation. Rates are highest during the cooler drier periods with case numbers beginning to rise towards the end of the rains when malaria is also a significant problem. Pneumonia is invariably reported as a leading cause of admission to hospital in all regions of the tropics, although accurate community-based incidence data are lacking. Attack rates in children are surpassed only by malaria and diarrhoea, and account for 18% of the 10 million deaths in children under the age of 5 each year. Equivalent estimates for adults are more uncertain. Rates of pneumonia in HIV-infected adults have been measured at 4000 per 100000 person years. HIV increases pneumonia risk between 5- and 10-fold; thus, between 2.2 and 3.3 million episodes of pneumonia (30–50%

Table 28.1 Predominant aetiological agents of pneumonia listed in order of frequency according to clinical presentation

Moderate severity pneumonia (inpatient management, not intensive care)	
Common	*Streptococcus pneumoniae*
	Haemophilus influenzae
Variable	*Mycoplasma pneumoniae*
	Influenza *type A*
	Chlamydia psittaci
	Legionella pneumophila
Rare	*Staphylococcus aureus*
Most severe pneumonia (intensive care)	
Common	*Streptococcus pneumoniae*
	Legionella pneumophila
Variable	*Haemophilus influenzae*
	Klebsiella pneumoniae (common S. Africa)
	Pseudomonas aeruginosa
	Burkholderia pseudomallei (common SE Asia)
	Staphylococcus aureus
Rare	*Mycoplasma pneumoniae*
	Chlamydia psittaci

with HIV coinfection) can be estimated to occur in adults in Africa each year (assuming 300 million adults, 10% HIV seroprevalence). Pneumonia case fatality was 60% in the pre-antibiotic era. With effective early therapy this may be reduced to 5%. Unfortunately, case fatality rates are still reported at 15–20%, reflecting the problems of late presentation and delays in therapy, common to all resource-limited settings.

Risk factors for pneumonia

- *Age*—small children and elderly adults are at particular risk. In regions with high HIV prevalence this pattern is lost as a consequence of increased pneumonia amongst young adults.
- *Cigarette smoking*—the most important risk factor for pneumonia in immunocompetent adults is cigarette smoking with an odds ratio of 6.
- *Pregnancy* is an important risk factor for pneumonia.
- *Coexistent medical problems*—HIV infection (most important), underlying lung disease, diabetes,

nephrotic syndrome, kwashiorkor, marasmus, measles and sickle cell disease/asplenia.
- *Social*—overcrowding, migrant labour, refugees, alcohol and drug abuse.
- *Environmental*—domestic smoke from biomass fuels (particularly firewood and animal dung) has been shown to increase the incidence of upper and lower respiratory tract infections in both adults and children, as have poorly ventilated dwellings and mining-associated dust exposure.

Clinical features

Symptoms of acute pneumonia

Presentation is typically acute with a 2- to 3-day history of cough, fever, dyspnoea and often some pleuritic pain. In adults purulent sputum production may not occur for several days after antibiotic therapy has been started. A more prolonged presentation may occur if the pneumonia has been partially treated or if there is an underlying chronic chest disease, in particular TB. In addition to fever, cough and dyspnoea, failure to feed is an important feature in infants. Streaky haemoptysis or 'rusty' sputum may occur—the latter suggestive of *S. pneumoniae* infection. Headache is common and may suggest meningitis, but this is unusual except in HIV-infected adults. Diarrhoea can occasionally be profuse and accompanied by abdominal pain leading to confusion with acute gastroenteritis. Elderly adults may have few if any symptoms at all.

Signs of acute pneumonia

Patients usually appear unwell and may be tachycardic and febrile. Nasal flaring—use of the accessory muscles of respiration—tachypnoea and lower chest wall in-drawing are particularly important to look for in children (Figure 28.1). Classically the signs of consolidation are dullness to chest percussion, bronchial breathing and aegophony (high-pitched transmission of speech sounds) but in the earlier phase of pneumonia, coarse inspiratory crackles consistent with retained secretions are more common. A pleural rub may be present and does not necessarily predict complicated pleural

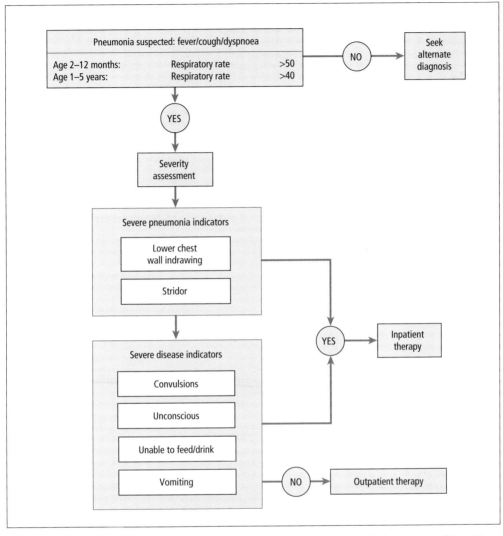

Figure 28.1 Pneumonia diagnosis and severity assessment in children. In regions with a high prevalence of bacterial pneumonia, use of respiratory rate alone will detect 80% of children who require antibiotics for pneumonia.

disease. Unusual presentations include acute psychosis, confusion, hypothermia, jaundice and abdominal tenderness.

Differential diagnosis of acute pneumonia

• *Tuberculosis*—this should always be considered in poorly resolving pneumonia and is the prime concern in more prolonged presentations.

• *Asthma*—an increasing problem in urban settings, often coexisting with pneumonia. Low-grade fever and poor air entry (obscuring the characteristic wheeze) are features of life-threatening severe asthma.

• *Diabetic ketoacidosis*—respiratory distress, clouded consciousness and a preceding history of weight loss may be overlooked as a case of HIV infection complicated by pneumonia. The smell of exhaled acetone, a more detailed history to elicit polyuria and polydipsia along with urinalysis, should identify the condition.

• *Poisoning*—this should be considered when the respiratory distress is out of proportion to the pulmonary findings and there is evidence of other system involvement, particularly neurological. Important poisons are aspirin, chloroquine, petrochemicals and herbicides either intentionally or accidentally ingested or inhaled.

• *Amoebic liver abscess*—the presence of a right-sided effusion should alert the clinician to consider an amoebic problem. Rarely, only consolidatory changes may be present in the right lower lobe.

• *Pulmonary eosinophilia*—as a consequence of migratory worms may present acutely. Bronchospasm may be present; more importantly, individuals are not unwell.

Investigations

To maximize the use of limited resources, investigations should be reserved for individuals with severe disease or cases where response to therapy has been suboptimal and when the information acquired is necessary for the case management process.

Radiology

In severe disease, radiology can be used to identify pneumothoraces, effusions and to rule out alternate diagnoses such as pericardial effusions or pulmonary oedema which require specific therapy. Bilateral interstitial pneumonia may suggest *Pneumocystis* pneumonia but this radiological pattern is found with both bacterial and TB infections, and thus has poor diagnostic precision. When pneumonia is slow to resolve, the presence of mediastinal/hilar lymphadenopathy should stimulate a search for tuberculosis. Cavities should also point towards tuberculosis or, occasionally, anaerobic/aspiration or staphylococcal pneumonia. The presence of pleural effusions in poorly resolving pneumonia should lead to pleural aspiration and examination for empyema.

Sputum Gram's stain

This is valuable when performed at presentation on a properly collected sample of sputum. The presence of 10–20 pus cells in a high power (×1000) field and no epithelial cells suggests an adequate specimen. The presence of Gram-positive diplococci (dark purple) in association with pus cells confirms a diagnosis of pneumococcal pneumonia and may be helpful in confirming appropriate management in severe disease (see also p. 13).

Sputum Ziehl–Neelsen stain

This should be carried out on all poorly resolving pneumonia and will identify 60–80% of *M. tuberculosis* infections. Culture for *Mycobacterium*, if available, increases the diagnostic yield. If numerous pus cells are seen on Gram's stain in the absence of organisms, Ziehl–Neelsen staining should be performed.

Trans-thoracic lung aspirate

This is a useful technique for recovering lower respiratory tract samples for staining and culture. Aspirates should only be taken from consolidated lung tissue, laterally to avoid the heart. When this is done pneumothoraces are uncommon (see also p. 13).

Pleural aspiration

Pleural effusions occur in 5–15% of cases of pneumonia. The majority will resolve with antibacterial therapy alone. Sampling of pleural fluid can be helpful in establishing a diagnosis and should always be carried out if empyema is suspected.

Other microbiological tests

Blood cultures have low diagnostic sensitivity and most basic laboratories do not have appropriate facilities, although recovery of an organism from blood is the gold standard (other than lung biopsy) for aetiological diagnosis. Serology and other immune-based diagnostics (e.g. immun-ofluorescence for *Pneumocystis jirovecii* pneumonia; PCP) are unlikely to be available and rarely contribute to management during the early crucial phase of pneumonia.

Other investigations

Haemoglobin measurements help to identify individuals who may require blood transfusion. Transcutaneous oxygen saturation measurements, if available, are a useful adjunct to determining the need for oxygen therapy. Biochemical assessment of renal and hepatic function are not essential (except in rare cases of renal failure requiring dialysis) but may provide prognostic information.

In regions of high HIV prevalence, the majority of pneumonia cases will be HIV-infected—rates range from 40% to 90%. If resources are available and national strategies emphasize identification of people with underlying HIV infection (e.g. to receive disease prophylaxis, antiretroviral therapy), pneumonia patients should be offered voluntary counselling and testing. In some instances, HIV testing can aid diagnosis and management (e.g. suspected PCP).

Management

Once pneumonia has been identified or suspected, an assessment of the severity of the condition is rapidly required (Figure 28.2). The threshold for admission to hospital may be more severe in tropical regions where inpatient facilities are crowded and an assessment of suitability for outpatient oral or inpatient parenteral therapy is required. Indicators of poor outcome in adults are listed in Table 28.2. Vomiting or profuse diarrhoea are relative contraindications to oral therapy as antibiotic absorption may be impaired.

Outpatient therapy

Oral amoxicillin (500 mg t.d.s.) or ampicillin (500 mg q.d.s.) are effective antipneumococcal agents and are a suitable first choice. Alternative agents include co-trimoxazole (promoted as a first choice in children by the WHO) and erythromycin. Chloramphenicol can also be used as it is well absorbed and has reasonable activity against *S. pneumoniae*. Individuals managed as outpatients should always be encouraged to re-attend to be assessed for tuberculosis if there are persisting respiratory symptoms.

Inpatient therapy

Basic resuscitation (ensuring airway patency and adequate respiratory and circulatory activity) should be rapidly followed by antimicrobial therapy. Parenteral penicillins (benzylpenicillin 1.8 g every 4–6 h or amoxicillin 0.5–1 g every 8 h) remain the agents of first choice. Chloramphenicol is valuable for *H. influenzae* infections or in individuals with penicillin allergy. A macrolide, tetracycline or ciprofloxacin can be added to therapy as oral agents (parenteral preparations are unavailable or expensive) in severe disease if an atypical organism is suspected.

In addition to antimicrobial therapy, other supportive treatment should be initiated. Supplemental oxygen, clearance of respiratory secretions (by changing posture, suctioning and provision of moist air), maintenance of appropriate hydration (with intravenous fluids if necessary) and adequate pain relief (preferably with non-opiate analgesics) may all be required. Assisted ventilation, when available, is necessary in some cases when respiratory muscle fatigue develops, heralded by a rising partial pressure of CO_2 and, more latterly, altered conscious level, blood pressure instability and decreasing respiratory effort.

Complications

An appropriate response to therapy is lysis of fever within 48–72 h of its commencement in association with an improvement in well-being and recommencement of oral intake. Failure of this pattern to emerge requires a reconsideration of the underlying diagnosis, therapy given and/or a search for an early complication—empyema, suppurative pericarditis, lung abscess, pneumothorax or meningitis. The late sequelae of

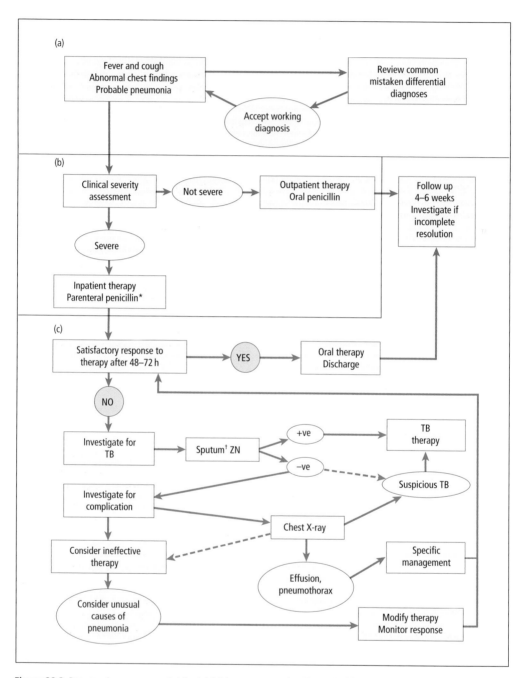

Figure 28.2 Pneumonia management: (a) establishing a presumptive diagnosis; (b) initiating empirical therapy and (c) testing and modification of initial diagnosis by assessing response to therapy.
* Erythromycin if penicillin allergic (if unavailable, use chloramphenicol).
† Sputum or pleural aspirate/lung aspirate/regional lymph node aspirate.

Table 28.2 Associations of severe disease and poor outcome in adult pneumonia. Two or more factors increase chance of dying four fold, and 5 or more factors increase chance of dying ten fold. This scheme has the advantage of being easily applied at the bedside in resource-poor settings but has not been prospectively validated in this setting.

Pre-existing factors (history)
Age >60 years
Pre-morbid illness

Examination
Low blood pressure and/or increased pulse
Multilobar disease
Increased respiratory rate (>30/min)
Confusion

Investigation
Low or high WCC
High urea
Low PaO$_2$
Bacteraemia

---

pneumococcal pneumonia (osteomyelitis, arthritis, endocarditis) are infrequent if appropriate antibiotics are given early, although HIV infection can be associated with complications and an increased risk of these metastatic infections. Following discharge from hospital, a follow-up visit in 4–6 weeks is advisable to ensure complete resolution of the pneumonia or further investigation for possible tuberculosis. The chest X-ray changes may take 4–6 weeks to resolve.

Prevention

Active vaccination

Polyvalent pneumococcal polysaccharide vaccines have been available for many years, but uncertainties over their effectiveness and their relative expense ($9 per dose) have limited their use. They are currently recommended for individuals with sickle cell disease but there are no other clear recommendations for use in the tropics. The vaccine is ineffective in HIV-infected adults and children under 2 years of age. The new

generation of protein conjugate pneumococcal polysaccharide vaccines are currently under evaluation in children in Africa, and the outcomes of these field trials are awaited before further recommendations are made. They have proved extremely effective in the USA at preventing pneumonic and invasive disease. Protection against *Haemophilus influenzae* type b (Hib) pneumonia in children is achievable by vaccination. Attempts to incorporate Hib vaccine in the EPI regimen are underway.

Chemoprophylaxis

Penicillin should be given on a daily basis to individuals with sickle cell disease or with asplenia to prevent pneumococcal infections. Daily co-trimoxazole is recommended for HIV-infected adults and children in the tropics. This approach is effective in reducing PCP in children under 1 year, but reduction of bacterial pneumonia in adults is less certain.

Future developments

Antibiotic resistance

Penicillin resistance amongst *S. pneumoniae* is on the increase globally and represents a major threat to cheap and effective therapy of lower respiratory tract infections. Alterations in the penicillin-binding proteins of pneumococci lead to incremental increases in resistance to penicillin. At present these changes are probably of little consequence for the treatment of pneumococcal pneumonia—achievable levels of penicillin in blood and pulmonary tissue with standard dosages will be bactericidal for most of the currently 'resistant' pneumococci (unlike the situation with meningitis). However, if pneumococci with higher grade resistance become established, current empirical antibiotic regimens will be ineffective. Moreover, penicillin resistance is associated with resistance to multiple antibiotics including macrolides and co-trimoxazole. The inevitable consequences are therapeutic failures and higher priced therapies. Local information on bacterial sensitivity patterns are essential to plan national and district level policy.

Pneumococcal vaccines

In addition to the protein conjugate, pneumococcal peptides (pneumolysin, pneumococcal surface proteins) are being studied as vaccine candidates or as components of the conjugate vaccines. These vaccines may be able to overcome the serotype-restricted nature of the polysaccharide vaccines and may be substantially cheaper to manufacture.

Further reading

Cutts FT, Zaman SM, Enwere G *et al*. Efficacy of nine-valent pneumococcal conjugate vaccine against pneumonia and invasive pneumococcal disease in The Gambia: randomized double-blind, placebo-controlled trial. *Lancet* 2005; 365: 1139–1146.

Ezzati M, Kammen D. Indoor air pollution from biomass combustion and acute respiratory infections in Kenya: an exposure-response study. *Lancet* 2001; 358: 619–624.

Madhi SA, Klugman KP. A role for Streptococcus pneumoniae in virus-associated pneumonia. *Nat Med* 2004; 10: 811–813.

Nuorti JP, Butler JC, Farley MM *et al*. Cigarette smoking and invasive pneumococcal disease. Active Bacterial Core Surveillance Team. *N Engl J Med* 2000; 342: 681–689.

Scott JA, Hall AJ, Muyodi C *et al*. Aetiology, outcome and risk factors for mortality among adults with acute pneumonia in Kenya. *Lancet* 2000; 355: 1225–1230.

www.who.int/Child-adolescent-health [Useful source of practical information for the management of childhood illnesses with several printable guideline documents for management of pneumonia.]

Chapter 29

Lung flukes

Lung flukes of the genus *Paragonimus* are zoonoses, but human infection can cause a chronic cough with haemoptysis which can easily be mistaken for tuberculosis. *Paragonimus westermani* is the most common cause of human disease.

Life cycle

Lung flukes are hermaphrodite trematodes. The stout adults, which are about 12 mm long, live as pairs in cavities in the lungs. Large brownish eggs (85–100 × 50–60 μm) are passed in the sputum or faeces and, if they reach water, develop in about 3 weeks to release a miracidium that infects certain species of freshwater snail in which the parasite undergoes asexual multiplication. Cercariae with knob-shaped tails emerge and encyst in freshwater crabs or crayfish.

The definitive hosts of the flukes are carnivores that eat crustacea; humans are incidental hosts infected by ingesting metacercariae in uncooked crab or crayfish meat or their juices. Human infections are most common in Asia, especially Korea where medicinal use of crayfish juice and in parts of China where eating live crabs dipped in rice wine ('drunken crabs') aid transmission (Figure 29.1). Other species of *Paragonimus* occur in Africa

Lecture Notes: Tropical Medicine, 6th edition.
By G.V. Gill and N.J. Beeching. Published 2009 by
Blackwell Publishing, ISBN: 978-1-4051-8048-1.

and the Americas. Paragonimiasis was common during the Biafran war in Nigeria and is found in native Indians in Ecuador and Colombia.

Clinical features

Patients with acute infections may present with malaise, shivers, sweats and urticarial skin rash or abdominal pain a few days or weeks after infection.

Lung disease

• Patients present with chronic cough productive of brownish-red sputum, sometimes with haemoptysis.
• Occasionally, there is breathlessness or chest pain.
• Radiology usually shows peripheral nodules or ring shadows; sometimes there is a crescentic shadow of a fluke within the ring. CT scans are useful.
• Pleural effusions or empyema are complications.

Ectopic disease

This is caused by aberrant migration of flukes from the gut. There are many possible presentations but these include:
• abdominal pain and inflammatory masses
• convulsions
• cerebral tumour-like presentations

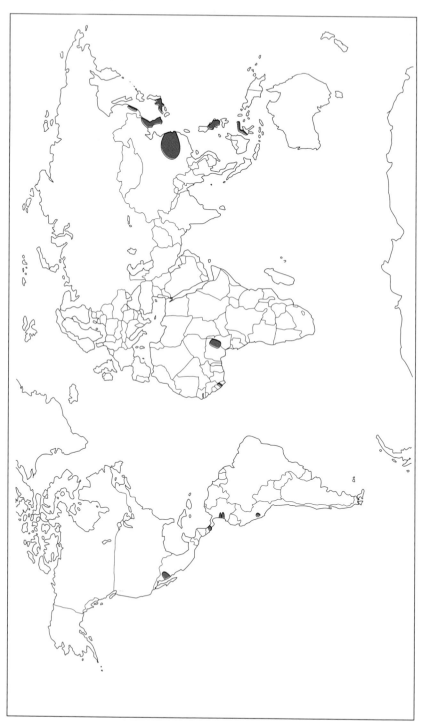

Figure 29.1 Distribution of lung fluke infections.

- mental disturbance; and
- migrating subcutaneous lumps (larva migrans).

Diagnosis

- Microscopy of sputum or stool. Concentrate stool using the formol-ether technique. Examine sputum for brownish flecks that may contain nests of eggs. Mucoid sputum is concentrated by adding 2–3 times the volume of 10% potassium hydroxide for 1h and then centrifuged for 3min at 1500 r.p.m. Examine the deposit using the low-power objective.
- Eggs can also be recovered by bronchoalveolar lavage.
- Serological diagnosis by EIA or dot enzyme immunoassay using antigens from flukes or metacercariae is available in some endemic areas.
- Radiological evidence and eosinophilia in early disease may aid diagnosis.

Treatment

Praziquantel is highly effective, given as 75 mg/kg/day in three divided doses for 2 days (150 mg/kg total dose) or as a single dose of 40 mg/kg. If available triclabendazole is an alternative, given as 10 mg/kg once or on two successive days. Treat cautiously if cerebral disease is suspected, as a sudden increase in intracranial pressure is possible. Use dexamethasone to control cerebral oedema.

Further reading

Keiser J, Engels D, Büscher G, Utzinger J. Triclabendazole for the treatment of fascioliasis and paragonimiasis. *Expert Opin Investig Drugs* 2005; 14: 1513–1526. [Useful review of praziquantel and triclabendazole treatment of both fluke infections.]

Rosenbaum SD. Paragonimiasis. Emedicine 2006 www.emedicine.com/ped/TOPIC1729.HTM [Short clinical review in Western setting with a few references available free online.]

Chapter 30

Tropical pulmonary eosinophilia

Tropical pulmonary eosinophilia (TPE) is an asthma-like disease caused by a hyperactive immunological response to 'human' filariae, usually *Wuchereria bancrofti* or *Brugia malayi* (see also Chapter 14). Microfilariae are destroyed in the pulmonary capillaries and antigen release recruits large numbers of degranulating eosinophils that release major basic protein and other chemicals. A granulomatous reaction may eventually progress to fibrosis and permanent lung damage, possibly due to antigenic similarity between the filarial worm enzymes and proteins found on human pulmonary epithelium.

Epidemiology

TPE is found commonly in India and in parts of West Africa. The disease usually occurs in children and young adults.

Clinical features

Patients present with a short history of cough, wheeze and shortness of breath, which is worse at night and often preceded or accompanied by malaise and low-grade fever. Signs are similar to

those of asthma but there is sometimes lymph node or splenic enlargement and, very rarely, seventh nerve palsy or other focal neurological signs.

Investigations

Chest X-ray may be normal but often shows diffuse alveolar mottling with small 1–2 mm nodules in the middle and lower zones. Hilar adenopathy is sometimes seen and less often there is a pleural effusion or areas of hyperacute pneumonitis.

The blood shows a marked eosinophilia, usually above 3×10^9/L and sometimes much higher. The erythrocyte sedimentation rate is raised. IgE levels are also greatly raised and tests for filarial antibodies show high titres. Microfilariae cannot usually be found in peripheral blood, even by sensitive filtration methods, but filarial antigen tests are positive.

Lung function testing shows restrictive changes and poor gas diffusion; obstructive changes are less common.

Diagnosis

Diagnosis is based on the high eosinophilia with high filarial antibody titres and the response to treatment. The differential diagnosis includes not only migrating helminths, especially *Ascaris* in children but also *Strongyloides stercoralis* or hookworms. These usually cause only temporary

Lecture Notes: Tropical Medicine, 6th edition.
By G.V. Gill and N.J. Beeching. Published 2009 by
Blackwell Publishing, ISBN: 978-1-4051-8048-1.

disability. Severe allergic asthma and bronchopulmonary aspergillosis should also be considered.

Treatment

TPE may remit spontaneously and recurs following treatment in 20% of cases. DEC 6 mg/kg in divided doses given for 12–21 days is the standard treatment. Symptomatic response within days is usual but lung function can remain impaired for months. Albendazole 400 mg twice daily for 3 weeks may be added to a second course of DEC in those who do not respond adequately.

Prevention

Control of *Aedes* mosquito breeding sites and reducing bites.

Further reading

Chitkara RK, Krishna G. Parasitic pulmonary eosinophilia. *Semin Respir Crit Care Med* 2006; 27: 171–184.

Vijayan VK. Tropical pulmonary eosinophilia: pathogenesis, diagnosis and management. *Curr Opin Pulm Med* 2007; 13: 428–433.

Chapter 31

Pyogenic meningitis

Bacterial meningitis is a major cause of morbidity and mortality in the tropics. It has been estimated that 1 in 250 children are affected before the age of 5 in urban West Africa (Dakar, Senegal) with up to 50% mortality. Further south in the 'meningitis belt', 1–2% of people may be affected during the cyclical epidemics of meningococcal disease that occur every 5–7 years. Viral meningitis and viral encephalitis occur in the tropics, but will not be considered further here (Chapter 33).

Epidemiology

The majority of cases of pyogenic meningitis are caused by the pneumococcus *Streptococcus pneumoniae* (many serogroups), the meningococcus *Neisseria meningitidis* (serogroups A, B, C, Y, W135, X) or *Haemophilus influenzae* type b (Hib). The latter rarely affects patients aged over 5 years, and all three are more common in children under 2 years. These young children are an important group of patients because they are least likely to respond to polysaccharide capsule-derived vaccines that have been produced for serogroups of each of the three main bacterial species. At the extremes of age, group B streptococci and staphylococci (both *Staphylococcus aureus* and coagulase

negative Staphylococci) are important in neonates, and various Gram-negative organisms are important in adults, who also become more susceptible to pneumococcal infections as age increases. The epidemiology of meningitis varies between countries, and it is important to determine the usual causative organisms wherever one is practising: for example, the most common cause of bacterial meningitis in adults in Vietnam is *Streptococcus suis*. HIV has led to a great change in the pattern of meningitis in much of Africa over the past decade with a huge rise in invasive pneumococcal disease as well as cryptococcal meningitis and a smaller rise in tuberculous meningitis but no specific increase in meningococcal disease. Antibiotic resistance is common in Hib throughout the world and in pneumococci in much of the tropics. Clinically significant resistance has yet to become common in meningococci but is beginning to be reported.

Meningococcal epidemiology

Epidemics have occurred with regularity in West Africa and Sudan for at least a century. Lapeysonnie defined the 'meningitis belt' in 1963 as an area with a high incidence and recurring epidemics between latitudes 4° and 16° North, south of the Sahara, with 300–1100 mm annual rainfall, comprising much of semiarid sub-Saharan Africa including the Sahel. This belt has high levels

Lecture Notes: Tropical Medicine, 6th edition.
By G.V. Gill and N.J. Beeching. Published 2009 by Blackwell Publishing, ISBN: 978-1-4051-8048-1.

of seasonal endemicity with large superimposed epidemics of infection of predominantly group A meningococci at irregular intervals. This zone has been extended further south in recent years to include other countries with at least 1 month of reduced humidity (Figure 31.1). Factors predisposing to meningococcal infection include overcrowding and poor hygiene, so that schools, urban slums, military barracks, prisons and similar large collections of people are at increased risk. Damage to the upper respiratory mucosa by tobacco or wood fire smoke, intercurrent viral infections such as influenza or external dust (e.g. the annual dry 'Harmattan' wind in Nigeria) facilitates invasion by meningococci. While group A meningococci are usually implicated in West Africa or in the previous epidemics related to the Hajj pilgrimage to Mecca, other strains—most recently W135 (and now group X and other novel strains)—became prominent after successful vaccination against group A. In South America, epidemics of group C strains have been described but should now be preventable by vaccination. In western countries where immunization against group C has been instituted, group B predominates and there is no effective vaccine against this strain. There does not seem to be increased risk of meningococcal infection in HIV-positive or similarly immunocompromised patients.

Pneumococcal epidemiology

There are many serogroups of pneumococci, the predominance of which varies from country to country, so that sophisticated microbiological surveillance is required in order to confirm the relevant mixture to be included in polyvalent vaccines. Host factors common in the tropics are well recognized to predispose to pneumococcal infection including haemoglobinopathies such as sickle and sickle–haemoglobin C (SC) disease, splenic dysfunction caused by these or because of removal after trauma, damage to the cribriform plate in the skull by trauma, and HIV infection. Recently, cyclical epidemics of specific serotypes of pneumococcal meningitis have been described, often coexisting with epidemics of meningococcal diseases. The standard of care for prevention in risk groups is the use of polysaccharide vaccines, although the evidence base is poor and even suggests that pneumococcal vaccine is harmful in some HIV-positive African populations. It is likely that conjugate vaccines will be more effective in both HIV-positive and HIV-negative groups.

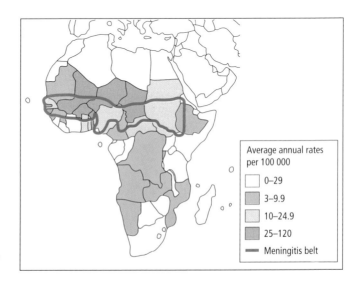

Figure 31.1 Meningococcal disease in Africa, 1993–2006 (Source: WHO, 2008).

Average annual rates per 100 000

- 0–29
- 3–9.9
- 10–24.9
- 25–120
- — Meningitis belt

Haemophilus influenzae type b epidemiology

Some countries in the tropics have virtually eliminated invasive Hib disease, including meningitis, by instituting early childhood immunization, as practised in the West. This has been shown in the Middle East and in the Gambia.

Vaccines

All three major causes of bacterial meningitis can be prevented by vaccines based on serogroup-specific antigens derived from their polysaccharide capsules. These vaccines require an intact 'cold chain' of refrigeration (<5°C) at all stages of transport from manufacturer to delivery at the point of health care. They are less immunogenic in the groups most at risk (under 2 years) and induced immunity is mainly T cell dependent and relatively short-lived. There is no vaccine for serogroup B meningococci, although trials of promising candidates are in progress.

New conjugate vaccines are more expensive but also more successful; proven examples are Hib vaccine and the group C meningococcal vaccine. Similar vaccines have been developed for other serogroups of meningococci (A, C, Y, W135) and for pneumococci.

Clinical features

The cardinal features of meningitis are no different in the tropics than elsewhere, and symptoms include headache, vomiting, fever, photophobia, loss of consciousness and fits, associated with the clinical signs of fever, neck stiffness and reducing level of consciousness. The index of suspicion is higher in children who may have less obvious features and who often have co-existing malaria parasitaemia. The rash of meningococcal disease develops rapidly and, in darker skins, it may be difficult to see unless the mucosal membranes are involved—always check in the mouth and conjunctivae. In some African groups, the meningococcal rash is slightly raised and can be palpated even if it is difficult to see.

The differential diagnosis in a tropical setting is wide (Box 31.1). The most important clinical decisions are whether the patient has cerebral malaria and/or meningitis, whether there is a space-occupying lesion (often an abscess related to severe otitis media) or whether the patient has TB or cryptococcal meningitis. Examination should focus on clues to underlying predisposing factors, including broken nose, laparotomy scars (for splenectomy) and features of haemoglobinopathy suggesting pneumococcal meningitis, or HIV suggesting pneumococcal or cryptococcal meningitis. Optic fundi may show miliary TB, HIV-related retinopathy (including CMV), haemorrhage caused by severe malaria, or tuberculomas as well as features of raised intracranial pressure in long-standing space-occupying lesions. Focal neurological signs suggest a space-occupying lesion, TB or late cryptococcal disease. Most TB meningitis present with a prolonged history but some cases do present acutely, and patients with cryptococcal meningitis and HIV may have little headache and minimal or no neck stiffness.

Box 31.1 Differential diagnosis of pyogenic meningitis.

- Malaria (cerebral or otherwise)
- Typhoid
- Pneumonia
- Urinary tract infection
- Otitis media/sinusitis
- Severe paediatric gastroenteritis
- Tetanus
- Trypanosomiasis
- Brucellosis
- Rickettsial disease
- Subarachnoid haemorrhage
- Cerebral abscess or other space-occupying lesion, including tuberculoma
- Causes of lymphocytic CSF (tuberculosis, cryptococcus, viral meningitis, etc.)
- Encephalitis
- Poisoning (alcohol, drugs, etc.) and other cause of coma
- Drug-induced extrapyramidal signs (phenothiazines, antiemetics)

Diagnosis

Lumbar puncture (LP) is mandatory whenever there is suspicion of meningitis. It should only be avoided if there is clear clinical evidence of a space-occupying lesion and, if omitted, the patient should be given antibiotics to cover the possibility of meningitis until it is considered safe to do an LP.

Diagnosis can be achieved with simple biochemical and microscopic tests. The patterns of white cells in CSF vary, and there is considerable overlap between the groups (Box 31.2). Abnormalities of cells persist in the CSF for several days, even after antibiotic treatment has been started. Some viral infections, especially mumps, may have neutrophil predominance in the early stages. Biochemical tests help to distinguish these, and a very high protein usually suggests bacterial infection or TB. In TB the CSF protein is sometimes high enough to form a 'spider-web' clot in the tube. The specificity of low CSF glucose for diagnosing bacterial infection is improved by

comparing it to simultaneous blood glucose, especially if the patient is diabetic or has other causes of altered blood glucose levels. Urine dipsticks can be used for CSF. Stains of CSF should include Gram's stain for bacteria, which is as sensitive as latex agglutination and other antigen detection systems, Ziehl–Neelsen or auramine (for TB), and India-ink stains for cryptococcal infection should always be considered if CSF is lymphocytic or even if there are no CSF white cells in an HIV-positive patient with suggestive symptoms. Cryptococcal antigen tests (if available) are very valuable.

Cultures for all the above organisms should be set up if facilities are available and large volumes of CSF (10 mL) need to be taken to maximize the chances of growing *Mycobacterium tuberculosis*. Molecular tests such as PCR-based tests on blood or CSF are valuable in a western setting for diagnosing meningococcal infection, particularly if the patient has already received antibiotics before arrival, but are not available in most tropical settings. Blood cultures should always be taken if facilities are available. Suggestive changes in other tests include neutrophilia in peripheral blood and a high C-reactive protein level, especially in children.

In many tropical settings, culture and more sophisticated tests are not available and Gram's staining will be negative. In such cases, the features that suggest pyogenic meningitis, rather than viral meningitis or other organisms, are summarized in Table 31.1. The sensitivity and specificity, and hence usefulness at the bedside, of these features vary from area to area. In a recent study in (mainly HIV-negative) Vietnamese adults, five features were more predictive of TB meningitis compared to bacterial meningitis: age, length of history, peripheral WBC count, total CSF WBC count and CSF neutrophil proportion. In a population of mainly HIV-positive adults in Malawi, patients with cryptococcal meningitis had longer histories, lower CSF WBC counts and lower proportions of neutrophils than those with bacterial meningitis.

Box 31.2 CSF patterns.

Pyogenic
- bacterial
- abscess

Lymphocytic with normal glucose
- most viruses (e.g. polio, enteroviruses, Coxsackie)
- rickettsiae
- HIV
- early TB
- miscellaneous (e.g. endocarditis, neoplastic)

Lymphocytic with low glucose
- partially treated bacterial meningitis
- cerebral abscess
- TB
- some viral (e.g. mumps)
- fungal (e.g. *Cryptococcus* and *Aspergillus*)
- brucellosis
- syphilis
- leptospirosis
- trypanosomiasis

Eosinophilic
- *Angiostrongylus cantonensis*
- *Taenia solium* (cysticercosis)
- Paragonimiasis

Amoebic (rare)
- *Naegleria* spp.

Management

The key features are to make a diagnosis, to assess severity of illness, to detect coexisting or underlying disease and to provide both supportive and specific therapy. For pyogenic meningitis alone, empirical or pathogen-specific antimicrobials should be given as early as possible, before the LP if there is going to be any delay in the procedure. All patients should be re-evaluated at least daily, especially when the CSF results become available. Patients with equivocal (lymphocytic) CSF findings are difficult; repeat LP may be required after 2–3 days. The important decision is whether to treat as TB or not, or whether the initial CSF changes were brought about by viral or partially treated bacterial meningitis or missed cryptococcal disease.

Meningococcal disease

This responds to short courses of chloramphenicol or penicillin and will also respond to third-generation cephalosporins. Uncomplicated meningococcal meningitis has a mortality of <10% and rarely needs more than 5–7 days of parenteral treatment, and there is increasing evidence that shorter regimens are equally effective. Meningococcal septicaemia (with or without meningitis) has a mortality of >40% in most tropical settings, requiring maximal intensive

Table 31.1 CSF changes predictive of bacterial causes if Gram's stain is negative (see also Table 3.5)

Opening pressure	High
Turbidity	Present
Total WBC	>2 × 10⁹/L (2000/mm³)
Neutrophils	>50% if total WBC >0.1 × 10⁹/L (100/mm³)
Glucose	<1 mmol/L (18 mg%)
CSF: blood glucose ratio	<40%
Protein	>2 g/L (200 mg%)
Gram's stain	Positive
Ziehl–Neelsen stain	Negative
India-ink stain	Negative
Culture	Positive
Antigen detection	Positive
Plus peripheral WBC >16 × 10⁹/L	

Abbreviation: WBC, white blood cell count.

care. Up to 10% of patients experience immune complex disease including uveitis, polyarthritis and pericarditis, typically in the second week of illness. This responds to inflammatory drugs including short courses of steroids.

Uncomplicated meningitis can also be managed with single doses of Triplopen or similar mixtures of long- and short-acting penicillins, or with Tifomycin, an oily suspension of chloramphenicol administered as 2–3 g once only (but divided into two injections because of volume) for an adult. The latter is becoming more difficult to obtain and is now being replaced by ceftriaxone, as cheaper generic formulations have become available. Ceftriaxone can be given i.m. or i.v. These regimens are useful for the management of large numbers of patients in an epidemic setting, provided that patients are reviewed daily for evidence of recovery.

Close contacts (family/household) may be given immediate chemoprophylaxis to prevent them from developing illness over the next fortnight. Suitable medications include sulfadiazine (only if the infecting strain is already known to be sensitive) but not penicillins. The alternatives include a single dose of ciprofloxacin (15 mg/kg orally in children, 750 mg orally in adults), rifampicin (20 mg/kg twice daily for children or 600 mg twice daily for adults, for 2 days) or ceftriaxone (50 mg/kg for children or 2 g for adults i.m. once only). 'Ring' vaccination of contacts is more appropriate in an epidemic situation (discussed later).

Pneumococcal disease

Antimicrobial therapy depends on local susceptibility patterns. In Papua New Guinea, much of sub-Saharan Africa and elsewhere, there may be at least moderate penicillin resistance, so that isolates need to be cultured to inform therapy, and empirical therapy should not be based on penicillin alone. In a western setting, large doses of third-generation cephalosporins (cefotaxime or ceftriaxone) are usually adequate, and are becoming more available in tropical settings. Ceftriaxone doses such as 2 g twice daily (i.m.

or i.v.) are recommended. Otherwise, monotherapy with chloramphenicol is often the only
available choice. Coexistent chloramphenicol
resistance is less common, and the commonly
recommended mixture of penicillin and chloramphenicol is wasteful of resources and confers
no improvement in survival or reduced morbidity in survivors. Meropenem is a safe (but expensive) alternative in proven chloramphenicol and
penicillin-resistant cases, or vancomycin can be
added. Pneumococcal meningitis has a mortality of over 50% in many tropical settings, and in
sub-Saharan Africa, the majority of these patients
are also HIV positive. Up to 40% of survivors will
have significant neurological deficits. Treatment
should last for at least 10 days for uncomplicated
disease and may need to extend beyond 14 days
in difficult cases.

Haemophilus influenzae disease

Found mainly in young children, clinically significant resistance to ampicillin and/or amoxicillin
and to benzyl penicillin is present in about 50%
of cases. Less marked chloramphenicol resistance is present in up to 10% of tropical cases.
The treatment of choice is a third-generation
cephalosporin or chloramphenicol alone.
Empirical ampicillin cannot be used until the
patient's own isolate is known to be sensitive.
Chemoprophylaxis of contacts is not usual in
tropical settings.

Empirical therapy

Unless there is good epidemiological (current
epidemic) and clinical (typical rash) evidence to
suggest meningococcal disease, the average adult
or child with pyogenic meningitis has to be managed to cover the three main bacterial pathogens,
including cover for *Salmonella* spp. in younger
children. Monotherapy with chloramphenicol or
a third-generation cephalosporin is the treatment
of choice. In resource-poor settings with multiresistant pathogens, it has been shown that two
doses of Tifomycin 48 h apart are as effective for
inpatient treatment as parenteral ampicillin plus

chloramphenicol for over a week, in terms of hospital mortality and serious sequelae in survivors.

Patients at extremes of age need extra cover for
other pathogens, for example, antistaphylococcal
cover (e.g. flucloxacillin) and/or antipseudomo-
nal cover (e.g. gentamicin) for neonates. Patients
with possible intracerebral abscess should receive
metronidazole to cover anaerobes as well as
chloramphenicol.

Use of steroids

Complications of bacterial meningitis are common and severe (Box 31.3). In parts of West
Africa, they may account for over one-third of
cases of deafness. There has been controversy
over the years about using high-dose steroids to
prevent this. Previous studies showed that post-
meningitis deafness could be reduced by dexamethasone given to western children with Hib
meningitis treated with cephalosporins. The
benefit was balanced by some morbidity from
gastrointestinal haemorrhage, and subsequent
studies of steroid use in children in low HIV
prevalence settings in the tropics have generally shown harm or no benefit. One large study
in Egypt showed that adults and children with
pneumococcal meningitis (not meningococcal or
Hib) had reduced mortality and subsequent deafness if given dexamethasone. In northern Europe,
only adult patients with proven or suspected
pneumococcal meningitis benefit from high-
dose dexamethasone (40 mg/day i.v. for 4 days)
given shortly before the first dose of antibiotics.
Similar benefit was only observed in patients with
confirmed *S. suis* meningitis in Vietnam (a low
HIV prevalence setting) despite late presentation

> **Box 31.3 Complications of bacterial meningitis.**
>
> - Cranial nerve palsy
> - Hemiplegia
> - Deafness
> - Subdural empyema
> - Abscess
> - Late hydrocephalus

and prior administration of antibiotics to some patients.

However, two large prospective trials have shown neither benefit nor harm from the use of high-dose dexamethasone in Malawi as an adjunct for treating pyogenic meningitis in children or adults with a high prevalence of HIV, many of whom presented late for hospital treatment. High-dose dexamethasone is expensive, and extra resources are required to administer it in a tropical setting. There is no evidence to support its use in definite or probable meningococcal disease or in most patients who have already received antibiotics of some sort in low HIV prevalence settings and no evidence to support its use in sub-Saharan Africa. However, empirical use for other forms of meningitis is likely to become more common in adults. In Vietnam, similar doses of dexamethasone reduced mortality from tuberculous meningitis but increased the number of survivors with severe disability.

Epidemic control (meningococcus)

The WHO has developed the definition of an 'alert threshold' for an epidemic of meningococcal meningitis as an incidence of >15 cases per 100 000 population for 1 week. Other features that should alert the clinician are a shift in the average age of patients affected, from younger than 5 years to teenagers or older, especially if in a high-risk situation (e.g. refugee camp or in the 'meningitis belt' during the dry season). If more than 3 years have elapsed since the last epidemic, the alert threshold is reduced to 10 cases per 100 000 (Table 31.2).

Early recognition is the key to management (Box 31.4). This should be followed by maximal attempts to confirm the diagnosis by culturing the organism to determine its antimicrobial sensitivities (to guide chemoprophylaxis) and serogroup (to guide vaccination). If facilities to do this are not routinely available, outside assistance is required. This is needed anyway to support enhanced surveillance and to enable provision of adequate supplies of drugs, vaccines, etc. Once an outbreak is declared, a decision must be made on how to get publicity to the affected population and how to conduct surveillance. Healthcare workers and educated lay persons need to be briefed, using simple case definitions on triaging the worried well as well as the sick at designated assessment centres, and clinical management protocols need to be prepared to guide the treatment of patients. The numbers may be large enough to require buildings to be made over specifically for this purpose.

Epidemics of group A disease can be controlled by vaccination—there is ample evidence to support this. The effectiveness depends on both early recognition of an outbreak and rapid mass administration of the appropriate vaccine. Mass chemoprophylaxis can also be used if the organism is sulfa-sensitive, or if a decision is made to use fluoroquinolone, but this is often not practical in a large population.

Box 31.4 Management of meningococcal epidemics.

Early recognition
- ('threshold' 15 cases/100 000 population/week)

Identify organism
- confirm clinical diagnosis and get CSF from cases
- establish strain and antibiotic sensitivity

Alert peripheral staff
- diagnostic algorithms and case definitions
- treatment algorithms

Alert authorities
- surveillance schemes
- temporary treatment centres

Prevent major outbreak
- mass chemoprophylaxis
- mass vaccination

Table 31.2 Meningococcal epidemiology

	Endemic	Epidemic
Incidence/100 000	<10	10–1000
Carrier:case ratio	High	Low
Secondary infections	Rare	Frequent
Peak age	<5	5–15
Usual serogroup	B or C	A, C or W135

Further reading

British Infection Society www.britishinfection society.org/guidelines/guidelines.aspx. [UK oriented algorithm for the management of adult meningitis that can be adapted for local use.]

Fitch MT, van de Beek D. Emergency diagnosis and treatment of bacterial meningitis. *Lancet Infect Dis* 2007; 7: 191–200. [Good overview from a group heavily committed to dexamethasone use in Western settings.]

Greenwood B. Pneumococcal meningitis epidemics in Africa. *Clin Infect Dis* 2006; 43: 701–702. [Summary of new challenges.]

Greenwood BM. Corticosteroids for bacterial meningitis. *N Engl J Med* 2007; 357: 2507–2509. [Key editorial on use of steroids in tropics.]

Hasbun R, Abrahams J, Jekel J, Quagliarello VJ. Computed tomography of the head before lumbar puncture in adults with suspected meningitis. *N Engl J Med* 2001; 345: 1727–1733. [Simple clinical features predict the absence of normality of computerized tomography of the head in adults in a Western setting.]

Molesworth AM, Cuevas LE, Connor SJ, Morse AP, Thomson MC. Environmental risk and meningitis epidemics in Africa. *Emerg Infect Dis* 2003; 9(10):1287–1293. [Article free online. History and geography of meningococcal epidemics in Africa, nice maps.]

Stephens DS, Greenwood G, Brandtzaeg P. Epidemic meningitis, meningococcaemia, and *Neisseria meningitidis*. *Lancet* 2007; 369: 2196–2210. [Superb summary of all aspects of meningococcal disease.]

Santaniello-Newton A, Hunter PR. Management of an outbreak of meningococcal meningitis in a Sudanese refugee camp in Northern Uganda. *Epidemiol Infect* 2000; 124: 75–81. [Case fatality rate of 13% and attack rate of 0.3% (group A meningococcus). They had better experience than other authors and estimated vaccine protective effect to be approximately 83%. The biovalent (A + C) vaccine they used had to be given subcutaneously. They emphasize the need for early epidemic recognition and immunization campaign.]

Thwaites GE, Chau TTH, Stepniewska K *et al.* Diagnosis of tuberculous meningitis by use of clinical and laboratory features. *Lancet* 2002; 360: 1287–1292. [Source reference on diagnostic methods and development of simple formula for bedside use in adults in Vietnam: age, length of history, WBC count, total CSF WBC count and CSF neutrophil proportion are five important variables that combine to distinguish TBM from bacterial meningitis.]

WHO www.who.int/topics/meningitis/en/ [World Health Organization website. Source of latest country-specific information and guidelines for diagnosis and treatment.]

Chapter 32

Cryptococcal meningitis

Organism and epidemiology

Cryptococcal disease is caused by the yeast-like fungus *Cryptococcus neoformans*. There are three varieties: var *gattii*, var *grubii* and var *neoformans*. Vars *grubii* and *neoformans* occur worldwide and are found in the environment related to avian droppings. Var *gattii* occurs predominantly in the tropics and is much harder to be found in the environment, but occurs in association with eucalyptus trees.

Cryptococcal disease occurs in both immunocompetent and immunocompromised hosts. Infection is acquired by inhalation and predominantly causes pulmonary disease or cryptococcal meningitis (CM). In the tropics prior to the AIDS epidemic, var *gattii* caused CM in immunocompetent individuals. However, most cases of cryptococcal disease in the tropics now occur in patients with HIV infection and are caused by var *grubii* or *neoformans*. CM occurs in HIV-infected individuals throughout the tropics, predominantly in those with CD4-cell counts of less than 100×10^6/L. It is one of the most common identified causes of death in HIV-infected Africans.

Clinical features

Cryptococcosis presents as pneumonia, cryptococcal meningitis or disseminated disease. Pneumonia is less common, often asymptomatic or mild and may resolve spontaneously. A small number of immunocompromised patients have a rapidly progressive pulmonary illness. CM presents as a subacute or chronic meningitis with headache, fever and alteration in mental state, often of several weeks' duration. The disease mimics tuberculous meningitis and may be indistinguishable clinically. Clinical signs include fever, cranial nerve palsies and visual disturbance associated with papilloedema; neck stiffness is relatively uncommon. Disseminated infection occurs in advanced immunosuppression, often presenting as fever. Skin lesions may occur and may contain the organism.

Diagnosis

A high index of suspicion should be maintained in those with HIV infection and unexplained fever or headache. Lumbar puncture classically demonstrates a raised CSF protein and white-cell count with a predominant lymphocytosis, although the cell count and protein can be normal in early CM or if the patient is very immunosuppressed. The CSF opening pressure is commonly raised. Cryptococci can be seen after Gram's staining

Lecture Notes: Tropical Medicine, 6th edition.
By G.V. Gill and N.J. Beeching. Published 2009 by Blackwell Publishing, ISBN: 978-1-4051-8048-1.

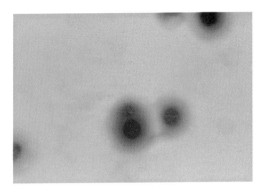

Figure 32.1 Budding yeast-like organisms of *Cryptococcus neoformans* in the cerebrospinal fluid stained with Gram's stain.

(Figure 32.1) or simply demonstrated in the CSF by the addition of a few drops of India ink. This outlines the capsule of the organism and makes it easier to distinguish the organism from white cells. India ink staining is positive in up to 70% of patients. The organism can also be cultured from the CSF, blood or, occasionally, skin lesions. Latex agglutination tests can detect cryptococcal polysaccharide antigen with a high sensitivity in the CSF or the blood and may be very useful if culture facilities are not available.

Treatment

Optimum treatment of CM is amphotericin B (1 mg/kg/day) in combination with flucytosine (100 mg/kg/day) for 2 weeks followed by fluconazole 400 mg daily for a further 8 weeks. However, there are often practical difficulties in the administration of amphotericin in resource-poor settings because of its renal toxicity and the need to monitor renal function. Flucytosine may also cause marrow suppression, which may be problematic in some HIV patients. Fluconazole (400 mg or more daily) may be used as initial therapy and has fewer side effects than amphotericin and flucytosine but takes much longer to sterilize the CSF and is associated with higher relapse rates.

Relapse is common in HIV patients following successful initial treatment. Secondary prophylaxis with fluconazole (200 mg/day) is effective in preventing relapse and needs to be continued for life or until the CD4 count has risen to above $200 \times 10^6/L$ for several months following antiretroviral therapy.

Many patients with CM have raised intracranial pressure, which is associated with a poor prognosis. There is no proven method of reducing this, but many clinicians advocate repeated lumbar punctures to reduce the intracranial pressure. In the absence of treatment of CM, the disease is uniformly fatal. Even with treatment, case fatality rates can be as high as 50% in some parts of the tropics. Initiation of antiretroviral therapy after successful treatment may be associated with cryptococcal immune reconstitution syndrome.

Further reading

Bicanic T, Harrison TS. Cryptococcal meningitis. *Br Med Bull* 2005; 72: 99–118. [Good up-to-date review on clinical and therapeutic aspects.]

Chapter 33

Encephalitis

Encephalitis (inflammation of the brain parenchyma) is, strictly speaking, a pathological diagnosis that should only be made with histological evidence at autopsy or from brain biopsy. Because of the obvious practical limitations of this, clinical definitions are often used. Most patients present with the triad of fever, headache and encephalopathy (reduced level of consciousness). Many also have focal neurological signs and seizures. However, patients occasionally present simply with abnormal behaviour, which may be mistaken for psychiatric illness.

Causes of encephalitis

Encephalitis can be caused by many viruses, other organisms and autoimmune processes (Table 33.1) However, viruses transmitted by insects (arboviruses; Chapter 40) make encephalitis especially common in the tropics.

Arboviral encephalitis

The arboviruses that cause neurological disease in humans come principally from three viral families (see Figure 40.1). The most important are the

flaviviruses, especially Japanese encephalitis virus. Flaviviruses exist in enzootic cycles, being transmitted by mosquitoes (in warm climates) or ticks (in cooler northern climates); most humans are coincidentally infected 'dead end' hosts. In addition, alphaviruses and bunyaviruses cause CNS disease in the Americas.

Japanese encephalitis

Japanese encephalitis is the most important cause of epidemic encephalitis worldwide. There are 35000–50000 cases estimated annually with 10000 deaths. More than half the survivors have severe neurological sequelae.

Epidemiology

The virus is transmitted naturally between birds by *Culex* mosquitoes, especially *Culex tritaeniorhynchus*, which breeds in rice paddy fields. Peri-domestic animals (especially pigs) act as amplifying hosts, and subsequently humans become infected (Figure 33.1). In southern tropical areas, the disease is endemic; in northern temperate zones, it occurs in summer epidemics (Figure 33.2). The geographical area affected is expanding, possibly because of increasing irrigation projects, and spread by birds. In endemic areas of rural Asia, the virus is ubiquitous and

Lecture Notes: Tropical Medicine, 6th edition.
By G.V. Gill and N.J. Beeching. Published 2009 by
Blackwell Publishing, ISBN: 978-1-4051-8048-1.

Table 33.1 Infectious causes of encephalitis

Arthropod-borne viruses (often epidemic and geographically localized)
Flaviviruses (Japanese encephalitis, West Nile, Murray Valley)
Alphaviruses (Venezuelan, Eastern and Western equine encephalitis; chikungunya)
Bunyaviruses (La Crosse encephalitis)

Non-arthropod-borne viruses (mostly sporadic and non-geographically localized)
Herpes viruses (Herpes simplex virus types 1 and 2, varicella zoster virus, Epstein–Barr virus)
Enteroviruses (Coxsackie, echovirus, enterovirus type 71)
Paramyxoviruses (measles, mumps, Nipah)
Rabies (Chapter 36)
Human immunodeficiency virus

Acute disseminated encephalomyelitis
Occurs several weeks after an acute infection (often viral) or vaccination

Other infectious causes of encephalitis
Usually distinguishable from viral encephalitis either because of their slower onset or because they are associated with other features (e.g. multiorgan failure, rash)
Trypanosomiasis, especially *Trypanosoma brucei rhodesiense*
Toxoplasma occasionally presents with diffuse encephalitis
Amoebic meningoencephalitis, e.g. *Naegleria fowleri, Balamuthia mandrillaris*
Typh us, especially African tick typhus (*Rickettsia africae*) and scrub typhus in Asia (*O. tsutsugamushi*)
Secondary syphilis and other spirochaetes (e.g. relapsing fevers)

almost all children are infected, but only a small proportion develops disease.

Clinical features

Following a non-specific febrile illness, which may include coryza, cough, vomiting, diarrhoea and headache, patients develop a reduced level of consciousness. This may be heralded by convulsions; status epilepticus is common. Focal neurological signs include upper and lower motor neurone signs; a 'Parkinsonian syndrome' with tremor, cogwheel rigidity and mask-like facies; rigidity spasms, flexor and extensor posturing and other signs of raised intracranial pressure. Other patients present with aseptic meningitis, febrile convulsions or a polio-like acute flaccid paralysis. The differential diagnosis includes other causes of encephalitis and non-viral causes of CNS disease (see Table 3.1).

Investigations

Typically, lymphocytes are present in the CSF (5–100/mm³), with a normal glucose level

and slightly elevated protein (50–100 mg/dL). However, the CSF may be normal if taken too early or too late in the disease. IgM antibodies appear in the serum and CSF after the first few days of illness and can be detected by ELISA or rapid diagnostic kits. Virus is sometimes isolated from CSF or brain tissue at postmortem, or detected by PCR in the CSF. CT or MRI may show characteristic midbrain changes.

Management

This is discussed at the end of this chapter.

Prevention and public health

Vaccines against Japanese encephalitis include a mouse brain–derived inactivated vaccine (requires three doses; occasional mild side effects), tissue culture–derived vaccines and a new Chinese live attenuated vaccine (safe and effective; single dose may be effective). Vector control measures such as treating rice paddy fields with neem cake (a natural insecticide) and intermittent irrigation of rice

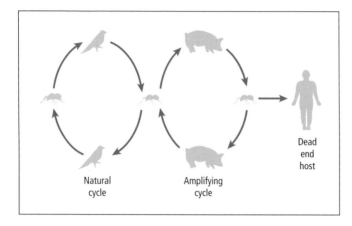

Figure 33.1 The transmission cycle of Japanese encephalitis virus. The virus is transmitted naturally between aquatic birds by *Culex* mosquitoes. During the rainy season, when there is an increase in the number of mosquitoes, the virus 'overflows' into pigs and other peri-domestic animals, and then into humans, from whom it is not transmitted further.

Natural cycle

Amplifying cycle

Dead end host

paddies to prevent *Culex* breeding probably have no major role in control. Individual protective measures include avoiding mosquito bites (easier for visitors than residents) and using DEET-containing spray, bed nets and protective clothing.

Future developments

The Chinese vaccine is being used increasingly in Asia, and newer approaches such as a chimeric vaccine and a tissue culture–derived vaccine are in advanced stages of development.

West Nile virus

This is a flavivirus widely distributed throughout Africa, Asia, the Middle East, southern Europe and has recently spread to North America. It is transmitted between water fowl by *C. pipiens*. West Nile virus was previously considered to be a cause of fever–arthralgia–rash syndrome, with occasional CNS disease. There have been recent epidemics of CNS disease in Romania (in 1996, 600 people) and in America (in 1999, 60 people and in 2002, 3500 people). Vaccines are in development.

St Louis encephalitis virus

This is a flavivirus found in the Americas. It previously caused large epidemics, 3000 cases/year,

but now only around 100 cases/year. It may be a good example of how arboviral disease can be controlled if there is enough money for sentinel surveillance and vector control (spraying).

Tick-borne encephalitis virus

The disease caused by this virus has many synonyms, for example Russian spring–summer encephalitis. The organism is a flavivirus transmitted between rodents and other small mammals by *Ixodes* ticks. It is also transmitted by ingesting infected goat's milk. The disease is found in a wide area from eastern Europe to the Far East and particularly affects forestry workers and hikers, who present 1–2 weeks after a tick bite. It is a biphasic illness with a high fever for 1 week followed by an afebrile period, then a meningoencephalitis or myelitis with upper limb, respiratory and bulbar flaccid paralysis. The CSF often shows neutrophils, and a peripheral leucocytosis and elevated ESR may mimic bacterial meningitis. A formalin-inactivated vaccine is available.

Murray Valley encephalitis virus

This is a flavivirus causing encephalitis in Australia and Papua New Guinea.

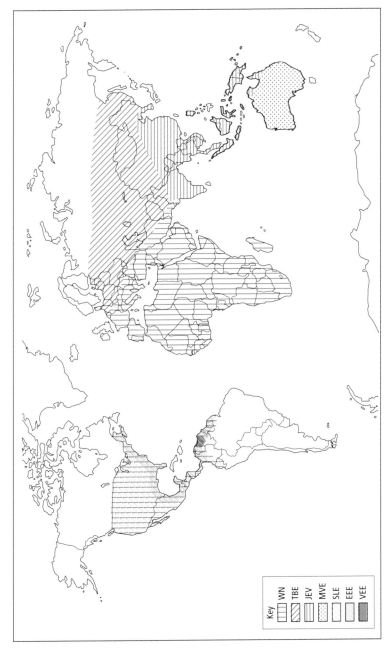

Figure 33.2 Map showing the approximate global distribution of CNS arboviruses. In North America, Western equine encephalitis has a distribution similar to St Louis encephalitis (SLE), and La Crosse has a distribution similar to West Nile (WN). EEE, Eastern equine encephalitis; JEV, Japanese encephalitis virus; MVE, Murray Valley encephalitis; TBE, tick-borne encephalitis; VEE, Venezuelan equine encephalitis.

Equine encephalitis viruses

Venezuelan, Eastern and Western equine encephalitis viruses are mosquito-borne alphaviruses transmitted between birds and/or small mammals by *Culex*, *Aedes* and *Culiseta* mosquitoes. They cause epidemics of encephalitis in horses and humans in the Americas.

La Crosse virus

A bunyavirus transmitted between chipmunks and squirrels, principally by *Aedes* mosquitoes. It causes up to 200 cases of encephalitis in the United States annually but has a low case fatality rate.

Management of patients with encephalitis

There is no specific antiviral treatment for most forms of viral encephalitis. Aciclovir is effective for herpes simplex virus type 1 and related viruses. In the West, it is therefore given as soon as encephalitis is suspected. In the tropics, where other causes are more common, aciclovir is often reserved for cases that are atypical for the common local arboviral cause (e.g. wrong age and wrong season) or for cases with typical radiological changes of herpes. Ideally, encephalitis patients in a coma should be sedated and ventilated on an intensive care unit. This allows airway protection, maximum medication to control seizures and hyperventilation to reduce raised intracranial pressure, but this is often not possible.

Whatever the viral cause, attention must be paid to the complications of encephalitis.

• *Pneumonia*—often caused by aspiration. Treat with broad-spectrum antibiotics.

• *Seizures*—sometimes these may be subtle motor seizures: look for twitching of a digit, the mouth or eye. Confirm with EEG if possible. Treat seizures with diazepam. Treat status epilepticus with phenytoin (using a cardiac monitor) or phenobarbital (see Chapter 59).

• *Raised intracranial pressure*—there may be elevated CSF opening pressure at lumbar puncture. Look for clinical signs of brainstem herniation syndromes (Chapter 3). Nurse patients at 30° with the neck straight, give osmotic diuretics (e.g. mannitol), hyperventilate.

• *Malnutrition*—despite nasogastric feeding, very common in patients who are ill for more than a few days.

• *Bedsores*—minimized by good nursing care. Placing rubber gloves (inflated with water) between the knees and below the heels can help prevent some sores.

• *Contractures*—encourage the family to keep joints supple; use splints (improvised if necessary) to keep joints in position.

Further reading

Davis LE. Acute viral meningitis and encephalitis. In: Kennedy PGE, Johnson RT, eds. *Infections of the Nervous System*. London: Butterworths, 1987: 156–176. [General review of viral meningoencephalitis.]

Solomon T. Exotic and emerging viral encephalitides. *Curr Opin Neurol* 2003; 16: 411–418. [Newer infections.]

Solomon T. New vaccine for Japanese encephalitis. *Lancet Neurol* 2008; 7: 116–117.

Solomon T, Dung NM, Kneen R *et al.* Neurological aspects of tropical diseases: Japanese encephalitis. *J Neurol Neurosurg Psychiatry* 2000; 68: 405–415.

Whitley RJ, Grann JW. Viral encephalitis: familiar infections and emerging pathogens. *Lancet* 2002; 359: 507–513. [Useful update on West Nile encephalitis.]

Chapter 34

Acute flaccid paralysis

Acute flaccid paralysis is defined as weakness in one or more limbs, or the respiratory or bulbar muscles, resulting from damaged lower motor neurones. Poliomyelitis was the most important cause, but since it has declined other causes have become more important.

Classically, in acute flaccid paralysis there is weakness with reduced tone (flaccid weakness) and reduced or absent reflexes. Differentiation from upper motor neurone weakness is usually straightforward, but it should be remembered that acute spinal shock (e.g. caused by trauma) can initially cause flaccid paralysis before spasticity develops.

Pathophysiology and clinical presentations

Broadly speaking, there are two pathophysiological processes that cause acute flaccid paralysis (Figure 34.1). These are direct viral damage of lower motor neurone cell bodies in the anterior horn of the spinal cord (e.g. polio, other enteroviruses, flaviviruses), and a para- or postinfectious immunologically mediated process damaging the motor nerves, and often sensory

nerves (e.g. Guillain–Barré syndrome), sometimes caused by antibodies directed against the gangliosides (glycolipids in the nerve cell membranes). Recognizing the clinical features of these two patterns helps in determining the likely cause (Table 34.1).

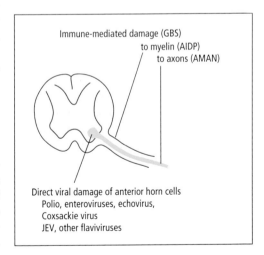

Figure 34.1 Pathophysiology of acute flaccid paralysis. Immune-mediated Guillain–Barré syndrome (GBS) occurs in two forms: in acute inflammatory demyelinating polyneuropathy (AIDP) the myelin is damaged; in acute motor axonal neuropathy (AMAN) the motor axons are targeted. Viruses such as polio and Japanese encephalitis virus (JEV) cause paralysis by directly attacking the lower motor neurones (the anterior horn cells).

Lecture Notes: Tropical Medicine, 6th edition. By G.V. Gill and N.J. Beeching. Published 2009 by Blackwell Publishing, ISBN: 978-1-4051-8048-1.

Table 34.1 Clinical features to distinguish causes of acute flaccid paralysis

	Direct viral damage to anterior horn cells (e.g. polio)	Immune-mediated damage to peripheral nerves (e.g. Guillain–Barré syndrome)
Paralysis onset	During (or straight after) febrile illness	Several weeks after febrile illness
Pattern of paralysis	Asymmetrical	Symmetrical
Time to reach maximum weakness	Short (e.g. 2–3 days)	Long (e.g. 7–14 days)
Sensory involvement	No	Often (depending on exact disease)
Cerebrospinal fluid	Increased lymphocytes (e.g. 100/mm³)	Increased protein (e.g. 100 mg/dL especially late in the disease)
Pain	Often limb muscle pain	Often back pain

Anterior horn cell damage causing acute flaccid paralysis

Polio

Infection with this enterovirus can be asymptomatic and can cause a mild non-specific febrile illness, viral meningitis or paralytic poliomyelitis, which can be spinal or bulbar. Paralytic poliomyelitis is biphasic, with a non-specific fever followed by a brief afebrile period before the CNS is invaded. This is heralded by further fever and an acute-onset asymmetrical flaccid paralysis of one or more limbs, which may be painful. Since the WHO campaign to eradicate polio using the oral polio vaccine, the number of cases dropped from more than 350000 cases in 1988 to approximately 1900 cases in 2002. Most of these came from South Asia (India, Pakistan and Afghanistan), West Africa (mainly Nigeria) and Central Africa (mainly Democratic Republic of Congo). However, since then the number of cases has risen again; for example, in 2004 there were 1255 confirmed cases from 16 countries. The setbacks have occurred in parts of the Asian subcontinent and Africa because of difficulty immunizing in areas of ongoing conflict, poor compliance with immunization because of mistrust in some communities, natural disasters disrupting infrastructure and issues over financing the programme.

Enterovirus 71

Enterovirus 71 has caused epidemics of acute flaccid paralysis in recent years (especially in Asia), often in association with hand, foot and mouth disease. Large outbreaks occur in some countries every 3–4 years. Many other enterovirus, Coxsackie virus and echovirus serotypes occasionally cause acute flaccid paralysis.

Japanese encephalitis virus

Japanese encephalitis virus, West Nile and other flaviviruses typically cause meningoencephalitis, but flaviviruses can also present with a pure flaccid paralysis that can be clinically similar to polio (Chapter 33).

Immune-mediated causes of acute flaccid paralysis

Guillain–Barré syndrome is now recognized as a group of disorders classified according to the predominant type of nerve injury (axonal or demyelinating) and the main nerve fibres involved (motor, sensory, cranial). Different anti-ganglioside antibodies are associated with different diseases.

Acute inflammatory demyelinating polyneuropathy (or 'classical' Guillain–Barré syndrome)

Acute inflammatory demyelinating polyneuropathy (AIDP) typically presents several weeks after a febrile illness with back pain, then symmetrical ascending flaccid paralysis and sensory changes. Recovery is usual. Treat rapidly progressing symptoms with intravenous immunoglobulin if available.

Acute motor axonal neuropathy (or Chinese paralytic syndrome)

Acute motor and axonal neuropathy (AMAN) typically follows diarrhoea caused by *Campylobacter jejuni*. Symmetrical weakness is present with no sensory changes. Residual weakness is common. Occurs in summer epidemics in China.

Other causes

- Exposure to rabid animal (paralytic rabies)
- Exposure to toxins
- Tick bites (tick paralysis is a slowly ascending paralysis that recovers when the tick is removed)
- History of a severe sore throat with neck swelling (diphtheritic neuropathy)
- Consumption of poorly preserved food (botulinum toxin)

Nerve conduction studies

Where available, nerve conduction studies may help distinguish further.

- *Anterior horn cell damage*—motor amplitude is reduced because motor cell bodies have been damaged.
- *Classical Guillain–Barré syndrome* (autoimmune demyelinating polyneuropathy)—motor and sensory nerves have reduced conduction velocities and delayed distal latencies because demyelinated nerves conduct more slowly.
- *AMAN* (Chinese paralytic syndrome)—motor amplitudes are reduced because motor axons have been damaged.

Further reading

Anonymous. Progress toward global poliomyelitis eradication, 1999. *MMWR Morbid Mortal Wkly Rep* 2000; 49: 349–354.

Bolton CF. The changing concepts of Guillain–Barré syndrome. *N Engl J Med* 1995; 333: 1415–1416. [Good explanation of acute motor axonal neuropathy as a form of Guillain–Barré syndrome.]

Solomon T, Willison H. Infectious causes of acute flaccid paralysis. *Curr Opin Infect Dis* 2003; 16: 375–379. [Annotated review of main infectious causes.]

Chapter 35

Spastic paralysis

Spastic paralysis is caused by damage to the upper motor neurones and is characterized by weakness with increased tone, brisk reflexes and extensor plantars.

Causes and anatomy

Some of the important causes of spastic paralysis are shown in Figure 35.1. The upper motor neurones can be affected anywhere along the corticospinal tract, but the associated features give a clue as to the site of damage as follows.

- A pure spastic paraparesis with no sensory changes is usually caused by damage in the brain where sensory and motor pathways are far apart (e.g. spastic diplegia in cerebral palsy, or frontal meningioma).
- In the spinal cord, sensory pathways lie close to the motor pathways and so are often also affected by any pathology. Look for dorsal column signs (loss of light touch, vibration and joint position sensation) and a sensory level.
- Intrinsic cord lesions are usually painless.
- Extrinsic lesions causing spinal cord compression often also press on the sensory roots as they leave the spinal cord, and thus cause pain in the distribution of those roots (radicular pain).

Lecture Notes: Tropical Medicine, 6th edition.
By G.V. Gill and N.J. Beeching. Published 2009 by Blackwell Publishing, ISBN: 978-1-4051-8048-1.

Assessment of the patient with spastic paralysis

Important features to determine include the following.
- Speed of onset—rapid in vascular disease, more prolonged in inflammatory, infectious and compressive disease.
- Past and current medical problems—cerebral palsy, tuberculosis, HIV, macrocytic anaemia.
- Urinary hesitancy, frequency or retention (the latter is a late feature).
- Constipation, incontinence, reduced anal tone and sensation.
- Presence of pain—extrinsic lesions compressing spinal roots cause radicular pain (e.g. tumours); abscesses give back pain and local tenderness.
- Examine for a gibbus of Pott's disease (see later), or naevus/hairy patch of spinal dysraphism (spina bifida occulta).
- Sensory level—nipples are T4, umbilicus is T10.

Important tropical causes of spastic paralysis

Tuberculosis

TB causes spastic paralysis in one of the following three ways:
1 TB of the vertebral bones leads to collapse (Pott's disease) and secondary cord compression

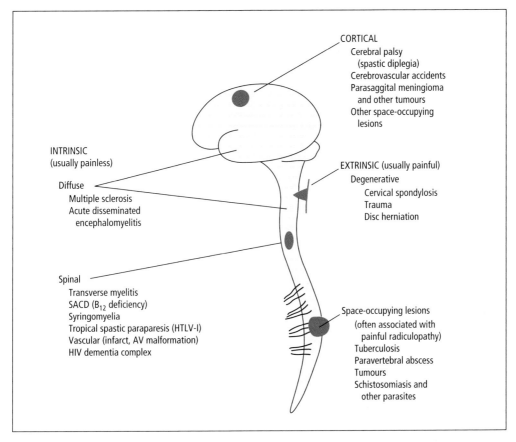

Figure 35.1 Causes of spastic paralysis. AV, arteriovenous; SACD, subacute combined degeneration of the spinal cord.

(a bony prominent sharp kyphosis caused by a collapsed vertebra is known as a gibbus).

2 Chronic TB meningitis leads to secondary arteritis and cord infarction.

3 A tuberculoma compresses the cord directly.

Many patients have a personal or family history of TB or evidence of the disease elsewhere. Investigate with a tuberculin test, ESR, chest X-ray, spinal X-ray, CT or MRI scanning if possible. Treatment consists of antituberculous therapy, and surgery if appropriate.

Spinal epidural abscess

Spinal epidural abscess is most frequently caused by *Staphylococcus aureus*. Patients present with the triad of fever, backache/tenderness and radicular

pain, followed by rapidly progressive spastic paraparesis, sensory loss and bowel and bladder dysfunction. There is usually a peripheral leucocytosis, elevated ESR and mild CSF pleocytosis with an increased protein level. An X-ray may show soft tissue changes and associated vertebral osteomyelitis. On myelography, the flow of contrast medium is blocked. MRI is the investigation of choice. Patients should be treated with emergency surgical drainage and antibiotics.

Transverse myelitis

Transverse myelitis is an acute inflammation of the spinal cord. Presentation is rapid and often a sensory level is present. It can be associated with many common infectious agents including many viruses and some bacteria (particularly *Mycoplasma pneumoniae*). It can also occur post most vaccinations. For many patients, it will be a monophasic illness and no cause may be found; however, some patients will go onto develop multiple sclerosis or Devic's neuromyelitis optica and others may have a connective tissue disorder. Tropical infections that are associated with transverse myelitis include HIV, schistosomiasis, syphilis, dengue, scrub typhus, leptospirosis and *Borrelia burgdorferi*.

HIV myelopathy

HIV myelopathy is a progressive myelopathy and is a frequent finding in patients with the AIDS–dementia complex. There is usually spasticity with increased or decreased reflexes, ataxia, incontinence and dorsal column signs. The MRI scan is usually normal, but at autopsy there is vacuolation of the spinal cord white matter, especially in the posterior and lateral columns of the thoracic cord. HIV myelopathy is thought to be caused directly by HIV-1 invasion. Other causes of myelopathy in AIDS include lymphoma, *Cryptococcus* and herpes viruses.

Subacute combined degeneration of the spinal cord

This is caused by vitamin B_{12} deficiency resulting from poor diet or impaired absorption secondary to

tropical sprue, *Diphyllobothrium latum* infection (fish tapeworm), gastrointestinal surgery or as part of pernicious anaemia. The disease leads to a mixture of upper motor neurone deficit (corticospinal tract damage), sensory deficit caused by dorsal column involvement and peripheral neuropathy, sometimes with optic neuropathy and dementia. Classical findings are extensor plantars with absent knee jerks. Neck flexion causes shooting pains down the arms (Lhermitte's sign). There is usually a macrocytic anaemia. The disease is treated with intramuscular vitamin B_{12} injections 1 mg/day for 6 days, then reducing to a maintenance dose (Chapter 57).

Tropical spastic paraparesis

Tropical spastic paraparesis is found in the Caribbean, Seychelles, equatorial Africa, Japan and parts of the Americas. Most cases are caused by human T lymphotrophic virus type 1 (HTLV-1), transmitted sexually, by exposure to blood products or by breast milk. The disease presents with progressive spastic paraparesis, impaired vibration and joint position sensation, and bowel and bladder dysfunction.

Chapter 36

Rabies

Rabies virus is a bullet-shaped RNA rhabdovirus that is widely prevalent among warm-blooded animals in many tropical countries. Worldwide, dogs are the main transmitters of rabies to humans; bats are involved in North America, certain South American countries, some areas of Europe and, more recently, Australia. Between 35 000 and 50 000 people die from rabies every year, with most deaths occurring in Asia.

On reaching the brain of an infected animal, the rabies virus spreads along peripheral nerves to reach the skin, and the lachrymal and salivary glands. An animal bite with virus-laden saliva is therefore the usual mode of infection, although the disease can also be acquired by salivary contamination of cuts, abrasions and mucous membranes, and occasionally by inhalation. Rarely, rabies has been transmitted by corneal transplants taken from donors dying from unrecognized rabies. The risk of rabies in a person bitten by a rabid animal varies widely up to 50%, depending on the site and nature of the bites and the animal species.

Rabies in the dog

This is usually furious: the dog rushes around emitting a high-pitched bark, and biting not only

Lecture Notes: Tropical Medicine, 6th edition.
By G.V. Gill and N.J. Beeching. Published 2009 by
Blackwell Publishing, ISBN: 978-1-4051-8048-1.

people but also objects. The animal may paw at its mouth, as if trying to dislodge a foreign body and salivate excessively. It nearly always dies within 15 days of becoming infective. This fact is made use of when a dog that has bitten someone is impounded. If the dog is alive 15 days after the bite, it is very unlikely to have been infective when it bit.

Dogs can be given a high degree of protection against rabies by an attenuated live vaccine.

Rabies in other animals

Dogs, foxes, wolves and jackals are the major reservoirs of rabies in most parts of the world, and cats can also transmit infection usually themselves suffering from a paralytic illness typical of 'dumb rabies'. In South America and the Caribbean, bats are very important vectors and cause enormous economic losses because of death of cattle from paralytic rabies. Bats can also cause human disease, not only from their bites but also from the inhalation of aerosolized bat secretions by speleologists exploring caves, mainly in the Americas.

Clinical features in humans

Once inoculated, the rabies virus travels centripetally along peripheral nerves to reach the spinal cord and brain. The incubation period is related to the inoculum size and the time taken to reach the brain: generally it is 2–8 weeks but may range between 9 days and a year or more. The incubation period is proportional to the distance the virus has to travel and therefore tends to be shorter in children, and after bites on the face and neck.

The disease may be heralded by pain, paraesthesiae or pruritus in the bitten area; these occur in 30–80% of cases. The illness proper usually begins abruptly with fever, insomnia, anxiety and other psychological disturbances. In the encephalitic (furious) form of the disease the patient suffers from intermittent episodes of confusion, agitation and aggression verging on mania, with intervening periods of calm and lucidity. Copious secretion of ropy saliva is characteristic and the patient may literally 'froth at the mouth'.

Painful spasms of the throat muscles, often precipitated by attempts to swallow, are accompanied by 'hydrophobia', an overwhelming terror of drinking. Spasms often become more widespread to involve the diaphragm and respiratory muscles: they may be accompanied by spitting, grimacing, vomiting, opisthotonos and seizures. Spasms may also be precipitated by air blowing on to the face (aerophobia). Death usually occurs within a week, with respiratory and bulbar paralysis.

Some 20% of patients suffer from a paralytic form of rabies. There is an ascending sensorimotor neuropathy with ocular, cranial and laryngeal palsies and sphincter disturbances: fasciculation may be seen in muscles. Hydrophobia is rare.

Diagnosis

Diagnosis during life

In most cases the diagnosis will be made on the characteristic clinical picture: laboratory tests for virus detection may not be available and currently lack sensitivity. Immunofluorescence of corneal impression smears or skin biopsies can detect viral antigen, especially late in the illness. Skin biopsies are taken from the nape of the neck so as to contain hair follicles and peripheral nerves. Attempts to culture virus from saliva, CSF or biopsies may not succeed in the later stages of illness because of the presence of neutralizing antibodies.

Diagnostic antibody tests do not become positive until about the eighth day and are difficult to interpret in vaccinated patients.

Rapid diagnostic methods based on nucleic acid amplification are being developed and look very promising: viral RNA can be detected in saliva and CSF as early as the second day of illness.

Postmortem diagnosis

Because of cross-infection hazards, a postmortem should only be performed if absolutely necessary. Staff should be immunized and must wear protective clothing and visors.

Immunofluorescence of fresh brain is the technique most widely used to demonstrate viral antigen. Rabies virus can be detected using tissue culture and mouse inoculation. PCR methods can also be applied. Histology, which is not routinely performed, shows a diffuse meningoencephalitis with extensive neuronal destruction and the presence of Negri inclusion bodies within brain cells.

Treatment

Rabies is almost invariably fatal and the disease causes great suffering. The main aim of treatment is to relieve symptoms with heavy sedation such as a mixture of a phenothiazine, a barbiturate and diamorphine. Intensive care may, in rare instances, have saved one or two lives.

Precautions with rabies patients

The patient's saliva is potentially infective. Everyone in contact with the patient should be protected as for barrier nursing, with the addition of visors. Staff should receive rabies immunization (four intradermal injections of 0.1 mL of human diploid cell vaccine, each given into a different limb on the same day).

Postexposure treatment

The aim is to eliminate or neutralize rabies virus during the incubation period. Management is aided by asking the patient 10 key questions (Table 36.1).

Table 36.1 Ten questions to ask the patient

> 1 Was the person bitten or licked on an open wound or mucous membranes by an animal?
> 2 Where on the body was the bite/lick?
> 3 Where did the incident take place and on what date?
> 4 What species was the animal?
> 5 Is rabies known or suspected in the species? In the area?
> 6 Is there a known and contactable owner?
> 7 (a) Was the animal behaving normally at the time?
>   (b) Had it been vaccinated?
>   (c) Is the animal being held under observation?
> 8 If the animal was a dog or a cat did it become ill while under observation?
> 9 If the animal has died, does laboratory examination of the animal's brain confirm rabies?
> 10 Has the bitten person previously received rabies vaccine? How much does the person weigh (relevant to rabies immune globulin dosage)?

First aid treatment

Wash and flush the wound vigorously with soap and water, detergent or water alone. Then apply ethanol 70% tincture or aqueous solution of iodine, or 0.1% quaternary ammonium compounds (with the latter, remove all traces of soap first).

Immediate treatment by or under the direction of a physician

1 Treat as in first aid treatment mentioned earlier
2 If indicated (Table 36.2), use topical rabies immune globulin (RIG) around the wound (see later).
3 Postpone suturing of wound; if suturing is necessary, use immune globulin locally.
4 Where indicated, institute antitetanus procedures and administer antibiotics and drugs to control infections other than rabies.

Postexposure immunization

See Table 36.2.

Active immunization
Purified inactivated cell culture or duck embryo vaccines are recommended as they are potent and safe. Costs can be reduced by intradermal administration.

Whichever vaccine is used, it must be started as early as possible after exposure and should never be withheld whatever time has elapsed.

Passive immunization
RIG should be given for high-risk exposures (Table 36.2) unless the patient has been previously fully immunized. The dose is 20 IU/kg body weight for human RIG and 40 IU/kg for equine RIG. Up to half the dose is given by infiltration in and around the wound, and the rest given by intramuscular injection at a site separate from the first dose of vaccine. If RIG is initially unobtainable, it may be given up to day 7. Equine RIG may cause allergic reactions and the usual precautions against anaphylaxis must be taken. Serum sickness occurs in 1–6% of patients, usually 7–10 days after injection. At the time of writing this preparation is not being manufactured.

Postexposure vaccine regimens

The following vaccines are recommended by the WHO:
- Human diploid cell vaccine (HDCV).
- Purified vero cell vaccine (PVRV).
- Purified primary chick embryo cell vaccine (PCECV).
- Purified duck embryo vaccine (PDEV).

Table 36.2 Treatment according to nature of exposure

| Nature of exposure | Status of biting animal (irrespective of previous vaccination) | | Recommended treatment |
	At time of exposure	During 15 days[a]	
1 Contact, but no lesions; indirect contact; no contact	Rabid		None
2 Licks of the skin; scratches or abrasions; minor bites (covered areas of arms, trunk and legs)	Suspected as rabid	Healthy	Start vaccine. Stop treatment if animal remains healthy for 15 days[a]
		Rabid	Start vaccine; administer rabies immune globulin if appropriate upon positive diagnosis and complete the course of vaccine
	Rabid; wild animal or animal unavailable for observation		Vaccine + rabies immune globulin, according to previous immunization history
3 Licks of mucosa; major bites (multiple or on face, head, finger or neck)	Suspect or rabid domestic or wild animal, or animal unavailable for observation		Vaccine + rabies immune globulin, according to previous immunization history. Stop treatment if animal remains healthy for 15 days[a]

Source: UK Department of Health (2000).
[a]Observation period applies to dogs and cats. Ten days recommended by WHO.

WHO recommended schedules

1 *Intramuscular administration (into the deltoid, never the buttock)*—for use with all recommended vaccines. One dose of vaccine on days 0, 3, 7, 14 and 28. Alternatively, two doses on day 0 (one into each deltoid), one dose on day 7 and one on day 21.

2 *Two-site intradermal method ('2-2-2-0-1-1')*—for use with PVRV, PCECV and PDEV. Days 0, 3 and 7: one intradermal dose given at each of two sites over the deltoid; days 28 and 90: one intradermal dose given at one site on the upper arm. The intradermal dose is one-fifth of the intramuscular dose.

3 *Eight-site intradermal method ('8-0-4-0-1-1')*—for use with HDCV and PCECV. Day 0: 0.1 mL of vaccine at each of eight sites (deltoid, lateral thigh, suprascapular region and lower quadrant of abdomen); day 7: 0.1 mL of vaccine at each of four sites (deltoid and thighs); days 28 and 90: 0.1 mL of vaccine at one site (deltoid).

Nerve tissue vaccines

These are less potent and are more likely to cause neuroparalytic complications. Suckling mouse brain (SMB) vaccine is often used in Latin America. Subcutaneous doses are usually given daily for 7 days, with booster doses at 10, 20 and 90 days. Vaccines prepared in fixed sheep and goat brains (e.g. Semple vaccine) carry an appreciable risk of postvaccinal encephalitis or polyneuritis.

Need for flexibility

These vaccination recommendations are intended only as a guide. Modification of standard procedures may be justifiable in areas of low rabies endemicity or where there is no indication of rabies infection in the animal species involved. Local expert advice should be obtained whenever possible. Vaccine use in the immunocompromised needs further investigation.

Pre-exposure immunization

This is recommended for travellers to endemic areas and those at special risk (e.g. veterinarians and animal handlers). Three doses of a cell culture or PDEV are given on days 0, 7 and 28. The vaccines may be given intramuscularly or intradermally; doses are according to manufacturers' instructions. The antibody response may be impaired by concomitant chloroquine administration, particularly if the intradermal route is used.

Prevention of rabies

In endemic areas this depends upon the mass immunization of dogs, import controls and the elimination of strays. Unvaccinated dogs (those not wearing a collar with a vaccination tag) should be regularly caught and destroyed. The best results are obtained by professional dog-catchers using bait. Attempts to control dogs by soldiers armed with assault rifles are invariably unsuccessful and dangerous.

Further reading

Anonymous. Human rabies prevention: United States, 1999. Recommendations of the Advisory Committee on Immunization Practises (ACIP). *MMWR Morb Mortal Wkly Rep* 1999; 48 (RR–1): 1–21. [Largely concerned with US practice; this discusses rabies epidemiology in bats, terrestrial carnivores and other wild animals. Extensively referenced.]

Department of Health. *Memorandum on Rabies Prevention and Control*. London: Department of Health, 2000. [Contains useful information on all aspects of rabies control: immunization, patient management, postmortem precautions and veterinary action.]

Willoughby RE, Kelly ST, Hoffman GM *et al.* Survival after treatment of rabies with induction of coma. *N Engl J Med* 2005; 352: 2508–2514. [Description of a rare case of successful rabies treatment, though with neurological damage.]

World Health Organization. WHO recommendations on rabies postexposure treatment and the correct technique of intradermal immunization against rabies. World Health Organization WHO/EMC/ZOO.96.6, 1997. [Essential reading; this gives straightforward advice on first aid, pre- and postexposure immunization and the use of rabies immune globulin.]

Chapter 37

Tetanus

Bacteriology and pathogenesis

Tetanus is caused by *Clostridium tetani*, a Gram-positive obligate anaerobe with a terminal spore, which is ubiquitous in the environment, particularly in soil. Spores are highly resistant to light and temperature; clinical disease occurs when spores are inoculated into wounds. Most cases of tetanus are related to acute injuries. Spores germinate under anaerobic conditions at the site of a wound and the growing bacteria produce two toxins: tetanolysin and tetanospasmin. Tetanospasmin undergoes proteolytic cleavage and binds and enters the pre-synaptic terminal. There, tetanospasmin cleaves the protein that allows fusion of synaptic vesicle with the membrane and thus prevents transmitter release. Tetanospasmin is able to travel retrogradely via axons to cell bodies and cross synapses, thus reaching the spinal cord, brain and autonomic nervous system. It primarily affects inhibitory glycine or γ-aminobutyric acid (GABA) neurones, leading to increased firing and lack of normal relaxation and causing the classical spasms of tetanus.

Clinical manifestations

The incubation period varies according to the site of injury and is shorter in severe disease, with an average incubation of 8 days for severe disease. There are several classical clinical subtypes which reflect the main site of action of toxin.

Generalized tetanus

This is the most common clinical form. It often commences with trismus ('lock jaw') in which the patients are unable to open their mouth or risus sardonicus, a grimace caused by spasm of facial muscles. The predominant feature is of repeated spasms which may involve the neck, thorax, abdomen or extremities. Generalized spasms with opisthotonos also occur. Spasms are precipitated by external or internal stimuli, may last for minutes and are painful as full consciousness is retained. Respiratory compromise may occur because of involvement of the glottis or diaphragm. The disease may continue to progress for up to 10 days after the first symptoms.

In severe tetanus, autonomic dysfunction may occur after several days. Hypertension, tachycardia, arrhythmias and hyperpyrexia may all occur and can be extremely difficult to manage. Recovery may take up to 4 weeks; case fatality rates can reach 60% with death usually occurring because of respiratory or autonomic involvement.

Neonatal tetanus

This is usually caused by infection of the umbilical stump. The risk of infection is related to the

Lecture Notes: Tropical Medicine, 6th edition.
By G.V. Gill and N.J. Beeching. Published 2009 by
Blackwell Publishing, ISBN: 978-1-4051-8048-1.

length of stump, the care and cleanliness with which the cord is ligated and cut and the cleanliness of the environment. Neonatal tetanus occurs only in the children of non-immune mothers. Symptoms and signs occur 1–10 days postpartum. Initially, generalized weakness and floppiness of the baby are noticed, with irritability and an inability to suck and feed. Subsequently, spasms, opisthotonos and hypersympathetic states occur. Up to 90% of affected infants die and mental retardation is common in survivors.

Localized tetanus

This is usually a mild form in which rigidity is limited to muscles near the site of injury. Weakness of the muscles may also occur because of the action of the toxin at the neuromuscular junction. Symptoms may be mild and persist for months. If the diagnosis is not made, progression to the generalized form may occur.

Cephalic tetanus

This is the rarest form and occurs in head injuries or with middle ear infection. The incubation period is normally 1–2 days and the major clinical manifestations are caused by involvement of cranial nerves with facial paresis, dysphagia and extraocular palsies. This form can also progress to generalized tetanus.

Diagnosis

The diagnosis is usually made clinically. Bacteriology is of little help; the organism is often not found, and a positive wound culture for *Cl. tetani* does not prove that the organism is toxin producing and causing disease. Blood and CSF findings are usually normal. The differential diagnosis is limited but includes strychnine poisoning, dystonic reactions, hypocalcaemia and seizures in adults, and metabolic or neurological causes of posturing in neonates.

Treatment

Tetanus should be treated by the administration of tetanus immunoglobulin (human tetanus

Ig 150 IU/kg i.m. or equine tetanus Ig 10^4–10^6 IU i.m.). Limited evidence suggests that there might be additional benefit from intrathecal administration of tetanus Ig, but this is rarely given in practice. Wounds should be débrided to prevent further germination of spores. Metronidazole or benzylpenicillin should be given to prevent multiplication of bacteria. Much of the care is supportive. External stimulation should be reduced to prevent precipitation of spasms: patients should be nursed in a quiet, dim environment. The airway should be protected; endotracheal intubation or tracheostomy is often necessary. Spasms can be treated by the use of high doses of benzodiazepines; baclofen is also effective. Some patients require paralysis with non-depolarizing neuromuscular junction blockers. The treatment of autonomic instability is difficult as manifestations can alter quite rapidly. Labetolol or verapamil may be useful for the management of hypertension; atropine or pacing may be needed for bradycardias and sympathomimetics, and fluids are sometimes necessary to treat hypotension. Intravenous magnesium reduces the need for muscle relaxants and drugs to control cardiovascular manifestations.

Neonatal tetanus is treated in a similar fashion to generalized tetanus.

Epidemiology and prevention

Although tetanus occurs worldwide, it is predominantly a problem of tropical and developing countries, being particularly common in the Philippines, Vietnam, the Asian Subcontinent, Indonesia and Brazil. There are an estimated 220 000 deaths annually with over 90% occurring under the age of five. However, there has been a significant reduction in the number of cases through the use of vaccination, particularly maternal vaccination, better obstetric practice and care of the cord.

Tetanus is a vaccine-preventable disease. Immunization with tetanus toxoid is very effective. Children should receive vaccination with tetanus toxoid as part of the routine diphtheria, tetanus and pertussis (DTP) immunization and receive boosters at 4–7 years and in adolescence. A single booster in adulthood leads to lifetime protection. For those first vaccinated in adulthood, routine booster doses should be given at 10-yearly intervals following primary immunization: five doses in total protects for life. Although if tetanus-prone injuries occur, a booster should be given if not immunized within the last 5 years. A single dose of tetanus toxoid in pregnancy leads to protective titres in a proportion of mothers and neonates: non-immunized mothers should ideally receive two doses 4 weeks apart during pregnancy.

Further reading

Farrar JJ, Yen LM, Cook T et al. Tetanus. *J Neurol Neurosurg Psychiatry* 2000; 69: 292–301. [A useful review of the subject.]

Sanya EO, Taiwo SS, Olarinoye JK et al. A 12 year review of cases of adult tetanus managed at the University College Hospital, Ibadan, Nigeria. *Trop Doct* 2007; 37: 170–172. [Gives a good insight into the current clinical spectrum of adult tetanus.]

Chapter 38

Brucellosis

Brucellosis (Malta fever, Rock fever) is one of the classical zoonoses (infections of animals transmitted to humans). It is an important cause of fever in many parts of the world and is often underdiagnosed because of lack of laboratory facilities.

Epidemiology

Brucellae are Gram-negative coccobacilli. At least six species infect a wide variety of land-based mammals, and new species have recently been described in marine mammals such as whales and seals. Three species are responsible for most human infections

1 *Brucella abortus*, usually a disease of cattle, is prevalent in Africa, the Indian subcontinent and temperate zones;

2 *Brucella melitensis*, whose normal ruminant host is sheep and goats but is also found in camels, is particularly prevalent in countries around the Mediterranean, the Middle East and Central and South America;

3 *Brucella suis*, whose natural host is pigs, is still a problem in the United States.

Brucella canis (natural host dogs) can rarely infect humans. The organisms are intracellular and can remain hidden in the reticuloendothelial system so that clinical incubation periods after infection range from several weeks to months.

Lecture Notes: Tropical Medicine, 6th edition.
By G.V. Gill and N.J. Beeching. Published 2009 by
Blackwell Publishing, ISBN: 978-1-4051-8048-1.

Despite this, brucellosis does not appear to be more common or more severe in patients with HIV. In animals, they are important causes of epididymitis, abortion and infertility, but host animals may appear symptomless.

Humans acquire infection from ingesting milk or dairy products such as laban, lassi, buttermilk and cheeses that have not been pasteurized. The products of abortion and placentae from infected animals are highly infectious, and farmers and veterinarians can easily become infected by aerosol transmission from the products of conception. Rarely, human brucellosis can be acquired via breast milk, sexual transmission or transfusion of blood products. Veterinarians and farmers sometimes have localized skin disease caused by direct contact with infected animal products. Brucellosis is not transmitted by eating the meat of infected animals unless it is eaten raw and has been externally contaminated. In endemic settings, brucellosis is mainly a problem for the rural poor. Brucellosis has been eliminated from much of northern Europe, where cases are related to travel and immigration from endemic areas.

Clinical features

The symptoms of brucellosis are of recurrent prolonged bouts of fever. If specific treatment is not given, undulating patterns of fever may last for several weeks, followed by an afebrile period and then relapse. Approximately half of all cases are associated with focal musculoskeletal symptoms, which may be the only clinical clue that differentiates brucellosis from other causes of fever such as typhoid, Q fever, malaria and so on. In an endemic area, it is the first clinical diagnosis for any patient who presents with fever and difficulty in walking. Fever is worse at night and may be associated with profuse sweating. Patients are depressed, anorexic and lethargic, although the onset of these symptoms is often insidious. A small proportion present with more pronounced neuropsychiatric disorder or low-grade meningoencephalitis, and 5–10% of men have orchitis which must be distinguished from mumps. Patients often have a dry cough, mimicking the presentation of typhoid. Epistaxis is an unusual but well-recognized presentation because of associated thrombocytopaenia, but other features of bleeding disorder such as haematemesis or malaena are very unusual.

The overall pattern of presentation varies with the age of the patient and the infecting species. *B. abortus* infections have a more insidious onset and are more likely to affect the axial skeleton and to become chronic. *B. melitensis* tends to have a more acute onset and is more likely to affect peripheral joints as well as the vertebrae. Children often present with fever and a single clinically affected joint, typically the hip or knee, and this may be mistaken for rheumatic fever or septic arthritis. *B. suis* infections have an acute presentation complicated by focal deep tissue abscesses.

Patients look unwell and are lethargic but do not look as toxic as those with enteric fever. The temperature is almost invariably raised but often returns to normal during a 24-h cycle. Up to 10% have cervical or other lymphadenopathy, which must be differentiated from glandular fever, HIV or tuberculous adenitis. One-quarter have mild to moderate splenomegaly. The chest is usually clear, even if the patient has a cough. Individual joints may show signs typical of septic arthritis with swelling, heat, tenderness and effusions. There may be local tenderness, especially on movement of vertebrae or sacroiliac joints, but deformity of the back or long tract neurological signs are very unusual and suggest TB rather than brucellosis.

Brucellosis is rarely fatal unless complicated by endocarditis (~1% of cases) but causes prolonged debilitation and loss of productivity.

Diagnosis

The full blood count shows low WBCs with lymphopaenia and mild thrombocytopenia. Occasionally, there is more pronounced reduction of platelets and haemoglobin. Mild elevation of alkaline phosphatase and transaminases is common. Blood culture is the most reliable method of confirming the diagnosis, but will only be positive in about two-thirds of *B. melitensis* cases and less than one-third of cases caused by *B. abortus*. If modern 'signalling' blood culture systems are used, they usually become positive within a week, but culture should be prolonged to 3 weeks to detect late positives. If basic culture facilities are all that are available, cultures should be prolonged to at least 6 weeks, with most of the positives occurring between days 7 and 21. Laboratory staff must be told that brucellosis is a possibility, both so that cultures are prolonged and so that they are aware of the significant hazard that *Brucella* poses to laboratory workers because of the risk of aerosol spread.

A single bone marrow culture has a better yield than three sets of blood cultures and is occasionally useful in patients with PUO who have been given antibiotics. Synovial fluid should be cultured for *Brucellae* in any case of septic arthritis in an endemic area, and aspirates or biopsies from abnormal tissues such as lymph nodes or liver should also be cultured. CSF usually shows mild elevations of lymphocytes and proteins, and organisms may be cultured.

Serological tests are still based on the old (Wright's) standard agglutination test (SAT). *Brucella* antigen supplied with the kit is added to successive dilutions of patient serum, and if visible agglutination occurs, the test is positive. These tests are notoriously affected by the 'prozone phenomenon', which causes false-negative results. This occurs because patients with brucellosis have immunoglobulin A (IgA) antibodies, which interfere with agglutination at low dilutions, and the blocking effect is only overcome at increasing serum dilutions. Thus, the result might be negative at dilutions of 1/40, 1/80, 1/160 and 1/320 and positive only at 1/640. Many inexperienced laboratories will only dilute serum to 1/160 and therefore miss the true positives.

As with all serological tests, a fourfold rise in titre between acute and convalescent samples (10–14 days later) is strongly suggestive of brucellosis, but this result is too delayed to guide the immediate management of patients with fever. In endemic areas, many patients have had previous exposure to brucellosis and have low titres of antibodies already, so the diagnostic 'cut-offs' for a single sample to be positive have to be set higher, typically at 1/160 or 1/320. In a non-endemic area, or for an expatriate who has recently been exposed for the first time in an endemic area, a titre of 1/80 would be strongly predictive of brucellosis. About 10% of blood culture–positive patients have negative serological results at first presentation, so a negative result does not entirely rule out brucellosis.

The SAT is affected by the antigen used and many different commercial kits are available. Some provide antigens for both *B. abortus* and *B. melitensis* but there is much cross-reaction and one cannot reliably distinguish these infections on the basis of serology alone. Mercaptoethanol can be added to patient serum to dissociate IgM and therefore indicate if IgG predominates (more suggestive of chronic infection), but this is only moderately reliable. The SAT has been adapted in some reference laboratories to be performed in microtitre trays, the so-called microscopic agglutination (MAT). All these tests cross-react with some other Gram-negative bacteria (*Yersinia*, cholera) and recent cholera immunization.

ELISA tests have also been developed and are used in some laboratories, but are not internationally standardized and are more expensive. Rose Bengal serological tests, designed for animal diagnosis, are used as screening tests on human sera in many tropical settings, but their specificity and sensitivity have not been fully validated for this purpose. Urinary dipsticks to detect antibodies are sensitive but not widely used, and assays for circulatory or urinary antigen remain experimental. Molecular techniques (PCR) to detect DNA are sensitive but are still not standardized for routine clinical diagnostic use.

Tissues such as bone, lymph node or liver contain non-caseating granulomas but the distinction from tuberculous granulomas is not always easy. Radiological bone changes are also seen later; typically, erosions at the edge of joints or the end plates of vertebrae, with associated sclerosis. Marked bony destruction is unusual and is more suggestive of TB. Isotope bone scans show hotspots in affected bones and joints and frequently reveal further foci of infection that are asymptomatic. The clinical and radiological features that discriminate between spine involvement with TB or brucellosis are shown in Table 38.1.

Table 38.1 Radiology of spine: differences from tuberculosis

	Brucellosis	Tuberculosis
Site	Lumbar + others	Dorsolumbar
Vertebrae	Multiple or contiguous	Contiguous
Discitis	Late	Early
Body	Intact until late	Morphology lost early
Canal compression	Rare	Common
Epiphysitis	Anterosuperior (Pedro-Pons' sign)	General: upper + lower disc region, centre, subperiosteal
Osteophyte	Anterolateral (parrot beak)	Unusual
Deformity	Wedging uncommon	Anterior wedge (gibbus)
Recovery	Sclerosis of whole body	Variable
Paravertebral abscess	Small, well localized	Common + discrete loss transverse process
Psoas abscess	Rare	More likely

Treatment

Three questions guide management, once a presumptive or definite diagnosis has been made.

1 Is the disease acute (duration <1 month) or relapsing or chronic (>6 months)?
2 Is there focal disease of bone or joints?
3 Has TB definitely been excluded?

Adults with acute non-focal disease should be treated for a minimum of 6 weeks. Patients with focal disease and/or chronic disease require 3 months of treatment. Monotherapy should not be used because, although clinical illness responds in the short term, early relapse occurs in more than 30% of cases. At least two antibiotics should be used for all cases. Patients in whom TB has not been excluded have to be treated for both infections simultaneously or should be given antimicrobials to which only brucellosis responds (i.e. streptomycin or rifampicin should not be used).

The time-honoured combination of an oral tetracycline for 6–12 weeks plus 1 g/day streptomycin intramuscularly for 2–3 weeks is the gold standard. The preferred form of tetracycline is now 100 mg doxycycline twice daily as it is easier to take and less likely to cause renal toxicity. Modern aminoglycosides such as gentamicin (5 mg/kg/day) can be substituted for streptomycin, but the optimal duration of therapy has not yet been confirmed. Pending further trials, the WHO recommends 14 days of gentamicin (7 days is known to be insufficient).

An alternative regimen is doxycycline with rifampicin, both given for 6 weeks or 3 months. The relapse rate after 6 weeks of this regimen is >10% compared to ~5% with doxycycline/streptomycin, and some national programmes discourage use of rifampicin for this purpose, reserving it for TB and leprosy treatment. Co-trimoxazole in high doses (three tablets twice a day for large adults) can be used but can cause anaemia and drug rashes, and should be supplemented with daily folic acid. It provides a good alternative to tetracyclines in young children when given with a second antibiotic, but in adults, co-trimoxazole plus doxycycline is more effective than cotrimoxazole plus rifampicin. There is some evidence that

children (<12 years) are adequately treated by 3 weeks rather than 6 weeks of therapy.

Pregnant women should not receive tetracyclines and are usually given rifampicin alone or with two tablets co-trimoxazole twice daily (avoid, or add folate supplements in the first trimester). The triple combination of doxycycline, rifampicin and gentamicin is superior to a double regimen and should be used for all infections with complications such as severe spondylitis, endocarditis or meningitis. Further drugs such as ceftriaxone may be added, and patients with endocarditis often need valve replacement as well. Fluoroquinolones have been disappointing for routine treatment, but some physicians add them as a third drug in difficult cases. Azithromycin does not appear to be useful.

Follow-up

Patients should be seen at 3 and 6 weeks to encourage adherence to antibiotic therapy. The most useful features are improvement in general mood and health, with return of appetite and weight. Serology is not very useful as it follows a variable pattern for months to years after successful treatment and does not predictably rise to warn that relapse is imminent. Relapse is conventionally defined as a further episode of brucellosis occurring less than 6 months after the first. This is usually a result of failure to take adequate antibiotics for long enough rather than being due to drug resistance, and should be treated with a further 3-month course of two antibiotics as for a first episode; some would insist on including streptomycin for re-treatment in order to be sure the drugs have been taken. Chronic brucellosis is difficult to define serologically and difficult to distinguish from chronic fatigue syndrome, depression or malingering. Immunity after brucellosis is not solid in humans, who may suffer from repeated infections. No vaccine is available for human use.

Public health aspects

Brucellosis is controlled by simple measures that require political commitment. The first is education of the public to eat or drink only pasteurized milk and dairy products, but this is often difficult to achieve in the face of tradition. Animal herds can be protected by administration of live vaccines, and such control has also been shown to reduce the incidence of human infection. Control of infected herds or flocks is usually based on 'test and slaughter' (i.e. if any animal in the herd tests positive, the whole herd is slaughtered). The public will comply with such measures only if they are offered adequate financial compensation.

Further reading

Centers for Disease Control and Prevention. Brucellosis: frequently asked questions. www.cdc.gov/ncidod/dbmd/diseaseinfo/brucellosis_g.htm. [Useful general detail on the web, including patient handouts and updated information of all sorts.]

Health Protection Agency (HPA) for general information and detail of deliberate release from British perspective, www.hpa.org.uk/.

Hoover DL, Friedlander AM. Brucellosis. In: Sidell FR, Takafuji ET, Franz DR, eds. *Medical Aspects of Chemical and Biological Warfare: Textbook of Military Medicine*. Office of the Surgeon General, Dept of the Army, USA, 1997: 513–521. Available online free at http://www.nbc-med.org/SiteContent/HomePage/WhatsNew/MedAspects/contents.html. [Convenient free textbook chapter.]

Pappas G. Treatment of brucellosis. *Br Med J* 2008; 336: 678–679. [Useful editorial accompanying Skalsky article. Six of the 11 references are to the author's own recent publications on epidemiology of human brucellosis and conundrums of diagnosis and treatment.]

Skalsky K, Yahav D, Bishara J, Pitlik S, Leibovici L, Paul M. Treatment of human brucellosis: systematic review and meta-analysis of randomized controlled trials. *Br Med J* 2008; 336: 701–704. [Excellent concise review with most references on supplementary website.]

World Health Organization (WHO) www.who.int/entity/zoonoses/diseases/brucellosis/en/index.html has some information. The most useful recent publication *Brucellosis in animals and humans* (WHO 2006), a comprehensive document on all aspects of brucellosis, is available at www.who.int/csr/resources/publications/Brucellosis.pdf.

Chapter 39

Typhoid and paratyphoid fevers

Typhoid and paratyphoid fevers are illnesses caused by *Salmonella enterica* serovar Typhi and serovars Paratyphi A, B and C. They cause a systemic septicaemic illness which is also called enteric fever. The many zoonotic salmonellas, which usually cause gastroenteritis, occasionally cause an enteric fever-like illness, especially severe in patients with HIV infection.

Typhoid and paratyphoid are most common where standards of personal and environmental hygiene are low, and only to this extent are these diseases tropical. There are 27 million cases estimated of typhoid fever worldwide each year with more than 200000 deaths. The incidence is more than 100/100000 population/year in the Indian subcontinent and South-East Asia and 10–100/100000 population/year in other resource-poor countries in Asia, Africa, the Caribbean, Central and South America. In endemic areas, the disease is most common in children and young adults (aged 2–35 years).

Organisms

The organisms are Gram-negative bacilli of the Enterobacteriacae. All possess somatic (O) and

Lecture Notes: Tropical Medicine, 6th edition.
By G.V. Gill and N.J. Beeching. Published 2009 by Blackwell Publishing, ISBN: 978-1-4051-8048-1.

flagellar (H) antigens. *S. enterica* ser. Typhi and ser. Paratyphi C possess a surface (Vi) antigen that coats the O antigen and potentially protects it from antibody attack. *S. enterica* ser. Typhi and ser. Paratyphi A and B infect only humans. *S. enterica* ser Paratyphi C may affect a variety of animals.

Mode of infection

Infection is usually by ingestion, with transmission in water (mainly *S. enterica* ser. Typhi) and food. Ingestion of 10^5 *S. enteric* ser. Typhi organisms may cause a relatively low attack rate with a long incubation period. Increasing the infecting dose to 10^9 organisms raises the attack rate to 95% and greatly shortens the incubation period. Conditions causing low gastric acidity allow a lower inoculum to cause infection. The most important reservoirs of infection are asymptomatic convalescent or chronic human carriers. Food-handlers, who are also carriers, are a potentially important source of transmission.

Typhoid fever

After ingestion, the organisms attach and then penetrate the small intestinal mucosa and are transported by the lymphatics to mesenteric lymph glands. There they multiply and enter the bloodstream via the thoracic duct and are carried to the bone marrow, spleen, liver and gall bladder. At these sites, the bacilli are able to survive and multiply inside macrophages. Eventually, the bacteria are rereleased into the bloodstream, and this second bacteraemia corresponds to the onset of symptoms.

There is a secondary invasion of the bowel via the infected bile. Macrophages collect in large numbers in the intestinal lymph follicles, particularly the Peyer's patches in the ileum. The strong inflammatory response in the Peyer's patches may lead to hyperplasia, necrosis and ulceration in 7–10 days if the inflammation does not resolve. Involvement of blood vessels may lead to bleeding and, if the whole thickness of the bowel is involved, perforation follows.

Elsewhere in the body, foci of inflammation with macrophages and lymphocytes, so-called typhoid nodules, are scattered in various organs, especially the liver, spleen, marrow and lymph glands. More diffuse organ involvement also occurs affecting the myocardium, kidney and lung. Late in the disease, there may be abscess formation most often affecting bone, brain, liver or spleen. Serious disease of the brain, lung and kidneys is not invariably accompanied by typhoid nodule formation, and the assumption is that some unidentified toxin must be the cause.

The natural course of the untreated disease is very variable. In a classical case, fever has returned to normal at the end of the third week and repair processes then begin. However, in some cases, fever and symptoms last for only a few days (particularly in preschool children) and in others may continue for many weeks. Death most commonly results from perforation, haemodynamic shock associated with either intestinal haemorrhage or severe toxaemia with altered consciousness and occasionally from other complications such as meningitis.

Clinical picture

The average incubation period is about 14 days but can vary from less than a week to more than 3 weeks. The only almost constant symptom is fever. The onset is usually gradual, and rigors are unusual. Fever increases day by day in the first week, often with an evening rise. A high and sustained fever (39–40°C) then continues for another week or more, falling by lysis in the third or fourth week.

Patients with typhoid usually feel very unwell, with malaise, generalized aches and pains and anorexia. Abdominal pain or discomfort, headache, diarrhoea or constipation and a non-productive cough are common symptoms.

Physical signs

These depend not only on the severity of the illness but also on the length of time the patient has been ill. In patients who seek medical aid early, there has usually been no significant dehydration from diarrhoea, and the patient often looks relatively well and is mentally alert. In contrast, the patient who presents after 2 weeks of illness is often very toxic, mentally stuporose and gravely dehydrated. The high fever may be accompanied by hepatomegaly, splenomegaly (often tender), mental changes including apathy, signs of bronchitis and meningism.

Rose spots are usually only seen with ease in fair-skinned patients. They are found from day 7 onwards and take the form of pink macules usually scanty and found mainly on the trunk. They fade on pressure from a glass slide. In occasional patients, the pulse rate is disproportionately slow compared with the fever and may not reach 100 b.p.m. even when the temperature is 40°C (so-called relative bradycardia).

Complications

These may develop as the illness progresses and can follow a clinically mild attack. The clinician must remember that typhoid patients may present with the complication rather than with the symptoms of typhoid fever, and these patients are often difficult to diagnose. The most important complications are as follows with the first three the most common.
• *Perforation*—This typically occurs in the third week. Toxic patients may show few signs of

peritonitis, except for abdominal distension, increasing toxaemia and a rising pulse. Surgery is preferable to conservative management, and excision or segmental resection is safer than simple suturing because the gut wall immediately surrounding the perforation may be too friable to hold sutures. Antibiotic therapy should be broadened to cover gastrointestinal organisms contaminating the peritoneum.

• *Haemorrhage*—Patients may have repeated small bleeds that resolve without specific treatment. Massive bleeding is typically a complication of the third week. Surgery is seldom needed provided that blood transfusion is available.

• *Severe toxaemia*—Some patients have severe disease characterized by delirium, obtundation, stupor or coma often accompanied by haemodynamic shock (not caused by gastrointestinal haemorrhage). For unexplained reasons, this complication has been reported more frequently in Indonesia, Papua New Guinea and West Africa than in other countries.

• *Haemolytic anaemia*—This may occur in patients with G6PD deficiency; typhoid depresses G6PD levels in normal as well as in deficient patients.

• *Typhoid lobar pneumonia*—This is a rare complication of the second and third week. Rusty sputum is not produced.

• *Meningitis*—This may be the only obvious manifestation of typhoid when it resembles any other pyogenic meningitis. It usually occurs in young children.

• *Renal disease*—This may present as renal failure or an acute nephrotic syndrome and is probably an immune complex nephritis. Recovery after successful chemotherapy is usual.

• *Typhoid abscess*—This is a late complication that can occur almost anywhere, especially in the spleen, liver, brain, breast and skeletal system.

• *Skeletal complications*—These are mainly suppurative arthritis and osteomyelitis. Both may be greatly delayed in onset. Zenker's degeneration of muscle or polymyositis may occur.

• *Other complications or sequelae*—Many are described including suppurative parotitis, acute cholecystitis, deep venous thrombosis, psychiatric disturbance and Guillain–Barré syndrome.

Diagnosis

Culture

Culture of the organism is the best way to confirm the diagnosis, but the technology to do this is often lacking in those hospitals in developing countries that most need it. Blood culture is the most useful, particularly in the first and second week. The average number of bacteria in the blood is low, so an adequate volume of blood should be taken for culture to increase the likelihood of a positive result. Bone marrow culture gives a higher culture-positive rate, probably because the concentration of organisms is 10-fold higher than in the blood and may even yield a positive culture after chemotherapy has been started. A string capsule used to sample duodenal contents can yield positive cultures, but in practice this method is not widely used. Aspirates from rose spots, CSF, or pus from abscesses may also yield positive cultures. Stool culture does not confirm the diagnosis, as the patient may be a chronic carrier. Faecal and urine cultures are mainly of value for the detection of carriers.

Serodiagnosis

The Widal test, which measures agglutinating antibodies to the somatic (O) and flagellar (H) antigens, is widely used. Although the test is relatively cheap and straightforward to perform, it lacks specificity and sensitivity. In endemic areas, low levels of antibodies are detectable in the healthy population, presumably because of prior exposure to the organisms and other non-typhoid salmonellae that share O and H antigens, and H antibody titres can remain high for a long time after typhoid immunization. In typhoid patients, titres often rise before the clinical onset, making it very difficult to demonstrate the diagnostic fourfold rise between initial and subsequent specimens. Furthermore, a significant number of culture-positive patients develop no rise in titre at all. However, if the test is interpreted intelligently, bearing all these facts in mind, a significant number of patients will be correctly diagnosed by the Widal test when all other methods have failed. Interpretation of the result is helped by knowledge of the background levels of antibodies in the local healthy population.

New antibody tests that detect different antigens to those used in the Widal test are being developed and appear promising.

Other laboratory findings

The WBC count is usually within the normal range, as is the differential count, but there may be leucopenia or leucocytosis and relative lymphocytosis is common. Biochemical tests usually show only minor changes such as slight elevation of transaminases and bilirubin. A considerable elevation of indirect bilirubin is often associated with haemolytic anaemia in patients with G6PD deficiency and in children. In severe cases, albuminuria is almost invariable. There may be evidence of DIC, although this rarely causes a clinical problem.

Treatment

The mainstay of treatment is effective antimicrobial chemotherapy. In endemic areas, many patients are managed as outpatients with oral antibiotics. Severely ill patients who may be mentally uncooperative require admission to hospital, good nursing care and careful supportive medical care, including attention to fluid and electrolyte balance.

Chemotherapy

Chloramphenicol used to be acknowledged everywhere as the drug of choice, with amoxicillin or co-trimoxazole as effective alternatives (Table 39.1). However, in recent years, MDR isolates of *S. enterica* ser. Typhi and ser. Paratyphi A resistant to all three antibiotics have been widely reported in the Indian subcontinent, countries of South-East Asia and some countries in Africa.

The fluoroquinolone antibiotics, third-generation cephalosporins and azithromycin have proved effective alternatives for treating MDR infections. Unfortunately, these antibiotics are expensive, in particular the cephalosporins.

Widespread use of fluoroquinolones has led to the emergence of strains with low-level and full resistance to these antibiotics. In some countries in Asia (Indonesia, Papua New Guinea), Africa (except Kenya and some countries in West Africa) and South and Central America most strains remain susceptible to chloramphenicol.

Relapses after chemotherapy occur in a variable proportion of patients (2–10%) and are usually rather less severe than the initial illness and respond to the same chemotherapy.

Fluoroquinolones

A 5- to 7-day course of a fluoroquinolone such as ciprofloxacin (Table 39.1) has proved extremely effective for the treatment of fully susceptible isolates, with rapid resolution of fever and symptoms. There have been concerns about the use of fluoroquinolones in children because of evidence of damage to the cartilage in the growing joints of animals. However, compassionate use of short courses of fluoroquinolones in children with multiresistant Gram-negative infections, where alternatives were unavailable, has proved safe.

Strains with low-level resistance to fluoroquinolones have appeared in the Indian subcontinent and South-East Asia. Infections with these strains may fail to respond to ciprofloxacin or ofloxacin therapy. There is some evidence that the newer fluoroquinolone, gatifloxacin is better for treating such infections. Microbiology laboratories can have difficulty in detecting these strains with the currently recommended methods. Resistance to the related antibiotic nalidixic acid, however, is a useful marker. Patients with enteric fever who are still sick after 5–7 days of an adequate dose of fluoroquinolone are likely to be infected with a resistant strain and should be changed to an alternative antibiotic. Fully fluoroquinolone-resistant strains are now appearing in the major cities in India.

Third-generation cephalosporins

Third-generation cephalosporins such as ceftriaxone, cefotaxime and cefixime are effective in treating MDR strains. However, the response to

Table 39.1 Choice of antibiotic to treat typhoid fever

Antibiotic	Dosage	Frequency	Route	Duration (days)		Side effects
				Non-severe	Severe or complicated	
Chloramphenicol	50–100 mg/kg/day; reduce dose to 30 mg/kg/day when fever ceases	4	o (i.m./i.v.)	14–21	14–21	Bone marrow depression
Amoxicillin	75–100 mg/kg/day	3	o/i.m./i.v.	14	14	
Co-trimoxazole (trimethoprim-sulfamethoxazole)	8 mg/kg/day trimethoprim +40 mg/kg/day sulfamethoxazole	2–3	o/i.m./i.v.	14	14	Nephrotoxic Allergy Not for children <2 years
Ciprofloxacin[a]	20 mg/kg/day	2	o/i.v.	5–7	10–14	
Ofloxacin[a]	15 mg/kg/day	2	o/i.v.	5–7	10–14	
Gatifloxacin[a]	10 mg/kg/day	1	o/i.v.	5–7	10–14	
Ceftriaxone	50–80 mg/kg/day	1–2	i.m./i.v.	7–10	10–14	
Cefotaxime	100–150 mg/kg/day	3–4	i.m./i.v.	7–10	10–14	
Cefixime	20–30 mg/kg/day	2	o	7–10	Not recommended	
Azithromycin	20 mg/kg/day	1	o	5–7	Not recommended	

Abbreviations: i.m., intramuscularly; i.v., intravenously; o, orally.
[a]Nalidixic acid-resistant isolates may not respond.

treatment is frequently slow with the fever and symptoms taking 7–10 days to resolve.

Azithromycin

There is emerging evidence that azithromycin is another effective alternative for MDR typhoid in adults and children. It has not been used yet in severe disease.

Chloramphenicol

A fairly prolonged course must be given to prevent relapse, such as a total of 14 days, or 12 days after fever has abated. It commonly takes 48 h before the fever shows a response and 5 days or more until the patient becomes completely afebrile in severe cases. A Herxheimer-type reaction is sometimes seen early in treatment and should be treated with steroids.

Amoxicillin

This is more expensive than chloramphenicol, but at least as effective if given in high doses. Ampicillin is inferior to chloramphenicol.

Co-trimoxazole

The clinical response is at least as rapid as with chloramphenicol.

Steroids

Adults and children with severe typhoid characterized by delirium, obtundation, coma or shock were shown to benefit in a study from Indonesia from the prompt administration of dexamethasone. The dosage given was 3 mg/kg by slow intravenous infusion over a period of 30 min followed by 1 mg/kg given at the same rate every 6 h for eight additional doses. Hydrocortisone given at a lower dose was not effective.

Carrier state

This commonly persists for some months into convalescence, and when it terminates spontaneously, such patients are called convalescent carriers. They are an obvious source of infection to others, but even more important are chronic carriers (1–3% of cases) in which a persisting focus of infection smoulders on in the gall bladder (faecal carriers) or in the urinary tract (urinary carriers) for more than 1 year. In most endemic areas, few carriers are identified because culture facilities do not exist. Persistent elevation of Vi antibodies often accompanies the carrier state.

The excretion of organisms by carriers is variable and erratic. Chronic faecal carriers may have chronic cholecystitis with or without gallstones or pathological abnormalities in the urinary tract, including *Schistosoma haematobium* infection in chronic urinary carriers. *Schistosoma mansoni* may be associated with a relapsing non-typhoid *Salmonella* septicaemia.

Treatment of chronic carriers

Ciprofloxacin 750 mg twice daily for 28 days has proved effective. If ciprofloxacin is unavailable and the strains are susceptible, two tablets of co-trimoxazole twice a day for 3 months or 100 mg/kg/day amoxicillin combined with 30 mg/kg/day probenecid, both for 3 months, may also be effective. Faecal carriers with gallstones only respond temporarily to chemotherapy, and cholecystectomy is needed to terminate the carrier state in such cases.

If the patient is intelligent and conscientious, and not a food-handler, the carrier state need not be treated at all for the fastidious maintenance of high standards of environmental and personal hygiene will prevent transmission of the infection to others.

Typhoid vaccine

Two vaccines are currently available. The live attenuated oral vaccine (Ty21a) requires three doses over 5 days with a booster recommended every 5 years. This vaccine is not recommended for children under the age of 6 years. The second, a purified Vi antigen vaccine, is given as a single dose intramuscularly; boosters are recommended every 3 years. It is not recommended for children under the age of 2 years. A new modified conjugate Vi vaccine and single dose attenuated oral vaccines are in development. These vaccines aim to be effective in very young children. The disadvantage of all these vaccines is their cost. The use of vaccination as a public health tool is now recommended by WHO in highly endemic areas where there are high rates of resistance to available antimicrobials.

If typhoid does develop in a vaccinated subject, it is no less severe than in the unvaccinated.

Paratyphoid A and B

These usually infect via contaminated foods in which the organisms have multiplied. For this reason, diarrhoea and vomiting may precede septicaemia. Many mild cases occur. Treatment is as for typhoid. Drug-resistant strains have become common in some areas of the Indian subcontinent.

Paratyphoid C

This commonly produces septicaemia without involvement of the gut, and abscess formation is common.

Further reading

Bhan MK, Bahl R, Bhatnager S. Typhoid and paratyphoid fever. *Lancet* 2005; 366: 749–762.

Bhutta ZA. Current concepts in the diagnosis and treatment of typhoid fever. *Br Med J* 2006; 333: 78–82.

Chapter 40

Arboviruses

Arbovirus (short for arthropod-borne virus) is an ecological description for viruses that are transmitted between vertebrate hosts by insects—principally mosquitoes, ticks, sandflies or midges. There are more than 500 arboviruses, in four viral families, but only a small number are medically important (Figure 40.1). Some arboviruses are named after the disease they cause (e.g. Yellow fever or O'nyong nyong—'joint weakening' in a Ugandan dialect); some after their insect vector (e.g. phleboviruses after 'phlebotomus'—sandflies) and some after the geographical area where the disease first occurred (e.g. Japanese encephalitis).

Vectors and hosts

Following infection with an arbovirus, most animals develop lifelong immunity to that virus. An arbovirus therefore needs a ready supply of immunologically naïve hosts. A few arboviruses (notably dengue) have evolved to use humans as the 'natural host'; however, most use small mammals or birds because of their high reproductive rate. For these 'enzootic' viruses, humans are coincidentally infected 'dead-end hosts' and do not transmit the disease. In some situations an 'amplifying host' increases the amount of circulating virus and acts as a link to human infection.

Lecture Notes: Tropical Medicine, 6th edition.
By G.V. Gill and N.J. Beeching. Published 2009 by
Blackwell Publishing, ISBN: 978-1-4051-8048-1.

Clinical syndromes

The majority of human infections with arboviruses are asymptomatic or cause a mild non-specific febrile illness. When an arbovirus causes disease, it usually leads to one of three clinical syndromes.
1 Fever–arthralgia–rash (FAR).
2 Viral haemorrhagic fever.
3 CNS infection.

Most viruses cause a single syndrome, but there can be overlap; for example, dengue viruses can present with a FAR syndrome (dengue fever), a haemorrhagic syndrome (dengue haemorrhagic fever) and even, occasionally, CNS disease. The most important haemorrhagic fevers are considered in Chapter 41 and CNS arboviruses are discussed in Chapter 33. FAR arboviruses are summarized below.

Fever–arthralgia–rash arboviruses

Chikungunya

Chikungunya occurs in Africa, India and South-East Asia. Humans and primates are the natural host, and *Aedes* and *Culex* mosquitoes transmit the disease. Since March 2005, the virus has caused large outbreaks in the Pacific islands, and Asia and has even reached southern Europe.

O'nyong nyong

O'nyong nyong occurs in Africa and is the only arbovirus transmitted by *Anopheles* mosquitoes.

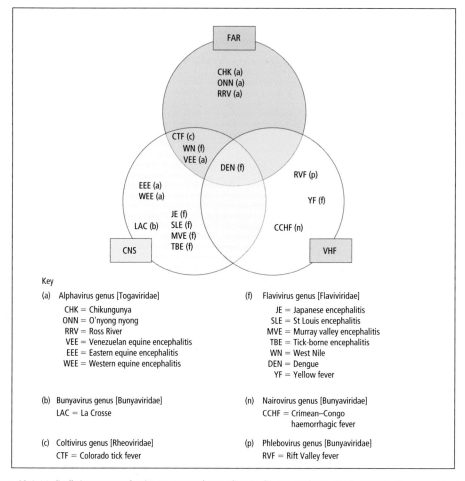

Figure 40.1 Medically important arboviruses grouped according to disease syndrome (top), and listed by genus (bottom). CNS, central nervous system; FAR, fever–arthralgia–rash; VHF, viral haemorrhagic fever. Viral families are indicated by [ ].

Humans are the only hosts and a common clinical feature is conjunctivitis.

Ross River

This occurs in Australia and is transmitted by *Aedes* and *Culex* mosquitoes. It can cause 'epidemic polyarthritis'.

Colorado tick fever

This is found in the Rocky Mountain states of the United States and is transmitted among small mammals by *Dermacentor* ticks. It causes CNS disease in 10% of children; haemorrhagic disease

is rarer. It is easily confused with the rickettsial disease, Rocky Mountain spotted fever.

Dengue virus

This is the most common FAR arbovirus and is discussed more fully in Chapter 41.

Further reading

Solomon T. Arboviruses. In: Dawood R, ed. *Travellers' Health*, 3rd edn. London: Oxford University Press, 2002: 151–170. [A leisurely discussion of concepts and diseases.]

Viral haemorrhagic fevers

Few diseases cause as much terror as the viral haemorrhagic fevers (VHFs), but this is often out of proportion to the actual harm they do. VHFs are caused by a diverse group of viruses from four viral families: the Arenaviridae, Filoviridae, Bunyaviridae and Flaviviridae (Table 41.1).

Epidemiology

The epidemiology can be simplified by considering three questions (Figure 41.1).

1 How is the virus transmitted in its natural cycle—via arthropods, directly or unknown?

2 How do human index cases become infected—via insects, directly or unknown?

3 Is there direct transmission between humans to cause nosocomial spread?

Pathogenesis

The pathogenesis varies according to virus, but usually includes a combination of vascular damage, coagulopathy, immunological impairment and end-organ damage. These lead to:

• increased vascular permeability—the major pathophysiological process for most VHFs, which

allows plasma to leak from the vessels into the tissue and causes shock, oedema and effusions

• haemorrhagic manifestations, which are sometimes relatively minor (e.g. petechiae) or can be major (e.g. gastrointestinal bleeding in Crimean–Congo haemorrhagic fever [CCHF])

• hepatic and renal failure

• encephalopathy.

Management

The management of VHFs includes the identification and treatment of suspected cases, limiting further spread (for the directly transmissible VHFs) and identifying others who may have been infected.

Identifying VHF in the febrile patient

Most patients with suspected VHF turn out to have malaria, typhoid or another non-transmissible disease. Unnecessary alarm can be avoided, and attention focused on likely cases of VHF, by considering the following (Figure 41.2):

• Most VHFs are acquired in rural rather than urban areas.

• Travel history should include details of activities that may have caused exposure.

• An interval of 3 weeks between possible exposure and onset rules out VHF.

Lecture Notes: Tropical Medicine, 6th edition.
By G.V. Gill and N.J. Beeching. Published 2009 by
Blackwell Publishing, ISBN: 978-1-4051-8048-1.

Table 41.1 Overview of the major viral haemorrhagic fevers

Virus	Genus, family	Geographical area	Natural cycle	Human disease
Lassa	*Arenavirus*, Arenaviridae	Western Africa	*Mastomys* rodent	Human–human spread occurs. 2–15% mortality. Treat with ribavirin
Ebola and Marburg	*Filovirus*, Filoviridae	Sub-Saharan Africa	Unknown	Nosocomial spread common. 25–90% mortality. No antiviral treatment
Hantaan and others (Haemorrhagic fever with renal syndrome)	*Hantavirus*, Bunyaviridae	Far East, Europe	Various rural rodents	No human–human spread. 1–15% mortality depending on virus. Treat severe disease with ribavirin
Crimean–Congo haemorrhagic fever	*Nairovirus*, Bunyaviridae	Eastern Europe, Asia, Africa	*Hyalomma* ticks and livestock	Human–human spread. 15–30% mortality. Treat with ribavirin
Rift Valley fever	*Phlebovirus*, Bunyaviridae	Africa, Middle East	*Aedes* and other mosquitoes and livestock	Human–human spread not documented, but possible. Most infections asymptomatic. 50% mortality for VHF. Treat with ribavirin
Dengue	*Flavivirus*, Flaviviridae	Tropics and subtropics worldwide	*Aedes* mosquitoes and humans	No human–human spread. Mortality <1% with adequate fluid treatment. No antivirals
Yellow fever	*Flavivirus*, Flaviviridae	Africa, South America	Various mosquitoes and monkeys	No human–human spread. 20–50% mortality. No antivirals

- Most early symptoms are non-specific but certain features should ring alarm bells; for example pharyngitis with ulcers or causing difficulty swallowing, retrosternal chest pain, conjunctival injection and prostration.
- Haemorrhagic manifestations may not be obvious—look for petechiae in the skin folds and axillae, gum bleeding and microscopic haematuria and perform a tourniquet test (see p. 298).
- Look, repeatedly if necessary, for a rising haematocrit (caused by plasma leakage), pleural effusions on decubitus chest X-ray, leucopenia, thrombocytopenia and proteinuria.

Diagnosis

The differential diagnosis of VHFs includes many causes of fever in the tropics (Table 41.2). Early laboratory diagnosis of the illness is by virus isolation, reverse transcriptase PCR or antigen capture ELISAs. Subsequently, IgM and IgG ELISAs are used. Because of the infectious nature of the directly transmissible VHFs, these tests must be carried out in biosafety level-4 facilities (high levels of staff protection only available in specialist centres).

Management

Encourage oral fluid intake with oral rehydration solution, and a straw if the patient cannot sit up. For patients with suspected Lassa fever, CCHF, Rift Valley fever (RVF) and haemorrhagic fever with renal syndrome (HFRS), ribavirin should be started as soon as possible (30 mg/kg loading dose, then 16 mg/kg q.d.s. for 4 days, then 8 mg/kg t.d.s. for 6 days). Hypovolaemic shock should be treated with crystalloids and colloids, and ionotropes may be needed. Pulmonary oedema and effusions are common because of the increased capillary permeability. Blood transfusions are not required

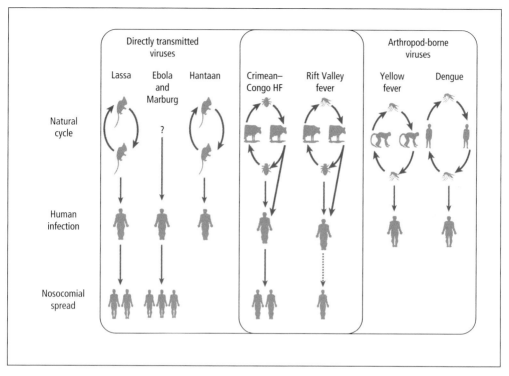

Figure 41.1 Ecological overview of viral haemorrhagic fevers showing natural cycle, transmission to humans and potential for nosocomial spread. Note the distinction between directly transmissible viruses (Lassa, Ebola, Marburg and Hantaan), arboviruses (yellow fever and dengue), and those transmitted by both routes (Crimean–Congo haemorrhagic fever and Rift Valley fever). (Modified from Solomon [2002], with permission from Elsevier Science.)

in most patients, but fresh frozen plasma may be needed.

Nosocomial spread is limited by isolating the patient, strict barrier nursing (with goggles and mask), proper decontamination and disposal of clinical waste and sharps and prompt disposal of bodies by specialized burial teams. Laboratory staff must be warned about possible hazardous specimens. The risks of respiratory spread are probably negligible. Negative pressure isolation units are used in the West, but not in the African countries where most cases occur. Here implementation of the measures outlined above has dramatically reduced nosocomial transmission. 'High risk' contacts who were exposed to blood, secretions or body fluids (usually before the diagnosis is suspected) should have their temperature checked twice daily for 3 weeks. Casual contacts

at low risk should be told to report if they have fever. Survivors can suffer severe psychological damage, and support is needed.

Lassa fever

Lassa fever is the directly transmissible VHF most likely to be seen in returning travellers, because of its wide distribution and long incubation period (5 days to 3 weeks). Lassa virus (genus *Arenavirus*, family Arenaviridae) is found across West Africa and is transmitted naturally between *Mastomys* rodents via their urine and faeces. Humans are infected by contact with these secretions (probably via inhalation of virus). Secondary human cases may occur by nosocomial spread. It is estimated that there are 100 000 cases and 5000 deaths annually, plus many unapparent infections.

	Directly transmissible VHF*					Non-directly transmissible VHF		
	Ebola/ Marburg	Lassa	South American VHFs	CCHF	RVF†	HFRS	DHF	Yellow fever

1. Obtain a travel history:

	Ebola/ Marburg	Lassa	South American VHFs	CCHF	RVF	HFRS	DHF	Yellow fever
Africa	+	+		+	+		+	+
Middle East				+	+		+	
Asian subcontinent				+			+	
Europe				+		+		
Far East						+	+	
Americas			+				+	+

2. Ask about activities that may have caused exposure to virus:

	Directly transmissible VHF					HFRS	DHF	Yellow fever
Exposure to human cases	Recent contact (<3 weeks) with any sick individual with unexplained fever and bleeding					−	−	−
Exposure to animal reservoir	? Monkeys ? Bats	Rodent excreta (urban)	Rodent excreta (rural)	Livestock		Rodent excreta	−	Monkeys
Activities undertaken	Jungle visits, caving	Cleaning basements, etc.	Farming, harvesting	Farming, abattoir work, rural activities		Rural, agricultural work	Urban mosquito exposure	Jungle mosquito exposure

3. Look for suggestive clinical features:

Early features	Pharyngitis Conjunctival injection Retrosternal chest pain Prostration	Rash Venepuncture oozing Petechial haemorrhages Mucosal bleeding	Facial oedema Small pleural effusions Abdominal pain Tender hepatomegaly
Late features	Shock Pleural effusions Ascites Pericardial effusions	Haematemesis DIC Hepatic failure	Renal failure Encephalopathy Acidosis

4. Consider investigative findings common in VHFs:

Leucopenia Thrombocytopenia Rising haematocrit	Proteinuria Haematuria Renal impairment	Prolonged TT, APTT Elevated transaminases

5. If malaria film and other tests negative, and patient deteriorating despite presumptive treatment, suspect VHF:

For a directly transmissible VHF, begin isolation procedure; alert medical, nursing, laboratory, cleaning and laundry staff, public health officials	For non-transmissible VHF, ensure standard safe practices are being followed. Inform public health authorities

6. Start intravenous ribavirin if one of the following is suspected:

−	+	+	+	+	+	−	−
Ebola/ Marburg	Lassa	South American VHFs	CCHF	RVF	HFRS	DHF	YF

Directly transmissible VHF	Non-directly transmissible VHF

Figure 41.2 Algorithm for identifying VHF patients. (Modified from Solomon [2002], with permission from Elsevier Science.) *Directly transmissible between humans. †Patients with VHF caused by RVF should be treated as infectious, although direct transmission between humans has not yet been shown. CCHF, Crimean Congo haemorrhagic fever; DHF, dengue haemorrhagic fever; HFRS, haemorrhagic fever with renal syndrome; RVF, Rift Valley fever; YF, yellow fever.

Table 41.2 Differential diagnosis of viral haemorrhagic fevers

Viral haemorrhagic fevers (in order of incidence)	*Arboviral causes of fever with rash*
Dengue haemorrhagic fever	**Alphaviruses**
Haemorrhagic fever with renal syndrome	Chikungunya
Yellow fever	O'nyong nyong
Lassa fever	Sindbis
Crimean–Congo haemorrhagic fever	**Bunyaviruses**
Argentine, Bolivian and Venezuelan haemorrhagic fevers	Oropouche
Rift Valley fever	**Phleboviruses**
Omsk haemorrhagic fever and Kyasanur Forest disease	Sandfly fever
Ebola and Marburg haemorrhagic fevers	**Coltiviruses**
	Colorado tick fever
Treatable causes of fever with rash/haemorrhage	*Non-arboviral causes of fever with rash*
Parasites	**Enteroviruses**
Malaria (rash/haemorrhage rate)	Coxsackie viruses
Bacteria	Echoviruses
Meningococcal	Enteroviruses 68–71
Typhoid	**Paramyxoviruses**
Septicaemic plague	Measles
Shigellosis	**Herpes viruses**
Any severe sepsis with DIC	Herpes zoster virus
Rickettsia	Human herpes virus 6 and 7
Tick and epidemic typhus	**Orthomyxoviruses**
Rocky Mountain spotted fever	Influenza A and B
Spirochaetes	**Rubiviruses**
Leptospirosis	Rubella
Borreliosis	
Causes of fulminant hepatic failure	*Miscellaneous*
Hepatitis viruses A–E	Drug reactions
Paracetamol and other drugs	Toxins
Reye's syndrome	Acute surgical emergencies (upper gastrointestinal bleeding)
Alcohol	

DIC, disseminated intravascular coagulation.

Clinically, Lassa fever usually presents as a non-specific febrile illness, followed by conjunctival injection, sore throat with a pharyngeal exudate, retrosternal chest pain, vomiting and diarrhoea. Some patients progress to facial and laryngeal oedema, a mild bleeding diathesis and shock. Sensorineural deafness is a late complication in 30% of patients. The disease should be treated with ribavirin. Control measures include rodent control.

South American haemorrhagic fevers

Related arenaviruses with epidemiological and clinical similarities to Lassa are found in South America: Junin, Machupo and Guanarito viruses cause Argentine, Bolivian and Venezuelan haemorrhagic fever respectively. Whitewater Arroyo virus is a recently identified rare cause of VHF in southern United States.

Ebola and Marburg haemorrhagic fevers

These are caused by Ebola and Marburg viruses (genus *Filovirus*, family Filoviridae), which are presumed to be zoonotic, but the natural reservoir remains unknown despite intensive investigations. Marburg virus first caused disease in 1967 in laboratory workers in Marburg, Germany, who were handling tissue from African green monkeys imported from Uganda. Occasional cases followed in Africa, then a large outbreak in the Democratic Republic of Congo in 1999. The first outbreak of Ebola occurred in 1976 in southern Sudan and the Democratic Republic of Congo (formerly Zaire). Subsequent outbreaks occurred in 1979, 1995 (Congo), 2000 (Uganda) and 2001–2003 (Gabon and Congo). Four biotypes have been identified: Ebola Zaire, Ebola Sudan, Ebola Côte d'Ivoire and Ebola Reston (which originated in the Philippines).

Naturally acquired human index cases of Ebola and Marburg always occur in rural areas (sometimes bat infested, and sometimes following contact with diseased primates). Secondary cases are infected by contact with blood or other fluids from primary cases and hence are mostly carers. The route of virus entry is uncertain, but is possibly via small cuts in the skin or conjunctivae. Reuse of unsterile needles and lack of barrier nursing were important factors in early nosocomial outbreaks.

Clinically, the incubation period is 4–10 days. Patients present with a febrile illness with myalgia, abdominal pain, sore throat, herpetic lesions in the mouth and pharynx, conjunctival injection, diarrhoea and a maculopapular rash. There is sometimes bleeding from the gastrointestinal tract, nose or injection sites. Petechiae, shock and neurological manifestations can occur. The case fatality rate is 30% (Marburg) and 60–90% (Ebola). Supportive treatment only can be given. Convalescent serum from survivors may help, and barrier nursing is essential. A range of experimental treatments are in development.

Haemorrhagic fever with renal syndrome

This is caused by four viruses (all members of the genus *Hantavirus*, family Bunyaviridae), which are transmitted naturally between various rural rodents in their excreta.

• Hantaan virus causes epidemic HFRS in the far East.

• Seoul virus causes a milder syndrome in the same geographical area.

• Dobrova virus causes severe HFRS in the Balkans (Europe).

• Puumula virus causes a milder variant across Scandinavia and northern Europe, with renal predominance (also called nephropathia epidemica).

Hantavirus pulmonary syndrome (a related condition with non-cardiogenic pulmonary oedema and shock) occurs in the Americas and is caused by Sin Nombre and other 'new world' hantaviruses. Humans are infected with hantaviruses by contact with rodent excreta. There is no evidence of human–human spread. Classically, HFRS patients have five phases: febrile, hypotensive phase (with haemorrhage), oliguric, diuretic and then convalescent. The illness should be treated with ribavirin. Prevention and control measures include minimizing human exposure to rodent excreta; for example, by rodent-proofing homes. Formalin-inactivated vaccines are used in Asia.

Crimean–Congo haemorrhagic fever

This virus is transmitted naturally between animals (small mammals and livestock) by ixodid ticks, especially of the *Hyalomma* genus. It is endemic throughout Africa, Asia, the former USSR, eastern Europe and the Middle East. There have been recent outbreaks in Afghanistan, Pakistan, the Russian Federation and South Africa. Humans are infected after being bitten by, or crushing, an infected tick; or by contact with blood from infected livestock or patients (hence barrier nursing is necessary). Unlike other VHFs, major haemorrhage is more important than vascular leakage in the pathophysiology and clinical presentation of CCHF. It is treated with ribavirin and prevention is by minimizing tick exposure.

Rift Valley fever

 RVF is endemic in the African Rift Valley and much of sub-Saharan Africa, Egypt, Saudi Arabia and Yemen. It is transmitted naturally between livestock by many mosquito species, especially *Aedes* and *Culex*. Epidemics are associated with increases in mosquito population following heavy rains, or irrigation projects. Humans are infected by mosquitoes and by contact with animal products. Direct transmission between humans has not been documented, but barrier nursing is advisable. RVF also causes disease in sheep and cattle (abortions). Clinically, it presents as a mild febrile illness in humans; 5% have haemorrhagic manifestations, meningoencephalitis or retinitis. Ribavirin treatment is probably effective, and control measures include livestock vaccination, personal protection of workers in the livestock industry and mosquito control.

Dengue haemorrhagic fever and yellow fever

These are discussed in Chapter 42.

Further reading

Centres for Disease Control and Prevention and World Health Organization. *Infection Control for Viral Haemorrhagic Fevers in the African Health Care Setting*. Atlanta: Centers for Disease Control and Prevention, 1998. http://www.cdc.gov/ncidod/dvrd/spb. [Very helpful manual for use in the field.]

Solomon T. Viral haemorrhagic fevers. In: Cook G, Zumla A, eds. *Manson's Tropical Diseases*, 21st edn. London: Saunders, 2000: 773–793. [Detailed discussion of the ecology, pathophysiology and clinical aspects of viral haemorrhagic fevers.]

Chapter 42

Dengue and yellow fever

While the most important viral haemorrhagic fevers numerically (dengue and yellow fever) are transmitted exclusively by arthropods, other arboviral haemorrhagic fevers (Crimean–Congo and Rift Valley fevers) can also be transmitted directly by body fluids. A third group of haemorrhagic fever viruses (Lassa, Ebola and Marburg) are only transmitted directly and are not transmitted by arthropods at all. The directly transmissible viral haemorrhagic fevers are discussed in Chapter 41.

Dengue

Dengue virus is numerically the most important arbovirus infecting humans with an estimated 100 million cases per year and 2.5 billion people at risk. There are four serotypes of dengue virus transmitted by *Aedes* mosquitoes, and it is unusual among arboviruses in which humans are the natural hosts. Dengue fever ('breakbone fever') has been around for many hundreds of years; dengue haemorrhagic fever (DHF) emerged as an apparently new disease in South-East Asia in the 1950s.

Epidemiology

Dengue has spread dramatically since the end of World War II in what has been described as a

Lecture Notes: Tropical Medicine, 6th edition.
By G.V. Gill and N.J. Beeching. Published 2009 by Blackwell Publishing, ISBN: 978-1-4051-8048-1.

global pandemic. Virtually every country between the tropics of Capricorn and Cancer is now affected (Figure 42.1).

Factors implicated in the spread of dengue viruses include poor control of its principal vector (*Aedes aegypti*) as well as reinfestation of this insect into Central and South America (it was largely eradicated in the 1960s). Other factors include intercontinental transport of car tyres containing *Aedes albopictus* eggs, overcrowding of refugee and urban populations, and increasing human travel. In hyperendemic areas of Asia, disease is seen mainly in children.

Aedes mosquitoes are 'peri-domestic'; they breed in collections of freshwater around the house (e.g. water storage jars). They feed on humans (anthrophilic), mainly by day, and feed repeatedly on different hosts (enhancing their role as vectors).

Clinical features

Dengue virus may cause a non-specific febrile illness or asymptomatic infection, especially in young children. However, there are two main clinical dengue syndromes: dengue fever (DF) and DHF.

Dengue fever

This is a classical fever–arthralgia–rash syndrome (Chapter 40) with retro-orbital pain, photophobia,

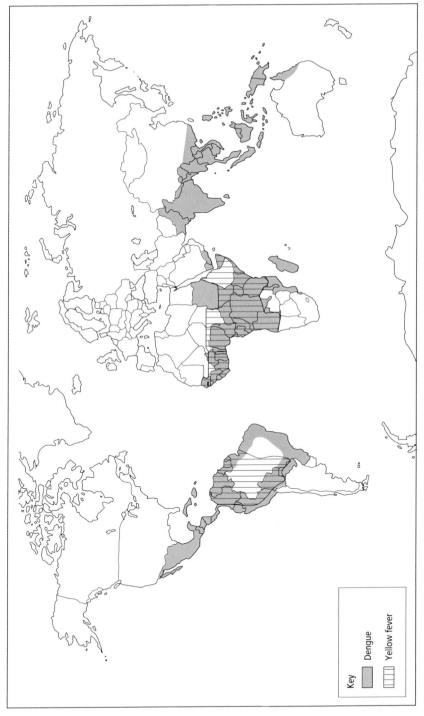

Figure 42.1 Map showing the approximate distribution of dengue and yellow fever viruses.

lymphadenopathy and, in about 50% of patients, a rash. This is usually maculopapular but may be mottling or flushing. In addition there may be petechiae and other bleeding manifestations including gum, nose or gastrointestinal haemorrhage, but these do not define it as DHF according to WHO criteria—see later (Table 42.1). About one-third of patients have a positive tourniquet test (a blood pressure cuff inflated to half way between systolic and diastolic pressure for 5 min produces 20 or more petechiae in a 2.5 cm² area on the forearm).

Dengue haemorrhagic fever

Initially, patients have a non-specific febrile illness, which may include a petechial rash. Then on the third to seventh day of illness, as the fever subsides, there is a massive increase in vascular permeability (this is the major pathophysiological process). This leads to plasma leakage from the blood vessels into the tissue, causing an elevated haematocrit, oedema and effusions. In addition there is thrombocytopenia and haemorrhagic manifestations. If a positive tourniquet test is the only such manifestation, then this is defined as DHF grade I (Table 42.1). If there is spontaneous bleeding, this is grade II. In grade III, the plasma leakage is sufficient to cause shock (defined in children as a pulse pressure <20 mmHg). In grade IV, the blood pressure is unrecordable. Collectively, grades III and IV are known as dengue shock syndrome (DSS). Patients with DHF are restless or lethargic and often have tender hepatomegaly or abdominal pain.

Investigations

Leucopenia and thrombocytopenia are common. In the first few days of illness, dengue virus can be isolated from serum or detected by PCR. After the fever subsides, IgM and then IgG antibodies can be detected by ELISA. New enzyme immunoassay kits allow rapid diagnosis in the field. A lateral chest X-ray may show a pleural effusion in DHF.

Management

Dengue fever

Most cases are self-limiting. Oral fluids should be encouraged, and paracetamol should be given. Patients may have a maculopapular recovery rash and prolonged lethargy and depression after recovery are common.

Table 42.1 WHO criteria for distinguishing DF and DHF grades I–IV. DHF grades III and IV are collectively known as DSS

	Plasma leakage[a]	Platelets (× 10⁹/L)	Circulatory collapse	Haemorrhagic manifestations
DF	No	Variable	Absent	Variable
DHF I	Present	<100	Absent	Positive tourniquet test (or easy bruising)
DHF II	Present	<100	Absent	Spontaneous bleeding[b] with or without positive tourniquet test
DHF III	Present	<100	PP < 20 mmHg[c]	Spontaneous bleeding and/or positive tourniquet test
DHF IV	Present	<100	Pulse and BP undetectable	Spontaneous bleeding and/or positive tourniquet test

Abbreviation: BP, blood pressure; DF, dengue fever; DHF, dengue haemorrhagic fever; DSS, dengue shock syndrome; PP, pulse pressure; WHO, world health organization.
[a]Identified by haematocrit 20% above normal or clinical signs of plasma leakage.
[b]Skin petechiae, mucosal or gastrointestinal bleeding.
[c]Pulse pressure less than 20 mmHg or hypotension for age.

Dengue haemorrhagic fever

For grades I and II DHF, oral fluids should be encouraged, vital signs closely monitored, as well as haematocrit and platelet count, which may warn of deterioration to grades III and IV. For grades III and IV (DSS), central venous pressure (CVP) should be monitored if possible. Intravenous crystalloid (10–20 mL/kg/h) should be given followed by intravenous colloid if shock persists. Patients should be watched carefully for fluid overload, and infusions reduced accordingly.

Other severe manifestations of dengue infection

These include hepatitis or fulminant hepatic failure (Reye-like syndrome) as well as neurological complications (metabolic encephalopathy, cerebral oedema or, occasionally, viral encephalitis).

Pathogenesis of DHF

Current evidence suggests that two mechanisms may be important:
1. *Antibody-dependent enhancement*—antibodies against one dengue virus serotype (from a previous infection) enhance the entry of a second dengue virus into macrophages, leading to a more severe infection.
2. *Viral strain differences*—for example increased virulence of South-East Asian strains of dengue-2 virus.

Prevention

Prevention is by control of *Aedes* mosquitoes. Methods include treating stored water with larvicides (e.g. temephos), educating people to remove collections of water around the house (e.g. in rubbish) and spraying with insecticide during epidemics.

Future developments include tetravalent vaccines (effective against all four dengue serotypes), which are in development, for example live attenuated vaccines and recombinant copy DNA infectious clone vaccines.

Yellow fever

Epidemiology

Yellow fever virus is naturally transmitted between primates by various mosquitoes in jungle cycles in Central America and Africa (Figure 42.1). *A. aegypti* transmits the virus to humans in urban cycles. The disease has re-emerged in South America since the 1970s, when the *Aedes* eradication programme was relaxed. There are an estimated 200 000 cases with 30 000 deaths annually.

Clinical features

The illness is biphasic and often mild. Severe disease is characterized by jaundice, fulminant hepatic failure and gastrointestinal bleeding. Faget's sign is the failure of the heart rate to increase with a rising temperature and is indicative of cardiac damage. Elevated liver function tests, leucopenia, thrombocytopenia and clotting abnormalities may occur. Liver histology reveals

---

Box 42.1 Differential diagnosis of dengue

Fever with arthralgia or rash
- *Arboviruses*—chikungunya, o'nyong nyong, Sindbis, West Nile, Ross River, Oropouche, sandfly fevers and Colorado tick fever.
- *Other viruses*—rubella, measles, herpes and enteroviruses.
- *Bacteria*—meningococcus and typhoid.
- *Spirochaetes*—leptospirosis, Lyme disease and relapsing fevers.
- *Rickettsiae*—tick and endemic typhus and Rocky Mountain spotted fever.
- *Parasites*—malaria.
Fever with haemorrhage
- *Arboviruses*—yellow fever, Crimean–Congo haemorrhagic fever, Rift Valley fever and Omsk haemorrhagic fever.
- *Other viruses*—hantaviruses, fulminant hepatitis (A–E); Lassa; South American haemorrhagic fevers, Ebola, Marburg.
- Any severe sepsis with disseminated intravascular coagulation (DIC).
- Drug reactions.

Councilman bodies, which also occur in Crimean–Congo haemorrhagic fever and Rift Valley fever.

Control

Yellow fever control consists of use of the highly effective 17D live attenuated vaccine. In recent years, there have been reports of adverse events, particularly in the elderly. For elderly travellers to yellow fever risk areas, the small risks of vaccination need to be balanced carefully against the risk of illness. Vector control is as for DF.

Further reading

Barnett ED. Yellow fever: epidemiology and prevention. *Clin Infect Dis* 2007; 44: 850–856. [General review, including risks of vaccination.]

Garg P, Nagpal J, Khairnor P, Seneviratne SL. Economic burden of dengue infections in India. *Trans R Soc Trop Med Hyg* 2008; 102: 570–577. [Describes the considerable economic burden of dengue; estimated to be US $27.4 million in the 2006 Indian epidemic.]

Gibbons RV, Vaughan DW. Dengue—an escalating problem. *Br Med J* 2002; 324: 1563–1566.

Halstead SB. Dengue. *Lancet* 2007; 370: 1644–1652.

National Travel Health Network and Centre. http://www.nathnac.org. [Excellent discussion on risks of vaccine and risk maps for infection with yellow fever, tick-borne encephalitis, etc for travellers.]

Solomon T, Mallewa MJ. Dengue and other emerging flaviviruses. *J Infect* 2001; 42: 104–115. [Includes important tick-borne viruses.]

Chapter 43

Relapsing fevers

Relapsing fevers are caused by various species of *Borrelia*. They fall into two main categories: epidemic or louse-borne relapsing fever (LBRF) caused by *Borrelia recurrentis* and endemic or tick-borne relapsing fever (TBRF) caused by numerous other species of *Borrelia*, depending on the geographical location. Untreated, these infections are characterized by a series of febrile episodes, often associated with systemic symptoms, separated by periods of relative well-being. TBRF is usually clinically milder and may be associated with up to 11 relapses, whereas LBRF is more severe but seldom gives rise to more than three relapses.

Epidemiology

LBRF, in common with many louse-borne infections, tends to occur in epidemics in situations of poor hygiene and overcrowding such as in prisons and among refugee, displaced and homeless populations. The disease is most common in the highland regions of Ethiopia and Burundi and, to a lesser extent, in other highland areas of Africa, India and the Andes. Humans are the reservoir host. The louse, most commonly the human body louse (*Pediculus humanus*) but also occasionally

the head louse (*P. capitis*) and, possibly, the crab louse (*Phthirus pubis*), becomes infected following a blood meal and remains infected for life. The louse provokes itching and is crushed when the host scratches, releasing *Borrelia* which enter the new host via abrasions and mucous membranes. Blood-borne and congenital infections may also occur.

TBRF occurs in geographically widespread endemic foci: central, eastern and southern Africa (*B. duttonii*); north-western Africa and the Iberian peninsula (*B. hispanica*); central Asia and parts of the Middle East, India and China (*B. persica*); and various regions of the Americas (*B. hermsii, B. turicatae* and *B. venezuelensis*). Animal reservoirs include wild rodents, lizards, toads and owls. Recently, *Borrelia* species have been identified in pigs and chickens in East Africa raising the possibility that domestic animals also may be implicated as reservoir hosts. Transmission to humans occurs following the bite of an infected argasid (soft) tick of the genus *Ornithodorus* via tick saliva or coxal fluid. Soft ticks favour cool, relatively humid environments such as caves or the mud walls or thatch of huts. They exhibit 'transovarial transmission': vertical transmission of *Borrelia* from one tick generation to the next without further exposure to a reservoir host. Human congenital infections may also occur.

A recent study in rural Senegal concluded that the incidence of TBRF was higher than that of

Lecture Notes: Tropical Medicine, 6th edition.
By G.V. Gill and N.J. Beeching. Published 2009 by
Blackwell Publishing, ISBN: 978-1-4051-8048-1.

any other bacterial disease and that TBRF was likely to be a common cause of disease in similar rural communities elsewhere in West Africa.

Pathology

Borrelia multiply in blood by simple fission and are taken up by the reticuloendothelial system. They have a predisposition for the liver (sometimes resulting in intrahepatic biliary obstruction), spleen and the CNS. Widespread vascular endothelial damage and platelet sequestration in the bone marrow occur. Myocardial and pulmonary damage are also common. Clinical severity tends to correlate with the level of spirochaetaemia. Relapses result from antigenic variation.

Clinical features

The incubation period is usually 4–8 days (range 2–15). Typically, there is a sudden onset of high fever accompanied by headache, confusion, meningism, myalgia, arthralgia, nausea, vomiting and, sometimes, dysphagia.

Dyspnoea and cough may be severe and, if productive, sputum may contain *Borrelia*. Hepatomegaly is common and is associated with jaundice in 50% of patients with LBRF and in less than 10% of those with TBRF. Splenomegaly is common and may be associated with an increased risk of rupture. Petechiae, erythematous rashes, epistaxis, conjunctival injection and haemorrhages are more common in LBRF. Complications include pneumonia, nephritis, parotitis, arthritis, cranial and peripheral neuropathies, meningoencephalitis, meningitis, acute ophthalmitis and iritis. Myocarditis may give rise to sudden and fatal arrhythmias. Most complications are more common and more severe in LBRF. Case fatality rates may reach 70% in epidemics of LBRF. In contrast, with the exception of children and pregnant women, case fatality rates rarely exceed 10% in untreated cases of TBRF.

Differential diagnosis

The differential diagnosis is wide and includes malaria, typhus, typhoid, meningococcal septicaemia/meningitis, dengue, hepatitis, leptospirosis, yellow fever and other viral haemorrhagic fevers.

Diagnosis

Borrelia are large spirochaetes measuring 10–30 × 0.2–0.5 μm. They are visible in Giemsa or Field stained blood films and may be a surprise finding in a patient with suspected malaria. Dual infections of malaria and *Borrelia* may occur and, usually the latter, may be overlooked. The spirochaetes are also visible unstained using dark field or phase-contrast microscopy. They may be concentrated above the buffy coat following centrifugation of anticoagulated whole blood. The acridine orange-coated QBC technique is also useful. Infected blood or CSF inoculated into mice or rats yields borreliae in the peripheral blood after 2–3 days. Serology is unreliable. Examination of the vector may also be useful. PCR assays are becoming available for diagnosis and speciation. In a recent study, PCR was shown to be at least twice as sensitive as microscopy for detecting *Borrelia* infections among children in Tanzania, and it led to the discovery of a new species of *Borrelia*.

Treatment

A single dose of antibiotic is effective in about 95% of cases of LBRF and in up to 80% of those with TBRF. However, the usual practice is to give a 5- to 10-day course to minimize the likelihood of relapses. Effective antibiotics include tetracycline, doxycycline, penicillin, erythromycin, chloramphenicol and ciprofloxacin. Ceftriaxone is recommended for patients presenting with meningitis or encephalitis. The choice will depend on drug availability, age, allergies, whether the patient is pregnant and one's confidence in the diagnosis.

A potentially fatal Jarisch–Herxheimer reaction occurs in 80–90% of patients treated for LBRF and in 30–40% of those treated for TBRF. This usually follows within a few hours of the first dose of antibiotic and is characterized by intense rigors, restlessness and anxiety. The temperature rises sharply accompanied by an initial rise in pulse rate and blood pressure. This is followed by marked vasodilation and sweating, sometimes resulting in collapse and shock. Patients must be closely monitored for this complication and may require intravenous fluids to maintain blood pressure. If available, meptazinol, an opioid antagonist, should be given to reduce the severity of the reaction. Antitumor necrosis factor alpha antibodies may also be effective. Steroids are of no benefit.

Prevention and control

Prevention of LBRF is largely a matter of improving hygiene, reducing crowding and delousing. Postexposure antibiotic prophylaxis with tetracycline or doxycycline may be recommended in high-risk situations. TBRF is best prevented by avoiding tick habitats.

Further reading

Kisinza WN, McCall PJ, Mitani H, Talbert A, Fukunaga M. A newly identified tick-borne *Borrelia* species and relapsing fever in Tanzania. *Lancet* 2003; 362: 1283–1284. [Illustrates how advances in molecular techniques are leading to some interesting new discoveries concerning the epidemiology and clinical importance of *Borrelia* infections.]

McCall PJ, Hume J, Motshegwa K *et al.* Does tick-borne relapsing fever have an animal reservoir in East Africa? *Vector Borne and Zoonotic Dis* 2007; 7: 1–8. [Reports interesting epidemiological findings on TBRF in East Africa.]

Parola P, Raoult D. Ticks and tickborne bacterial diseases in humans: an emerging infectious threat. *Clin Infect Dis* 2001; 32: 897–928. [This article reviews and illustrates various aspects of the biology of ticks and the tick-borne bacterial diseases—rickettsioses, ehrlichioses, Lyme disease, relapsing fever borrelioses, tularaemia and Q fever—particularly those regarded as emerging diseases.]

Raoult D, Ndihokubwayo JB, Tissot-Dupont H *et al.* Outbreak of epidemic typhus associated with trench fever in Burundi. *Lancet* 1998; 352: 353–358. [This epidemic highlights the appalling conditions in central African refugee camps and the failure of public health programmes to serve their inhabitants.]

Vial L, Diatta G, Tall A *et al.* Incidence of tick-borne relapsing fever in West Africa: longitudinal study. *Lancet* 2006; 368: 37–43. [Highlights the importance of TBRF as a common cause of fever in parts of rural West Africa.]

Chapter 44

Rickettsial infections

There are many species and subspecies of *Rickettsiae* that can infect humans. They may also infect rodents, and are transmitted to humans by the bites, body fluids or faeces of various arthropods. The illness is very variable in intensity, but is characterized by fever and rash. Therefore, there is often a wide differential diagnosis. In this chapter, only the three main types of typhus seen worldwide are considered: louse-borne typhus, scrub typhus and African tick typhus.

Louse-borne typhus

This is caused by *Rickettsia prowazekii*, which is transmitted to humans from the infected faeces of the human body louse, *Pediculus humanus*, usually by being scratched into the skin. Louse-borne typhus may be epidemic, and occurs particularly in malnourished migrant populations with poor hygiene (e.g. in refugee camps). The disease can occur in wide geographical areas; indeed it was common in Europe in the nineteenth century and was a frequent cause of death in concentration camps in World War II.

Clinical features

The disease incubates for about 12 days following which there is high fever, myalgia, headache and prostration. The conjunctivae may be suffused and delirium is common. A rash appears on about the third or fourth day—it is central and macular, although the lesions may later become petechial or purpuric. Pneumonia and/or meningoencephalitis frequently occur later, as can sometimes myocarditis. Untreated, the disease has a high mortality. Diagnosis is usually made clinically, especially in epidemic situations. The Weil–Felix serological test can still be useful, but modern, specific serological and PCR techniques are better.

Treatment

Together with full supportive medical and nursing care, the disease usually responds well and rapidly to either tetracycline or chloramphenicol as listed below:

- tetracycline 500 mg four times daily (adult dose) orally or intravenously for 1 week
- chloramphenicol 500 mg four times daily (adult dose) orally or intravenously for 1 week
- doxycycline 200 mg/day for 7 days

Preventive measures are important in epidemics. In addition to delousing procedures, doxycycline 200 mg given as a single dose to all those at risk may be useful.

Lecture Notes: Tropical Medicine, 6th edition.
By G.V. Gill and N.J. Beeching. Published 2009 by Blackwell Publishing, ISBN: 978-1-4051-8048-1.

Scrub typhus

This is also known as mite typhus or Tsutsugamushi fever. It is caused by *Orientia tsutsugamushi* (previously known as *R. orientalis* or *R. tsutsugamushi*). It is a zoonosis of rodents, and humans are infected by the bites of infected larval mites. Scrub typhus occurs in wide parts of South East Asia, Oceania and northern parts of Australia.

Clinical features

The incubation period is 5–10 days, and a small eschar may be noted at the site of the mite bite. There is an abrupt fever, as well as headache, myalgia and prostration, as in louse-borne typhus. The rash is also similar. Lymphadenopathy may be generalized or local (related to the eschar). Hepatosplenomegaly may also occur, as may pneumonia and myocarditis. Delirium is frequently marked, although neuropsychiatric features are not as prominent as in louse-borne typhus and the overall mortality is lower. Diagnosis is usually clinically based. The Weil–Felix test is insensitive in this form of typhus.

Treatment

Tetracycline and chloramphenicol are effective in regimens as in other forms of typhus (see earlier). However, the simplest and the most optimal treatment is doxycycline 200 mg orally once daily for 3–7 days.

Resistance to both tetracycline and chloramphenicol has been reported in northern Thailand, and here rifampicin or ciprofloxacin may have to be used. Preventive measures include avoidance of mite-infested areas, impregnation of clothing with permethrin and prophylactic doxycycline (200 mg weekly while in high-risk areas).

African tick typhus

There are various forms of tick typhus (e.g. Rocky Mountain spotted fever, Siberian tick typhus and Queensland tick typhus). African tick typhus occurs in wide areas of Africa, but particularly in central and southern parts. The causative organism is usually *R. conorii*, although in Zimbabwe it is often *R. africae* which has a reservoir in cattle, domestic cattle and even in the hippopotamus and rhinoceros. Various tick species are involved as both vectors and reservoirs. The infection is usually caught by travellers and campers in veld areas or grasslands.

Clinical features

The illness mimics a mild attack of scrub typhus. There is usually a noticeable eschar with local lymphadenopathy, and a mild fever with toxaemic symptoms. A central maculopapular rash later spreads to the limbs. The disease is brief and complications are rare. There is almost no mortality. Diagnosis is usually clinically based.

Treatment

Mild cases may not require treatment. If necessary, tetracycline or chloramphenicol can be used as earlier, or doxycycline 200 mg daily for 3–7 days. Azithromycin is also effective, but less widely available. Preventive measures include tick-avoidance strategies such as appropriate clothing and insect repellents.

Further reading

Watt G, Parola P. Scrub typhus and tropical rickettsioses. *Curr Opin Infect Dis* 2003; 16: 429–436. [Comprehensive and well-annotated but brief review.]

Chapter 45

Leptospirosis

Leptospirosis is a zoonotic infection that can cause a variety of different clinical pictures in man ranging from asymptomatic infection to fulminant hepato renal failure (Weil's disease). It has a worldwide distribution (except for the Polar regions) but can cause particular problems in the tropics.

Microbiology

The causative organism belongs to the genus *Leptospira* which is part of the Spirochaete family (that also includes *Treponema* and *Borrelia*). The nomenclature of the individual *Leptospira* is complex and undergoes frequent change. Historically, there were two species (*L. interrogans* and *L. bireflexa*) but these have recently been reclassified. There are about 250 serovars that are potentially pathogenic.

Epidemiology

Rodents and other small mammals are the most important animal reservoir. They are usually infected during infancy and continue with chronic renal infection for life. They excrete the organism in the urine to infect other mammals

or humans. Larger mammals such as dogs and cattle may become chronic carriers or they may develop symptomatic infection that may be fatal. Excreted organisms may remain viable in soil or water for weeks and the incidence of infection is often higher after heavy rainfall. Those most at risk therefore have direct contact with soil, water or animals. Therefore, at particular risk are farmers, veterinary workers, sewage workers and the military. In a Western setting, infection is often acquired recreationally by canoeists or triathletes.

Pathogenesis

Infection is caused by *Leptospira* penetrating either the skin through minor cuts and abrasions or mucous membranes. It is not established whether they can penetrate intact skin. They are disseminated via the bloodstream and are therefore widely distributed through the body where they produce a vasculitis, the exact mechanism of which remains obscure.

Clinical features

This is incredibly variable. Many of those infected will have an asymptomatic seroconversion. Others may have a mild non-specific febrile illness and some others may have one of the more easily appreciated syndromes. The average incubation period seems to be about 10 days

Lecture Notes: Tropical Medicine, 6th edition.
By G.V. Gill and N.J. Beeching. Published 2009 by Blackwell Publishing, ISBN: 978-1-4051-8048-1.

although, of course, it is always difficult to establish exactly when infection occurred, and a range of incubations from 2 to 26 days has been reported. The majority of symptomatic cases then present with sudden onset of fever, rigors, myalgia and headache. Nausea, vomiting, diarrhoea and cough are also common features. On examination, the most characteristic finding is conjunctival suffusion and muscle tenderness but they probably only occur in a minority of cases. Other physical findings include more rarely lymphadenopathy, hepatosplenomegaly, chest signs and a rash. Clinical features of meningitis may also be present. Although the illness is often described classically as 'biphasic', in practice such a pattern is rarely recognized. However, as the immune response appears the patient may deteriorate and develop one of the more specific syndromes associated with *Leptospira* infection. These include the following:

• Aseptic meningitis—this may occur in up to 50–80% of cases and is difficult to distinguish from other causes of aseptic meningitis.

• Weil's disease—this is the classical presentation of jaundice, thrombocytopenia and renal failure. Despite the jaundice, liver function is usually relatively well preserved.

• Pulmonary syndrome—this has been described especially in South America and may vary from mild respiratory symptoms and signs to severe pulmonary haemorrhage and adult respiratory distress syndrome. A recent review in Peru suggested that nearly 4% of patients with serologically confirmed *Leptospira* infection had severe pulmonary manifestations and would not have been otherwise diagnosed if they had not been part of the study.

• Cardiac syndrome—recently severe cardiac involvement has been described in India with myocarditis leading to cardiac failure.

Several of these syndromes may coexist.

Diagnosis

Clearly, the differential diagnosis during the non-specific febrile phase is wide and would include malaria, typhoid, influenza, rickettsial infection (especially scrub typhus) and arbovirus infection (including dengue fever). Routine laboratory investigations are similarly non-specific—white cell count may be elevated or lowered (usual range 3000 to $25\,000 \times 10^6$/L) often with a left shift. About half the patients will have elevations of liver transaminases (fairly mild) and creatinine kinase. The urine will often be abnormal with proteinuria, white cells, casts and occasional microscopic haematuria. In Weil's disease, renal function will deteriorate and the bilirubin may be very high. Chest X-ray may show non-specific shadowing. The platelet count may sometimes be reduced. The CSF may show an elevated white cell count with neutrophils or lymphocytes, minimal to moderately elevated protein concentrations and normal glucose.

Because of the non-specific nature of the clinical picture and the laboratory findings, a high index of suspicion must be maintained if the diagnosis is not to be missed.

Leptospira can be seen microscopically in blood or urine but sensitivity and specificity is low and these techniques are rarely used in practice. The organism can also be isolated in blood cultures from specimens taken from the patient in the first 10 days of illness and before antibiotics have been administered. Urine cultures may become positive a week into the illness and remain positive for some time afterwards. A urinary antigen test was reported but does not seem to have been developed further.

Most patients have their infection identified serologically. The traditional gold standard test has been the MAT test that uses live organisms and can be technically difficult to perform. Therefore most laboratories would first use a screening test such as an ELISA for IgM antibodies—these are usually detectable on day 5 of illness. PCR methods are in development but are not widely used.

Treatment

Leptospirosis is sensitive to many antibiotics and many have been used to treat it (e.g. ceftriaxone, penicillin, doxycycline and azithromycin). It is controversial about how effective antibiotics are unless they are given very early in the natural history of the condition and there is also doubt about whether mild disease needs to be treated. In endemic areas, it is common for leptospirosis to be misdiagnosed as a rickettsial infection or visa versa; therefore oral doxycycline 100 mg bd is a sensible option as this will treat both conditions empirically whilst serological diagnosis is awaited. If the patient is very unwell, then intravenous penicillin 1.2 g 6 hourly or ceftriaxone 1 g once daily should be used. There are no trials on duration of therapy but 10 days is usually recommended.

Prevention

Risk of infection can be reduced by avoiding high-risk exposure. A human vaccine has been used but is not widely available. A vaccine is used in veterinary practice. A study from 1984 showed significant benefit of weekly doxycycline 200 mg amongst US troops in the jungles of Panama.

Further reading

Chakurkar G, Vaideeswar P, Pandit SP et al. Cardiovascular lesions in lepto-spirosis: an autopsy study. *J Infect* 2008; 56: 197–203. [Well-illustrated reports and discussion.]

Edwards CN, Levett PN. Treatment and prevention of leptospirosis. *Ex Rev Anti-infect Ther* 2004; 2: 293–298.

Phimda K, Hoontrakul S, Suttinon C et al. Doxycycline versus azithromycin for treatment of leptospirosis and scrub typhus. *Antimicrob Agents Chemother* 2007; 51: 3259–3263. [Both drugs equally effective – doxycycline cheaper and more readily available, but causes more side effects.]

www.leptospirosis.org/medical/ [General information source and good links.]

Chapter 46

Melioidosis

Epidemiology

Melioidosis is caused by the Gram-negative bacillus, *Burkholderia pseudomallei*. In endemic areas, the organism can be easily found in the soil and surface water such as in rice paddies, but only certain strains are pathogenic to humans. Melioidosis was initially recognized as a serious problem during the Vietnam War and now causes clinical disease in a relatively geographically constrained area of South-East Asia. In Thailand, the most affected country, 3000–5000 new cases are diagnosed annually. Clinical cases are also regularly reported from Vietnam, Malaysia, Singapore and northern Australia, although sporadic cases occur over a far greater geographical area including India, China, the Caribbean and Brazil.

Pathogenesis

Infection is acquired primarily by inoculation of contaminated soil or water but may also be acquired by inhalation. Most infection is asymptomatic; organisms may remain latent within the macrophages and can cause disease many years after infection. Localized abscesses may develop at the site of inoculation which can lead to bacteraemia and dissemination of the organism. Up to 70% of

Lecture Notes: Tropical Medicine, 6th edition.
By G.V. Gill and N.J. Beeching. Published 2009 by Blackwell Publishing, ISBN: 978-1-4051-8048-1.

patients have predisposing diseases. Diabetes mellitus is the most common, but chronic renal impairment, chronic lung disease, excess alcohol intake, steroid therapy and malignancy are also important. There is no association with HIV infection.

Clinical features

Many individuals are found to have positive serology without having had obvious clinical symptoms. Acute presentations can be with localized or septicaemic disease. The most common form of localized disease is pneumonia, but abscesses may also be found in the skin and soft tissue or organs such as the spleen and liver. Localized disease may lead to subsequent bacteraemia. Septicaemic disease is associated with a poor prognosis: an obvious focus of disease cannot always be found. If patients survive the initial stages of septicaemic disease, dissemination can occur to cause abscesses in a number of different sites.

Diagnosis

Definitive diagnosis of melioidosis is by culture of the organism from blood or pus. Molecular techniques are available but are of limited utility in routine diagnosis. Serological tests can detect rising titres of IgG or a raised specific IgM in acute infections but are far less sensitive than culture in endemic areas.

Treatment

Melioidosis is both difficult and expensive to treat. *B. pseudomallei* is intrinsically resistant to a large number of antibiotics. Initial treatment should be with parenteral ceftazidime or a carbopenem for a minimum of 10 days. Ceftazidime is sometimes combined with co-trimoxazole (trimethoprim/sulfamethoxazole), although the value of this is uncertain. Amoxicillin clavulanate may also be used but has higher treatment failure rates. Several weeks of intravenous therapy may be needed to produce clinical improvement in patients with visceral abscesses. The response of symptoms to treatment is slow: fever may often persist for over a week and does not imply failure of antibiotic therapy.

Oral maintenance therapy is required following the completion of parenteral therapy to prevent relapse: relapse rates may reach 25% in severe disease. The combination of doxycycline and co-trimoxazole is cheap and effective if compliance can be maintained. Amoxicillin clavulanate is less effective and more expensive. Twenty weeks' therapy is advocated to reduce the relapse rate to less than 10%. Aggressive supportive therapy is required for individuals with septicaemic disease: the use of granulocyte colony stimulating factor along with meropenem appears to have reduced mortality in Australia. Abscesses should be surgically drained when feasible.

Prognosis

There is a very high mortality rate (up to 50%) in septicaemic melioidosis, even with adequate treatment. Long-term follow-up is necessary to detect relapse.

Further reading

Cheng AC, Currie BJ. Melioidosis: epidemiology, pathophysiology, and management. *Clin Microbiol Rev* 2005; 18(2): 383–416. [Detailed review.]

White NJ. Melioidosis. *Lancet* 2003; 361: 1715–1722. [A comprehensive review.]

Chapter 47

Tropical ulcer

Tropical ulcer is a term used to describe ulcers of the ankle and lower leg occurring in the tropics and subtropics that are not typical of other leg ulcers of more definitive aetiology (e.g. Buruli ulcers, diabetes and leprosy).

Clinical features

The vast majority of tropical ulcers occur below the knee, usually around the ankle. They are often initiated by minor trauma, and subjects with poor nutrition are at increased risk (Figure 47.1). Once developed the ulcer may become chronic and stable, but also it can run a destructive course with deep tissue invasion, osteitis and risk of amputation. Unlike Buruli ulcer (Chapter 48), tropical ulcers are typically painful.

Microbiology

There is no single agreed causative organism for tropical ulcers, although early lesions may be colonized or infected by *Bacillus fusiformis*, anaerobes and spirochaetes. Later, tropical ulcers may become infected with a wide variety of organisms, notably staphylococci and/or streptococci.

Epidemiology

Tropical ulcer is seen throughout the tropics and subtropics. Prevalence rates of up to 7% were reported from rural Ethiopia in the early 1990s, but frequency has generally declined since then. Tropical ulcer has been described as a disease of the 'poor and hungry', and it may be that slowly improving socioeconomic conditions and nutrition account for its decline. Urbanization of populations is another factor, as tropical ulcer is usually a rural problem. More widespread use of shoes and socks also provides protection from initiating trauma. Despite this susceptible individuals still develop tropical ulcers. Sometimes 'outbreaks' can occur; one was recorded in Tanzania in sugar cane workers (cutting the crop in bare

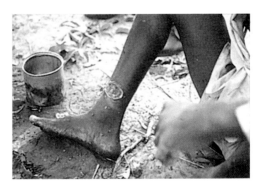

Figure 47.1 A chronic tropical ulcer in a poor and malnourished young Nigerian patient.

Lecture Notes: Tropical Medicine, 6th edition.
By G.V. Gill and N.J. Beeching. Published 2009 by Blackwell Publishing, ISBN: 978-1-4051-8048-1.

feet). Tropical ulcer can also occur in visitors to the tropics—the disease was very common amongst Allied prisoners of war working on the Thai–Burma railway in the early 1940s. The men often suffered very severe ulcers which frequently required amputation.

Treatment

Antibiotics should be given in adequate dosages. For early ulcers, penicillin is usually sufficient, although later broad-spectrum antibiotics are likely to be needed. Improved nutrition and vitamin supplementation are helpful. The important principle of dressings is that they must be non-adherent (e.g. saline soaks and petroleum jelly-impregnated gauze), otherwise they will stick to the ulcer surface and when removed they will disrupt granulation tissue. For sloughy ulcers, honey, sugar paste or paw paw (papaya) are useful inexpensive dressings. Large infected ulcers may require curettage and débridement under anaesthetic. Skin grafting can occasionally be helpful. In extreme cases, amputation may be inevitable.

Prevention

Trauma avoidance is important, in particular wearing adequate footwear. General good health and nutrition also reduce ulcer risk. Adequate and prompt treatment of ankle and leg skin breaks is also important.

Complications

- Deep tissue invasion—often with bone involvement, and potentially leading to amputation.
- Chronic ulceration—particularly if poorly treated, tropical ulcers may become chronic. In former Far East Prisoners of War of World War II, they have been recorded for over 50 years since original development of the ulcer.
- Recurrent ulceration— may occur in the same site when a 'paper-thin' scar forms over the ulcer.
- Squamous cell carcinoma—may occasionally develop, usually in very chronic cases, and at the edge of the ulcer.
- Tetanus—by entry of tetanus bacilli through the ulcer.

Further reading

Parry E. Tropical ulcer and the rural health team. *Africa Health* 1996; 18: 20–21. [A useful review of tropical ulcer and its individual and community effects, as well as good discussion of preventive strategies.]

Chapter 48

Buruli ulcer

Buruli ulcer is a highly destructive ulcerating condition caused by *Mycobacterium ulcerans*. Any part of the body may be affected, particularly areas exposed to minor trauma such as the limbs. *M. ulcerans* ranks third among mycobacterial infections affecting immunocompetent humans.

Microbiology

M. ulcerans, a slowly growing acid- and alcohol-fast organism, belongs to a large group of environmental mycobacteria. Three different genetic strains have been identified, but their relationship to virulence remains uncertain. Local immuno-suppression, ulceration and necrosis are caused by mycolactones—soluble polyketide toxins that also appear to be responsible for the painlessness that is characteristic of uncomplicated lesions. There is some evidence that intercurrent helmintic infections may also predispose to ulceration.

Background and epidemiology

Buruli ulcer has been reported from several parts of Africa, notably the Buruli region of Uganda,

Lecture Notes: Tropical Medicine, 6th edition.
By G.V. Gill and N.J. Beeching. Published 2009 by Blackwell Publishing, ISBN: 978-1-4051-8048-1.

Ghana, Papua New Guinea, the Americas, South-East Asia and China. Buruli ulcer has also been described among koala bears and Australian golfers. Predominantly a disease of children, infection is thought to occur following a penetrating injury—usually minor—resulting in inoculation of the organism, which is found naturally in soil or stagnant water. It has been postulated that transmission may also follow the bite of an infected water bug. *M. ulcerans* has also been identified in mosquitoes captured during an outbreak in Australia. Whether this is of any epidemiological or clinical significance is unclear. Person–person transmission is very rare.

Clinical features

A non-ulcerative lesion usually precedes ulceration. Four non-ulcerative presentations are recognized.

1 *Papule*—painless, sometimes itchy, non-tender palpable intradermal lesion (seen in Australia but rare in Africa).

2 *Nodule*—painless palpable firm lesion, 1–2 cm in diameter, situated in the subcutaneous tissue and usually attached to the skin (uncommon in Australia).

3 *Plaque*—painless well-demarcated, elevated, dry-indurated lesion more than 2 cm.

4 *Oedematous*—diffuse extensive non-pitting swelling, ill-defined margin, firm, usually painful, with or without colour change over the affected skin.

Table 48.1 Differential diagnosis of Buruli ulcer

Papule	Nodule	Plaque	Oedema	Ulcer
Granuloma annulare	Boil	Cellulitis	Actinomycosis	Cutaneous diphtheria
Herpes	Cyst	Haematoma	Cellulitis	Guinea worm
Insect bites	Leishmaniasis	Insect bites	Elephantiasis	Leishmaniasis
Leishmaniasis	Lipoma	Leishmaniasis	Necrotizing fasciitis	Necrotizing fasciitis
Pimple	Lymphadenitis	Leprosy	Onchocercoma	Neurogenic ulcer
Pityriasis	Mycosis	Mycosis	Osteomyelitis	Tropical ulcer
Psoriasis	Onchocercoma	Psoriasis		Tuberculosis
				Sickle cell disease
				Squamous cell carcinoma
				Syphilis
				Venous ulcer
				Yaws

Modified from *Diagnosis of* Mycobacterium ulcerans *disease* [Buruli ulcer], WHO/CDS/CPE/GBUI/2001.4.

In due course, the overlying skin breaks down and an ulcer forms with a necrotic centre, often spreading very rapidly in all directions. The following features are clinically very characteristic.
• The ulcer is usually painless, a factor contributing to the delay in health care seeking behaviour.
• The skin at the edge of the ulcer is deeply undermined.
• Satellite ulcers often communicate with the original ulcer by a subcutaneous tunnel, so the skin between adjacent ulcers is often unattached to the underlying tissues. The extent of the damage is always much greater than it looks from the surface.

Regional adenitis and systemic symptoms are unusual and, if present, are suggestive of primary or secondary bacterial infection. Complications such as tetanus and primary or secondary osteomyelitis may occur. Eventually, after months or years, healing may result in scarring, ankylosis and contractures. Currently, 25% of those affected develop long-term complications that may include amputation or loss of sight. HIV infection does not appear to be associated with an altered clinical course.

Differential diagnosis

Differential diagnosis is shown in Table 48.1.

Investigations

The slough from the ulcer usually contains numerous acid-fast bacilli on Ziehl–Neelsen stain but may be negative. Culture is time consuming, expensive and too frequently gives rise to false-positive results to make it worthwhile. PCR has been used as an epidemiological tool and is now increasingly used in diagnosis.

Management

Small pre-ulcerative papules, nodules and plaques can be surgically excised. Necrotic ulcers should also be excised with care to remove all affected tissue by extending the margin into healthy tissue. Excision is followed by primary closure or split-skin grafting. Surgery and physiotherapy may be required for patients with contractures.

In the past, medical treatment with antimycobacterial agents has been disappointing. However, supervised combination therapy using oral rifampicin (10 mg/kg) plus intramuscular streptomycin (15 mg/kg) daily for 8 weeks has recently been shown to be highly effective in Benin when used in conjunction with surgery depending on the size of the ulcer at presentation, with an overall treatment success rate of

96%. Antibiotic combination treatment without surgery achieved a cure rate of 47% and was most successful in patients with nodules, papules, plaques and ulcers <5 cm. Recurrence occurred in <2% overall. Antibiotic combination treatment, by reducing ulcer size, also makes larger ulcers more amenable to surgery and grafting. *In vitro* sensitivity has also been demonstrated for macrolide and quinolone antibiotics.

Topical treatment—with nitric oxide, phenytoin powder or local heat treatment—has been used successfully in treatment particularly of smaller lesions.

Prevention and public health aspects

Long trousers and other mechanical barriers reduce the likelihood of infection. There is no specific vaccine available at present, although BCG offers some protection. A prospective vaccine candidate is the environmental mycobacterium *M. vaccae*.

The Global Buruli Ulcer Initiative, launched by the WHO in 1998, is an important initiative targeting this neglected disease. The following control strategies are being promoted:
• Health education and staff training in the communities most affected.
• Development of educational materials adapted to the needs of the countries.
• Community-based surveillance system to increase early detection and referral for treatment in collaboration with diseases such as leprosy and Guinea worm.
• Assessment of local health services and resources currently available for the diagnosis and treatment of Buruli ulcer in endemic areas.

• Strengthening of the capacity of health systems in endemic areas by upgrading surgical facilities and improving laboratories.
• Rehabilitation of those already deformed by the disease.

Further reading

Anonymous. Buruli ulcer: progress report, 2004–2008. *Wkly Epidemiol Rec* 2008; 83: 145–154. [Up-to-date review summarizing some of the key developments made in recent years.]

Chauty A, Ardant M-F, Adeye A. Promising clinical efficacy of streptomycin-rifampin combination for treatment of Buruli ulcer (*Mycobacterium ulcerans* Disease). *Antimicrob Agents Chemother* 2007; 51: 4029–4035. [Recent publication indicating successful implementation of WHO 2003; revised guidelines for management of Buruli ulcer.]

Extensive information is also available from the WHO at http://www.who.int/gtb-buruli/ [Click on 'information resources'. This will lead you to further links providing a wealth of useful information.]

van der Werf TS, van der Graaf WT, Tappero JW, Asiedu K. *Mycobacterium ulcerans* infection. *Lancet* 1999; 354: 1013–1018. [Highly recommended, this concise review includes some good clinical photographs and an excellent figure illustrating pathogenesis.]

Wansbrough-Jones M, Phillips R. Buruli ulcer: emerging from obscurity. *Lancet* 2006; 367: 1849–1858. [Comprehensive review explaining the current understanding of *M. ulcerans* and its relations with human beings.]

Chapter 49

Myiasis

The term myiasis refers to a variety of conditions characterized by insect larvae invading the subcutaneous tissues or body cavities. There are only three common syndromes: the Tumbu fly, the Bot fly and Chiggers.

Tumbu fly

This is also sometimes known as the 'Putzi fly' in central and southern Africa. It is caused by the larvae of *Cordylobia anthropophaga*, which mostly inhabits sub-Saharan Africa. The fly lays its eggs on clothing (often on a washing line), and these hatch with body warmth when the clothes are worn. The larvae invade the skin and develop over the next 2 weeks causing a 'blind boil'. The lesion is painful and often 'prickles' as a result of larval movement. The small dark 'head' of the boil is actually the respiratory spiracles of the larva. Multiple lesions are often present.

Treatment is to partly suffocate the larva by putting petroleum jelly or other oil or grease over the spiracles. The larva will become activated and will partly extrude from the lesion when it can be grasped with forceps and removed intact. Care must be taken as maceration of the larva causes a severe inflammatory reaction. Prevention is by hot-ironing all clean clothes after drying.

Bot fly

This is *Dermatobia hominis* and is found in Central and South America. The Bot fly deposits eggs directly on the skin, rather than via clothes as does the Tumbu fly. The lesion that develops is similar; however, removal is more difficult. Occasionally, mechanical extraction of the larva can be done, but its shape often makes this difficult and incision under local anaesthetic is often needed. After infiltration of lidocaine, a cruciate incision should be made over the lesion, taking care not to incise the larva itself. Following this, extraction with forceps is usually easy. An interesting reported alternative is to put strips of raw fatty bacon over the lesion. Within a few hours the larva emerges and can be grasped with forceps. The lesions of both the Bot and Tumbu flies are usually microbiologically sterile, but sometimes secondary infection can occur, and antibiotics may be required.

Chiggers

Chiggers (or 'jiggers') are caused by *Tunga penetrans*, a flea that is widely distributed around the tropics—including much of Central and South America, Africa and the Asian Subcontinent.

Lecture Notes: Tropical Medicine, 6th edition.
By G.V. Gill and N.J. Beeching. Published 2009 by Blackwell Publishing, ISBN: 978-1-4051-8048-1.

The gravid jigger flea invades exposed human skin—almost always the feet, and usually the interdigital clefts or the base of the toes. The flea encapsulates itself and produces eggs about 10 days later. A papular—and often later pustular—lesion develops which is painful and itchy. Excoriation helps to expel the eggs. Secondary infection and even ulceration can occur and multiple 'jigger' lesions may be present.

The flea should be carefully removed with a sterile needle, following which the lesion usually heals. Late ulcerative lesions will require antibiotics. The main aspect of prevention is good foot care and wearing shoes.

Body cavity myiasis

A variety of syndromes of myiasis exist in which various larvae invade body cavities—including wounds, urethra, vagina, anus, eye and ear. Nasal myiasis is the most common caused usually (but not always) by the Old World screw fly (*Chrysomia bezziana*). Cold-like symptoms develop followed by nasal obstruction and epistaxis. The fly maggots can usually be seen with a nasal speculum. Application of 15% chloroform in vegetable oil to the nasal cavity causes the larva to appear, when it can be removed with forceps. In occasional advanced cases, invasions of the nasal sinuses and even the brain can occur.

Further reading

Brewer TF, Wilson ME, Gonzalez E, Felsenstein D. Bacon therapy and furuncular myiasis. *JAMA* 1993, 270: 2087–2088. [An interesting alternative to the more invasive method of incision for bot fly larvae.]

Chapter 50

Cutaneous larva migrans

Cutaneous larva migrans is an intensely itchy and slowly moving linear rash under the skin of the foot and ankle. It represents the subcutaneous meanderings of invading dog hookworms, and is one of the most common exotic diseases imported to western countries (usually after tropical beach holidays).

Parasitology

The disease is caused by the larvae of animal hookworms—most commonly the dog hookworm *Ancylostoma braziliense*. Eggs are shed in the faeces of canine hosts to the soil or sand. Humans walking barefoot, or lying on the soil or sand, can become infected by larval invasion through intact skin. Sometimes infection can arise from towels or clothes which have been in contact with infected sand. Humans are an incidental host, and infection represents a cul-de-sac of the life cycle. The larvae therefore travel aimlessly under the skin, causing the typical clinical eruption, until they eventually die.

Clinical features

A typical cutaneous larva migrans rash is shown in Figure 50.1. The rash is a very itchy serpiginous red track, which is often excoriated. The larva advances by only a few millimetres a day, so the rash is relatively static. This is in contrast to the very rapidly moving linear rash of larva currens caused by *Strongyloides stercoralis* (Chapter 52). Although the foot and ankle are by far the most common sites for cutaneous larva migrans, it can occur on other parts of the body in contact with the ground. 'Hookworm folliculitis' is an uncommon form of the disease characterized by pustular folliculitis of the buttocks.

Treatment

There is no constitutional disturbance and the rash will heal spontaneously within a few weeks.

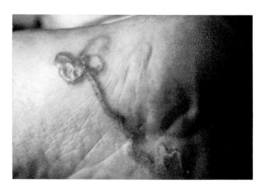

Figure 50.1 Typical rash of cutaneous larva migrans in a holidaymaker returned from a beach holiday in the Caribbean.

Lecture Notes: Tropical Medicine, 6th edition.
By G.V. Gill and N.J. Beeching. Published 2009 by Blackwell Publishing, ISBN: 978-1-4051-8048-1.

However, it is aesthetically unpleasant and the severe itch can be debilitating. Also, some larvae can survive for several months. Older treatments included local freezing of the head of the larval track with an ethyl chloride spray, or occlusive application of 10% or 15% tiabendazole in emulsifying ointment. Neither were highly effective and oral treatments are better. Current options are as follows:

• *Albendazole*—A single dose of 400 mg is usually completely effective, and if available this is the drug of choice.

• *Ivermectin*—This is also highly effective in a single dose (12 mg for adults).

• *Tiabendazole*—This is less effective than albendazole and ivermectin, and also more prone to side effects (e.g. dizziness, nausea and vomiting). The dose is 25 mg/kg twice a day for 3 days.

Prevention

Contamination of soil and sand by dog faeces is the cause of the disease. Beaches are a particular hazard, so banning dogs from beaches is an effective option (widely practised in Australia, but difficult to enforce in most developing countries). Programmes to deworm dogs regularly will also be effective, provided the uptake is high. On an individual basis, wearing shoes or sandals on beaches helps, as well as avoiding lying on dry sand (preferably using sand washed by the tide). It can be seen that both these practices significantly detract from the pleasures of a tropical beach, and many may prefer to risk infection from these annoying but benign parasites.

Further reading

Caumes F. Treatment of cutaneous larva migrans. *Clin Infect Dis* 2000; 30: 811–814.

Chapter 51

Scabies and lice

Scabies

Scabies is a common skin condition globally, but it is seen particularly frequently and severely in tropical countries. Infection rates of 10% overall, and up to 50% in children, have been reported from some areas. It is caused by infestation with the mite *Sarcoptes scabiei*. Infection occurs by direct skin contact, and there is often a 4- to 6-week period before clinical symptoms occur. The mite burrows beneath the skin, causing an inflammatory reaction, and an intensely itchy generalized rash ensues. The classical diagnostic lesion is the interdigital burrow from which the mite can be sometimes extracted with a sterile needle. In practice, however, the diagnosis is frequently made clinically and empirical treatment given.

The classical eruption is not always seen in tropical countries. Secondary infection and/or allergic hypersensitivity to the mite can alter the rash significantly. Thus, infected papules, widespread vesicles and papular urticaria may occur. In all types of rash, excoriation often alters its appearance. The important clinical principle is to always think of scabies when presented with an intensely itchy generalized rash in the tropics (especially in

a child). A history of nocturnal itch in other family members is good supportive evidence.

'Norwegian scabies' or 'crusted scabies' occurs sometimes in immunologically compromised patients (e.g. HIV or lepromatous leprosy), and represents a massive proliferation of infecting mites (perhaps analogous to the hyperinfection syndrome of *Strongyloides stercoralis*). The skin becomes scaly or 'crusted' and is frequently not as itchy as classical scabies. Crusted scabies also occurs sporadically for no obvious reason, and is relatively common in Australian aborigines.

Scabies treatment is usually topical and is applied from the neck down to all parts of the skin, with particular attention to crevices and the genitalia. For severe cases, a second treatment 5–7 days later should be given. All household contacts must be treated at the same time. The preparations available are as follows.

- *Benzyl benzoate 25%*—old-fashioned but still effective and cheap; however, best avoided in children under 4 years of age.
- *Sulphur 6% ointment*—a better alternative for young children (<4 years).
- *Permethrin 5% cream*—more effective than benzyl benzoate and the treatment of choice, if available.
- *Ivermectin 200μg/kg*—a single oral dose is effective especially in difficult cases.

The itch may continue for some weeks after effective treatment, and can be controlled with

Lecture Notes: Tropical Medicine, 6th edition.
By G.V. Gill and N.J. Beeching. Published 2009 by
Blackwell Publishing, ISBN: 978-1-4051-8048-1.

calamine lotion. Preventive measures for scabies include general principles of hygiene, and also the use of Tetmosol (5% tetraethylthiuram monosulphide) soap or rubbing oils.

Lice

Lice infestations in humans include *Pediculus humanus* (the body louse), *Phthirus pubis* (the pubic or crab louse) and *Pediculus capitis* (the head louse). Transmission is by close contact (usually head–head for head lice).

P. humanus can transmit louse-borne relapsing fever, louse-borne typhus and trench fever, but only the local effects are considered here. Body lice cause generalized itch and often a maculopapular rash which may become secondarily infected. Pubic and head lice cause local itch and sometimes excoriation, but their importance is frequently more aesthetic than medically important.

A variety of insecticidal preparations are available for treatment. These include lotions, dusting powders or shampoos of malathion, permethrin and DDT. Head lice can sometimes be managed physically with a 'lice comb' (a fine-toothed comb that removes the eggs or 'nits' from the shaft of the hair). This process can be aided by the use of hair conditioner.

Body lice will recur if clothing is not treated by heating to about 70°C for 30 min. It should also be remembered that there are wide geographical variations in the susceptibility of lice to drug treatment, and local information on resistance patterns should be sought.

Further reading

Gibs S. Basic dermatologic treatment for tropical district hospitals. *Trop Doct* 1997; 27: 142–145. [A useful practical guide to the management of common skin conditions in the tropics.]

Heukelbach J, Feldmeier H. Scabies. *Lancet* 2006; 367: 1767–1774. [An up to date and comprehensive review, including a section on developing world aspects.]

Chapter 52

Strongyloidiasis

Strongyloides stercoralis is a highly advanced nematode worm that inhabits the small bowel of human hosts. It occurs in widespread areas of the tropics and subtropics and has also been reported in more temperate climates (e.g. southern parts of North America, southern Europe and even the United Kingdom).

Most infections cause minor symptoms or none at all. However, because of its 'autoinfective' life cycle, strongyloidiasis can become permanently established in human hosts without the need for reinfection. In this situation, a more chronic clinical syndrome may occur. Of particular importance in such cases is the potential for fatal 'hyperinfection' if host immunity is reduced. Strongyloidiasis has been recorded in patients with HIV infection, but the association appears weak or absent, and the condition is not generally regarded as a classical HIV-associated infection. There is, however, a well-established association with HTLV-1 infection.

A related worm *S. fülleborni* has been reported to infect children, and to be associated with a condition known as 'swollen belly syndrome' in young children in Papua New Guinea.

Usual life cycle

Adults live in the small intestine of humans only. The females, 2 mm long and very slender, live in the mucosa. They lay eggs that soon release microscopic larvae which usually escape at the non-infective (rhabditiform) stage in the faeces. Adult male worms are rapidly expelled and reproduction is probably usually parthenogenetic.

In the hospitable environment of warm moist soil, the larvae develop into free-living male and female worms within a week. The free-living females produce another generation of rhabditiform larvae, which develop into infective filariform larvae under certain environmental conditions. Humans are infected by penetration of the intact skin. Larvae may persist in the soil for many weeks, and the free-living cycle may be repeated many times. *Stercoralis stercoralis* is the only common soil-transmitted helminth infecting humans in which the worms can multiply in the free-living stage. After penetrating the skin, the larvae are carried to the lungs, migrate through the alveoli to reach the bronchial tree and are swallowed to reach their normal habitat. Probably, it takes less than 4 weeks from initial infection to maturity.

Autoinfection cycle

The rhabditiform larvae, after their release into the bowel lumen, sometimes change into

Lecture Notes: Tropical Medicine, 6th edition.
By G.V. Gill and N.J. Beeching. Published 2009 by
Blackwell Publishing, ISBN: 978-1-4051-8048-1.

the infective filariform stage. They may then reinfect the same host by either penetrating the perianal skin or the bowel wall. They then migrate through the tissues and the lungs and re-establish themselves in the intestine as new adult worms. This is how infection can persist for more than 40 years, even in the absence of external reinfection, such as in about one in five of ex-prisoners of war of the Japanese who worked on the infamous Thai–Burma railway during World War II.

Clinical features

Many infections are asymptomatic. However, both acute and chronic stages of infection can have symptoms that are quite distinct from each other. Untreated acute infections may resolve spontaneously, or become chronic because of the autoinfective cycle. Immunologically, acute strongyloidiasis is characterized by a marked IgE and blood eosinophil response, but these are less constant in the chronic form of the disease, presumably because of the host becoming immunologically tolerant.

Acute infection

1 An itchy eruption at the site of larval penetration (patients seldom recollect this).
2 Cough and wheeze because of larvae in the lungs (also uncommon).
3 Abdominal pain and diarrhoea. Pain is usually vague and ill defined; diarrhoea can be marked. Occasionally, steatorrhoea and even bloody diarrhoea occurs.
4 Weight loss (usually associated with diarrhoea).

Chronic strongyloidiasis

1 *Larva currens* ('creeping eruption')—This is a characteristic, virtually pathognomonic skin eruption (Figure 52.1). It is caused by the migration of larvae through the skin during autoinfection. The eruption is typically:
- a serpiginous wheal (a raised line) surrounded by a flare
- evanescent (comes and goes in a few hours)

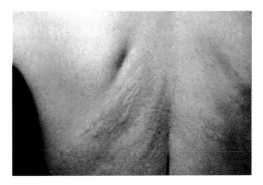

Figure 52.1 The 'larva currens' rash of strongyloidiasis in a former prisoner of World War II of the Japanese. The serpiginous wheals come and go in a few hours and travel rapidly over the central body areas. The rash is due to tissue larval migration of *Strongyloides stercoralis*.

- very itchy
- confined to the trunk between the neck and the knees
- tends to appear in crops at irregular and unpredictable intervals.

2 *Intestinal symptoms*—These are usually vague, taking the form of irregular bouts of looseness of the stools. Diarrhoea is not constant, and the patient may only recognize that his or her bowels were abnormal in retrospect, when the infection has been eliminated. Bloody diarrhoea is not a feature of uncomplicated chronic strongyloidiasis. Very occasionally, a 'sprue-like' syndrome of diarrhoea and weight loss occur.

Hyperinfection syndrome

Hyperinfection syndrome is a rare complication of *Strongyloides stercoralis* infection—usually the chronic form of disease. It occurs when host immunity is significantly and usually abruptly reduced, allowing rapid and disseminated migration of filariform larvae into tissues not involved in the normal human life cycle. Conditions reported to be associated with hyperinfection include the following:
- systemic steroid treatment
- other immunosuppressives treatment
- leukaemia and lymphoma
- postirradiation treatment

- severe malnutrition
- diabetic ketoacidosis
- lepromatous leprosy.

Of all the causes, corticosteroid treatment is the most common. A well-reported scenario for hyperinfection is post-renal transplant (resulting from steroid and other immunosuppressant therapy).

Features of the hyperinfection syndrome are as follows:

1 Severe and often bloody diarrhoea
2 Bowel inflammation with multiple microperforations
3 Bacterial peritonitis and paralytic ileus
4 Gram-negative septicaemia
5 Pulmonary exudates, haemoptysis, pleural effusions and hypoxia
6 Encephalitis and bacterial meningitis.

The diagnosis of hyperinfection is essentially clinical and a high index of suspicion is needed. Eosinophilia is usually absent, but larvae are generally easy to find in stool and other body fluids (e.g. peritoneal and/or pleural exudates, bronchoalveolar lavage samples). Treatment is with standard antihelmintic drugs (see later) as well as full supportive therapy (e.g. fluids, antibiotics); however, the outcome is poor. For patients in endemic areas who are likely to need steroid treatment (e.g. severe asthmatics), there is a case for regular diagnostic screening for strongyloidiasis, with appropriate eradication if the disease is found.

Diagnosis

Diagnosis of strongyloidiasis is notoriously difficult. The following strategies may be useful:

- direct stool microscopy
- stool microscopy after concentration
- stool culture
- microscopy of duodenal juice
- duodenal biopsy
- serological tests (e.g. ELISA)
- clinical suspicion
- therapeutic trials.

Except in hyperinfection, larvae in the stool are frequently scant and appear intermittently. This is especially true with chronic *Strongyloides* infections. Even with concentration techniques, there are well-documented cases of patients with up to 12 consecutive negative stool samples although subsequently shown to have strongyloidiasis. Stool culture with charcoal may be helpful, but duodenal aspirates can be especially helpful, although difficult to obtain. Flexible gastroduodenoscopy is an option (as well as an aspirate for microscopy, a duodenal biopsy for histological examination should be taken). However, such techniques are not frequently available in tropical countries, although an option is the Enterotest capsule (sometimes known as the 'hairy string' test). This is a small, weighted capsule containing a hairy nylon thread, the end of which is taped to the cheek while the capsule is swallowed. The capsule dissolves in the stomach, releasing the thread, which is carried through to the duodenum, usually in 2–3 h. The string is withdrawn and the part which has entered the duodenum is stained yellow with bile. The duodenal juices are squeezed into a Petri dish between the thumb and forefinger of a gloved hand, and the fluid is then examined microscopically. Finally, a variety of serological tests have been developed, the best of which is probably the ELISA method which is highly sensitive and specific.

Despite all these techniques, diagnosis may remain in doubt and clinical features should remain part of the diagnostic process. High eosinophilia, unexplained diarrhoea and a typical larva currens rash are all highly suggestive evidence of *Strongyloides* infection in at-risk subjects. In such cases, and even in the absence of supportive parasitology, a therapeutic trial may be worthwhile and is often rewarding.

Treatment

There are three possible therapeutic agents. If available, ivermectin is now generally regarded as the most effective therapy.

1 *Ivermectin*—The dose is 200 μg/kg/day for 3 days, although single doses of 6 mg (again, daily for 3 days) have been effective. A single 1-day dose may be as effective. A veterinary parenteral preparation of ivermectin is available, and a case

of *Strongyloides* hyperinfection syndrome has been reported to have been successfully treated with 12 mg of subcutaneous ivermectin given as a single dose.

2 *Albendazole*—The usual dose is 400 mg/day for 3 days, but there is evidence that 400 mg twice daily is more effective. A 7-day course should be given in chronic cases.

3 *Tiabendazole*—This is a more traditional treatment, but it is less effective than albendazole or ivermectin and prone to side effects (nausea, vomiting, dizziness and occasional neuropsychiatric problems). However, it may be the only drug available in many developing countries. The dose is 25 mg/kg twice daily for 3 days (usually 1.5 g twice daily). It should be given as syrup, or tablets that are chewed before swallowing.

Epidemiology and control

The occurrence of strongyloidiasis in the tropics is variable—with intense infection in some parts and apparent absence in others. The variability is partly climatic—prevalence is increased in wetter and humid areas. The free-living cycle of *Strongyloides* does better in such conditions than, for example, hookworm. Diagnostic problems may account for the apparent absence or rarity in some areas.

Because infection enters the human host by larval soil transmission through intact skin, encouragement to wear footwear is the mainstay of control strategies. The only case of strongyloidiasis recorded in Britain was in a young woman who was in the habit of walking barefoot in the local park.

The major control method for prevention of the hyperinfection syndrome is to screen people who need, or are likely to need, steroid or immunosuppressive therapy. Asthmatics are the most common group, but others include those with ulcerative colitis, collagen vascular disease, leukaemias, lymphomas, other malignancies and those on transplant waiting lists. Amoebiasis and tuberculosis should also be screened for in such individuals. Like strongyloidiasis, these conditions may also be seriously exacerbated by immunosuppressive therapy.

Further reading

Chiodini PL, Reid AJ, Wiselka MJ, Firmin R, Foweraker J. Parenteral ivermectin in *Strongyloides* hyperinfection. *Lancet* 2000; 335: 43–44. [An important report on the successful treatment of a case of hyperinfection with subcutaneous ivermectin.]

Concha R, Harrington W, Rogers AI. Intestinal strongyloidiasis – recognition, management and determinants of outcome. *J Clin Gastroenterol* 2005; 39: 203–211. [Useful general up to date review.]

Lewthwaite P, Gill GV, Hart CA, Beeching NJ. Gastrointestinal parasites in the immunocompromised. *Curr Opin Infect Dis* 2006; 18: 427–435. [Good review of immunosuppression and gastrointestinal parasite infection in general, including strongyloidiasis and its relationship with steroid treatment, HIV and HTLV-l infection.]

Suputtamongkol Y, Kungpanichkul N, Silpasakorn S, Beeching NJ. Efficacy and safety of a single-dose veterinary preparation of ivermectin versus 7-day high-dose albendazole for chronic strongyloidiasis. *Int J Antimicrob Agents* 2008; 1: 46–49. [Recent clinical trial of single dose ivermectin versus prolonged albendazole, showing superiority of ivermectin with an approximate 90% cure rate.]

Chapter 53

Guinea worm infection (dracunculiasis)

Guinea worm infection, a subcutaneous parasitic disease caused by *Dracunculus medinensis*, was a major cause of disability in Asia and Africa but is now confined to a few African countries and is expected to become the second disease after smallpox to be eradicated by public health efforts (Figure 53.1).

Life cycle

Larvae of guinea worm are drunk in water containing their intermediate host, the freshwater copepod (water flea) *Cyclops*. The larvae then penetrate the gut wall and develop within subcutaneous tissue into adults over about 3 months. Adult female worms grow to about 50–100 cm long and, as they become distended with millions of larvae, they migrate to dependent parts of the body after about 1 year. Here they secrete enzymes that allow them to emerge through the skin and discharge huge numbers of larvae once the skin is immersed in water. The active larvae that emerge swim for 2–3 days and must be ingested by a suitable *Cyclops*, within which they develop for a further 2 weeks before they become infective to humans.

Lecture Notes: Tropical Medicine, 6th edition.
By G.V. Gill and N.J. Beeching. Published 2009 by
Blackwell Publishing, ISBN: 978-1-4051-8048-1.

Clinical features

Patent human infections are usually highly seasonal and are often most frequent in the height of the dry season when water is scarce. Developing worms do not usually cause symptoms, but as guinea worms emerge, they cause burning pain that motivates patients to immerse the limb in water, thus encouraging transmission. Sometimes, emerging worms provoke allergic responses including urticaria or even asthma. A blister forms at the point of emergence; this is usually on the foot or lower leg but sometimes the arm, scrotum or indeed any part of the body. After discharging larvae, the worm dies and may gradually extrude or become absorbed. However, the process often takes many weeks and local ulceration with spreading secondary bacterial infection can cause disability for months, especially if there are multiple worms. Abscess formation is common. Worms migrating near a joint sometimes cause arthritis with effusion and, rarely, aberrant migration of a worm to the spinal cord causes paraplegia. The prolonged disability caused by guinea worm disrupts children's schooling and agricultural work.

Diagnosis

This is clinical. The white cloud of larvae extruded from a female worm immersed in water is characteristic. Dead calcified worms are sometimes seen on X-rays.

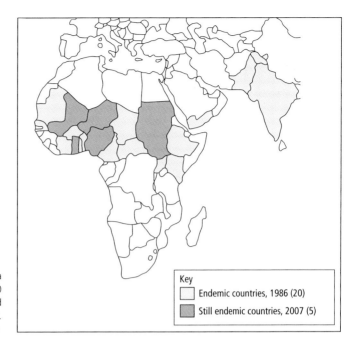

Figure 53.1 Distribution of guinea worm infection—endemic in 20 countries in 1986 (light colour) and only 5 countries (dark colour) in 2007. (From Carter Center, with permission.)

Key

☐ Endemic countries, 1986 (20)

▨ Still endemic countries, 2007 (5)

Treatment

There is no specific drug treatment. Courses of albendazole or metronidazole have been recommended as a means of reducing the inflammatory response, but they are of marginal benefit. If the uterus has emerged, discharge the larvae by immersion in water and take care to dispose of the water hygienically. The traditional method is to tie the end of the emerging worm to a small stick and wind the worm out slowly over many days, taking care not to rupture the worm as this can cause severe allergic responses. Ulceration requires antiseptic dressings. Tetanus immunization should be checked and updated if necessary. Surgical removal of the worm before it emerges, by extraction through small transverse incisions, reduces the risk of infection and disability. However, surgical facilities are usually lacking in the poor villages where the disease occurs.

Control

Provision of a safe drinking water supply is the key to control. Wells must be protected to prevent

contamination by people bathing infected limbs. Even straining water through cloth or unglazed pottery will filter out *Cyclops* and prevent infection. Filters made of monofilament nylon cloth for individuals, or within oil drums for a community, have proved useful in eradication projects. Efforts at prevention have been highly successful; from a peak of perhaps 50 million infections annually in the 1950s, there were about 10 000 infections in 2007 and the disease has been eradicated from Asia. Transmission is now concentrated in parts of West Africa, and in the south of the Sudan. The WHO is hoping for global disease eradication in the near future.

Further reading

Barry M. The tail end of guinea worm—global eradication without a drug or vaccine. *N Engl J Med* 2007; 356: 2561–2564. [Nice illustrated editorial with key references; free.]

Website of the Carter Center www.cartercenter. org/health/guinea_worm/index.html. [Useful resource from this centre which has taken the lead in final eradication efforts.]

Chapter 54

Histoplasmosis

There are two main types of histoplasmosis. 'Classical' histoplasmosis is caused by the dimorphic fungus *Histoplasma capsulatum* var *capsulatum*, and occurs in many parts of the world outside Europe. Central and South America are areas of particularly high occurrence, although it also occurs in the United States, the Asian subcontinent and the Far East. Cases imported to temperate countries have been recorded. African histoplasmosis is caused by *H. capsulatum* var *duboisii* and is confined to Africa—usually Central and West Africa.

Classical histoplasmosis

Clinical features

The fungus is present in bat and bird excreta and is a particular hazard for cave explorers in endemic areas. Infection is by inhalation, following which a number of clinical syndromes can result.

- *Asymptomatic*—Many infected individuals develop no illness but may have serological evidence of past exposure.
- *Acute pulmonary histoplasmosis*—This is a febrile bronchitic illness occurring 10–14 days after exposure. There is usually systemic malaise and

myalgia, and the chest X-ray shows generalized diffuse pulmonary shadows and sometimes hilar lymphadenopathy. The illness may resolve spontaneously with no treatment.

- *Chronic pulmonary histoplasmosis*—Sometimes the disease can cause asymptomatic single or multiple pulmonary nodules, often found on routine chest radiography. More importantly, and usually in patients with underlying chronic lung damage, focal consolidation and cavitation can occur, often in the lung apices, and this can mimic pulmonary tuberculosis (cough and haemoptysis may occur).
- *Acute disseminated histoplasmosis*—In this form of the disease liver, spleen, bone marrow and lymph glands are infected. Patients are usually ill and febrile with weight loss, lymphadenopathy and/or hepatosplenomegaly. This form of the disease is often associated with AIDS.
- *Chronic disseminated histoplasmosis*—Sometimes, years after exposure, various organ-specific syndromes resulting from histoplasmosis can present. These include oral ulceration, hypoadrenalism, meningitis and endocarditis.
- *Atypical presentations*—These include polyarthritis or polyarthralgia, erythema multiforme, erythema nodosum and hypoadrenalism.

Diagnosis

Lecture Notes: Tropical Medicine, 6th edition.
By G.V. Gill and N.J. Beeching. Published 2009 by
Blackwell Publishing, ISBN: 978-1-4051-8048-1.

This is ideally made by finding the fungus in body secretions or tissues (e.g. sputum, buffy coat layer, lymph node aspirates, bone marrow samples and biopsies of liver or pulmonary nodules). If culture facilities are available, the yeast can be grown from sputum or blood. There are a variety of serological tests available, as well as an intradermal histoplasmin skin test.

Treatment

Treatment should be reserved for severe cases or immunocompromised patients. Ideally, 200–400 mg/day itraconazole should be given. Fluconazole is probably also effective, but there is less experience. Amphotericin B is more difficult and toxic to use, but it is widely available. The dosage is 0.6–1.0 mg/kg/day by slow intravenous infusion. In AIDS patients, relapses are inevitable and, if possible, patients should receive long-term itraconazole or fluconazole as secondary prophylaxis.

African histoplasmosis

The portal of entry and source of the fungus is poorly understood. The most common presentation is with skin nodules or ulcers, enlarged lymph nodes or lytic lesions in bones. Disseminated disease can occur with lung and gastrointestinal involvement. Diagnosis is usually made histologically from biopsy specimens, and treatment is as for classical histoplasmosis. Although African histoplasmosis has been recorded with HIV infection, the association is much less certain than with acute disseminated histoplasmosis caused by *H. capsulatum* var *capsulatum*.

Further reading

Alonso D, Munoz J, Letang E *et al*. Imported acute histoplasmosis with rheumatologic manifestations in Spanish travelers. *J Travel Med* 2007; 14: 338–342. [Report of both imported cases to temperate climates and also atypical clinical presentations.]

Wheat J, Sarosi G, McKinsey D *et al*. Practical guidelines for the management of patients with histoplasmosis. Infectious Diseases Society of America. *Clin Infect Dis* 2000; 30: 688–695. [Useful summary of treatment options.]

Chapter 55

Other fungal infections

Mycetoma (Madura foot)

Mycetoma is defined as chronic swelling, induration and sinus formation with the discharge of fungal grains, involving the skin, subcutaneous tissue and bone, usually of the foot. The clinical syndrome is caused by a variety of different fungi (Eumycetes) and also by aerobic actinomycete bacteria. Differentiation is important because of the differing response to treatment. *Actinomycetes* are Gram-positive organisms with branching filaments whose width is generally less than 1 mm. Fungal hyphae stain with special fungal stains (periodic acid–Schiff [PAS] or methenamine silver) and are usually more than 2 mm in diameter; chlamydospores may also be seen.

Epidemiology

These are saprophytic organisms introduced through the skin by a thorn prick. They are not contagious but can also occur in animals. The diseases are widely distributed in tropical areas from 18°N to18°S, commonly among barefoot farmers. Some areas, particularly in the Sudan and India, have a high incidence. The chief agents of mycetoma differ in different areas (e.g. Mexico 80%

Nocardia brasiliensis; India chiefly *Madurella mycetomatis* and *Streptomyces somaliensis*).

Clinical features

Mycetoma presents with painless (80%) swelling usually involving the foot, less commonly the hands, back or head. After several years, nodules form in the skin and break down to form discharging sinuses from which pus and coloured fungal grains emerge. There are no systemic effects unless secondary infection occurs. The condition progresses slowly and relentlessly but lymphatic spread is late and is more likely in actinomycotic infection. Eumycetomas are better circumscribed with a palpable edge, while actinomyectomas are more diffuse.

Diagnosis

The colour, size and consistency of grains obtained from deep within a sinus together with microscopy after they are crushed in 10% sodium hydroxide gives a provisional diagnosis. Cultures are necessary and are best obtained by deep biopsy, and the material is sent for histology. Antibiotic sensitivities should be obtained for actinomycotic infections. Use of serological techniques has generally been disappointing but may occasionally be used to follow the effects of treatment in actinomycetoma. Radiological examination may show large

Lecture Notes: Tropical Medicine, 6th edition.
By G.V. Gill and N.J. Beeching. Published 2009 by
Blackwell Publishing, ISBN: 978-1-4051-8048-1.

erosions of bone, especially in eumycotic infections, while many small cavities and extensive bone sclerosis are more likely to be caused by actinomycotic disease.

Treatment

Drug treatment has generally been disappointing in true fungal infections despite organisms that are sensitive to antifungal drugs *in vitro*. However, successful treatment of *M. mycetomatis* infections with prolonged use of itraconazole or ketoconazole have been recorded, particularly if disease is limited. Many actinomycotic infections respond to treatment with antibiotics. Co-trimoxazole (trimethoprim/sulfamethoxazole) alone or in combination with an aminoglycoside (amikacin or streptomycin) is most commonly used. Amoxycillin–clavulanate may also be effective. Treatment may need to be continued for many months until clinical improvement occurs and repeat biopsies are culture negative.

Surgery may be useful, particularly in eumycetoma. Ideally, the affected area should be completely excised, with care taken not to rupture the 'capsule' that often surrounds the infection. Small nodules are often successfully treated in this way. Below-knee amputation may be needed, but sometimes the heel can be conserved. In poor farmers, amputation is often best left until the limb has become useless. Recurrences are quite common after surgery and so surgery should be both preceded and followed by chemotherapy.

Chromoblastomycosis

These are warty violaceous, often ulcerated, chronic skin lesions usually involving the leg and causing itching. Further spread is by scratching or via lymphatics. The condition is usually found in Latin America or Africa. Several different fungi are responsible (e.g. *Fonsecaea pedrosoi*). They are saprophytes of wood and transmitted by skin trauma.

Diagnosis

Diagnosis is by finding the chestnut brown thick-walled fungal cells often in a wall-like pattern, or branching hyphae in skin smears or histological sections.

Treatment

Treatment is unsatisfactory. Itraconazole and terbinafine in combination may be effective: 5-flucytosine may also be used. Surgical treatment tends to spread infection but cryosurgery is useful for small lesions, and long-term use of local heat packs has been successful.

Sporotrichosis

This infection is caused by *Sporothrix schenckii*, a worldwide saprophyte of decaying vegetation, sphagnum moss and soil. It typically affects farmers and florists. Cats and other animals can inoculate the organism by scratching. An epidemic in South African Witwatersrand miners was caused by infected wooden pit props.

Clinical features

Infection manifests as a pustule or nodule typically on a finger or hand, often followed by spread along lymphatics causing nodular ulcerating lesions. Osteoarticular, disseminated and pulmonary forms are uncommon except in the immunosuppressed.

Diagnosis

Diagnosis is by microscopy and culture of material from pus, crusts or biopsies. Yeast forms, hyphae or asteroid bodies (from antigen–antibody complexes on the fungal surface) can be demonstrated often with a background of polymorph leucocytes. The differential diagnosis of the 'sporotrichoid' lesions along lymphatics includes cutaneous leishmaniasis, nocardiosis, tuberculosis and atypical mycobacterial infection, especially *Mycobacterium marinum* (fish tank granuloma).

Treatment

Itraconazole (100–200 mg daily) is the treatment of choice. Saturated potassium iodide orally is also effective, starting with 1 mL three times daily and rising to 15 mL/day as tolerated. Treatment should be continued for at least 3 months.

Further reading

Hay RJ, ed. Tropical fungal infections. In: *Ballière's Clinical Tropical Medicine and Communicable Diseases*. London: Baillière Tindall, 1989. [An older but still useful review that includes the fungal infections mentioned above.]

Kauffman CA, Hajjeh R, Chapman SW. Practice guidelines for the management of patients with sporotrichosis. For the Mycoses Study Group, Infectious Diseases Society of America. *Clin Infect Dis* 2000; 30: 684–687.

Welsh O, Vera-Cabrera L, Salinas MC. Mycetoma. *Clin Dermatol* 2007; 25: 47–71. [Review of the disease and current treatment.]

Chapter 56

Haemoglobinopathies and red cell enzymopathies

Defects in the haemoglobin or enzymes within red cells interfere with their normal function and cause a range of clinical features depending on the type and degree of abnormality.

Haemoglobinopathies

Sickle cell anaemia

Sickle cell anaemia was the first condition for which a molecular basis was identified, and is the result of a β-globin chain mutation that alters the structure and function of haemoglobin. When the circulating red cells containing sickle haemoglobin (HbS) encounter conditions of low oxygen tension, the haemoglobin polymerizes and deforms the cells, which eventually take up a sickle shape (Figure 56.1). Polymerization, and therefore the clinical features of sickle cell anaemia, can be affected by many factors including temperature and hydrodynamics. Although normal red cells have a diameter of 7 μm, they are very flexible and able to squeeze through small capillaries such as those in the spleen, which are only 3 μm wide. Sickled red cells stick in these small vessels, and in combination with

the platelet and coagulation activation associated with sickle cell anaemia, cause microthrombi and ischaemia of the tissues. These pathological events precipitate the anaemia, chronic organ damage and pain crises and consequent organ failure, and chronic bony deformities which are so characteristic of sickle cell anaemia. In an individual with sickle cell anaemia, 80–95% of the haemoglobin will be HbS with the remainder being made up of HbF. In carriers of the sickle cell gene (sickle cell trait; HbAS), only about 30% of haemoglobin is HbS, the rest comprising predominantly HbA.

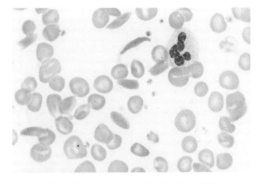

Figure 56.1 Sickle cells. (From Bain B. *Blood Cells: A Practical Guide*, 3rd edn. Oxford: Blackwell Publishing, 2002.)

Lecture Notes: Tropical Medicine, 6th edition.
By G.V. Gill and N.J. Beeching. Published 2009 by Blackwell Publishing, ISBN: 978-1-4051-8048-1.

Epidemiology and protection against malaria

The distribution of sickle cell disease follows that of malaria transmission. Carriers of the sickle cell gene have up to 10 times better protection against malaria than those with normal haemoglobin (see p. 62). This protection is in part due to accelerated acquisition of malaria immunity. The highest frequencies of the carrier state are generally found in Africa (e.g. up to 30% of all births are HbAS in parts of Nigeria, Ghana and central Africa), but frequencies are also high in parts of eastern Saudi Arabia and east central India.

Clinical features

At all ages, chronic haemolysis of abnormal red cells means that sickle cell anaemia is associated with steady state haemoglobin levels of 6–8 g/dL. The response to this anaemia is pronounced bone marrow expansion visible as bossing of the frontal bones in the skull (Figure 56.2) and overgrowth of the maxillae. In young children, clinical features include stunting, bony deformities, pain and swelling of the small bones in the hands and feet (dactylitis), acute sequestration of red cells in the spleen, aplastic crises and strokes. Before the introduction of early detection and systematic care for young children with sickle cell anaemia, the mortality in under-fives exceeded 95%. Much of this mortality can be prevented by neonatal screening programmes, which provide close monitoring of infants and young children during the critical first few years of life. The lives of older children and adults are punctuated by acute severe episodes of pain in the bones of the trunk and limbs, as well as organ-related complications such as sickle chest syndrome. Splenic atrophy due to microthrombi results in increased risk of infection particularly by encapsulated organisms. The chronic and unpredictable nature of sickle cell anaemia makes it difficult for patients to achieve adequate schooling and commit to regular employment. The carrier state, HbAS, is not normally associated with any clinical problems. Conditions that are clinically similar to sickle cell anaemia can result from a combination of HbS with other haemoglobin variants (e.g. HbSC, HbS thalassaemia and HbSD).

Diagnosis

Often the family history and clinical findings clearly point towards a diagnosis of sickle cell disease, and during an acute crisis, abundant sickled red cells can be seen on a blood film. The presence of sickle haemoglobin (e.g. HbAS, HbSS and HbSC) can be confirmed by a simple sickle slide or solubility test. Haemoglobin electrophoresis will distinguish between HbAS and HbSS. High-performance liquid chromatography and isoelectric focusing may be available in specialist centres.

Management

Individuals with sickle cell anaemia are best managed by a multidisciplinary team as they may require various specialist inputs including haematology, ophthalmology, nephrology, obstetrics, orthopaedics and physiotherapy. In steady state, it is usual practice to give sickle cell patients folate supplements (5 mg/day), because their high rates of haemopoiesis put them at risk of deficiency. They should also receive prophylactic oral penicillin (250 mg twice a day) and be monitored closely for signs of infection. Severe pain crises are generally managed in hospital with intravenous fluids and adequate, often opiate, analgesia. If the crisis was precipitated by an infection, this

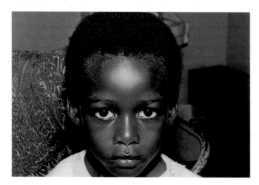

Figure 56.2 Frontal bossing in a child with sickle cell anaemia.

should also be treated. Because of the increased risk of thrombosis in sickle cell disease, blood transfusions should be given only for emergencies such as sequestration or aplastic crises and should not aim to increase the haemoglobin above steady state levels. The manual or automated replacement of the patient's blood with normal blood from donors to reduce the level of HbS to 30% (exchange transfusion) is beneficial only for specific clinical indications such as respiratory distress syndrome or incipient stroke.

β Thalassaemia

β Thalassaemia is a genetic defect that results in insufficient production of the β-globin chains needed to form HbA ($\alpha\alpha\beta\beta$) which makes up 97% of normal adult haemoglobin. The amount of β chain produced can vary from none (β0) to almost normal levels (β+), and the degree of anaemia and compensatory bone marrow overactivity determines the clinical severity.

Epidemiology

β Thalassaemia is present in all ethnic groups but has the highest incidence in the Mediterranean basin (15–20%) and South East Asia and Africa (5–10%).

Clinical features

Classification of β thalassaemias is based on clinical criteria.
- β Thalassaemia trait—clinically well with normal haemoglobin in steady state.
- β Thalassaemia intermedia—symptoms of anaemia (Hb ~7–8 g/dL) but not completely transfusion dependent.
- β Thalassaemia major—dysmorphic and transfusion dependent (Hb ~2–3 g/dL).

Diagnosis

Clinical features and family history should indicate the diagnosis, but definitive investigations require measurement of HbA_2 levels, which are usually increased, or molecular studies. The blood film shows hypochromic microcytic red cells with more target cells than are seen in iron deficiency. If there is severe anaemia, then marked bone marrow overactivity may be evident by the presence of many polychromatic red cells (seen as reticulocytes if a special staining technique is used) or even nucleated red cells.

Management

Management varies with the severity of the anaemia. To prevent death in β thalassaemia major in the first few years of life, regular transfusions must be given. This will soon lead to iron overload and death in the second decade if these are not accompanied by an iron chelation programme which involves overnight subcutaneous infusions of desferrioxamine. This is an expensive treatment and may not be affordable for poorer patients. Deferiprone is an oral iron chelator which can be used when desferrioxamine is contraindicated or inadequate.

Enzymopathies

G6PD deficiency

Epidemiology

The enzyme glucose-6-phosphate dehydrogenase (G6PD) is present in red cells and protects them from oxidant damage (e.g. infection, drugs and fava beans). G6PD deficiency is common and associated with over 160 different X-linked genetic defects (therefore occurs predominantly in males) which alter enzyme stability. Early red cells have higher levels of enzyme than older cells. The degree of haemolysis, and hence clinical severity, is dependent on the quantity and half-life of the abnormal enzyme. Like HbS, G6PD deficiency has a protective effect against malaria and has its highest prevalence in the Mediterranean basin (35–40%) and Africa (25%).

Clinical features

G6PD deficiency can cause neonatal anaemia and jaundice with a risk of kernicterus. In older children and adults, oxidant stress caused by drugs (e.g. primaquine, sulphonamides and nitrofuran), infections or fava beans (Mediterranean variety) causes sudden haemolysis. The severity is dependent on the levels of G6PD, which are genetically determined. The African type (G6PD A–) tends to be mild and self-limiting, whereas the Mediterranean variety can cause life-threatening haemolysis.

Diagnosis

During an acute haemolytic episode caused by G6PD deficiency, the blood film appearances are very characteristic. The haemoglobin in the red cells appears to be pushed into the middle or to one side of the cell ('bite' and 'helmet' cells; Figure 56.3). Screening tests such as the methaemoglobin reduction test can detect an 80% reduction in G6PD levels and can be performed by district hospitals in resource-poor countries where G6PD is common. Enzyme assays and genetic analyses are the definitive investigations, but need a specialist laboratory. Enzyme assays for G6PD deficiency should be carried out in the steady state 6–8 weeks after an acute attack. During the haemolytic episode, the cells that are deficient in G6PD are destroyed leaving only cells with normal levels of enzyme, so an enzyme assay carried out during acute haemolysis will, therefore, not detect a deficiency.

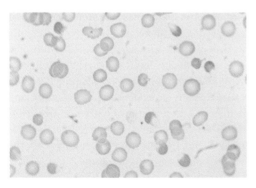

Figure 56.3 Red cell appearances during acute haemolytic crisis caused by G6PD deficiency. (From Bain B. *Blood Cells: A Practical Guide*, 3rd edn. Oxford: Blackwell Publishing, 2002.)

Table 56.1 Common drugs that can cause haemolysis in G6PD-deficient individuals

Analgesics—acetylsalicylic acid
Antimalarials—primaquine, dapsone
Antimicrobials—sulphonamides, nitrofurantoin
Others—vitamin K analogues, probenecid, PAS

Abbreviation: PAS, periodic acid–Schiff.

Management

As many episodes of G6PD haemolysis are self-limiting, particularly in Africa, transfusions are rarely required. In very severe cases, such as those associated with fava bean ingestion, acute renal failure necessitating dialysis may supervene. Once a patient has been identified as G6PD deficient, he or she should be advised to avoid drugs that may precipitate a haemolytic episode (Table 56.1).

Further reading

Bain B. *Haemoglobinopathy Diagnosis* (2e), Oxford: Blackwell Publishing Ltd, 2006. Print ISBN: 9781405135160. Online ISBN: 9780470988787. [Details and rationale of standard methods for laboratory diagnosis of haemoglobinopathies, covering a range of tests; includes a self-assessment exercise.]

Davies SC, Cronin E, Gill M et al. Screening for sickle cell disease and thalassaemia: a systematic review with supplementary research. *Health Technol Assess* 2000; 4: iii–v, 1–99. [A detailed overview of the methods and rationale for establishing newborn screening programmes for haemoglobinopathies and of the evidence for its efficacy.]

Kwiatkowski DP. How malaria has affected the human genome and what human genetics can teach us about malaria. *Am J Hum Genet* 2005; 77: 171–192. [More than 200 references relating to malaria and red cell abnormalities.]

Mason PJ, Bautista JM, Gilsanz F. G6PD deficiency: the genotype–phenotype association. *Blood Rev* 2007; 21: 267–283, 2007. [Good overview of complex relationship between genetic mutations and resultant clinical picture.]

Roberts DJ, Brunskill SJ, Doree C, Williams S, Howard J, Hyde CJ. Oral deferiprone for iron chelation in people with thalassaemia. Cochrane Database Syst Rev. (3):CD004839, 2007. DOI: 10.1002/14651858.CD004839.pub2 [Systematic review of use of oral chelator.]

Serjeant GR. The emerging understanding of sickle cell disease. *Br J Haematol* 2001; 112: 3–18. [Comprehensive review of all aspects of sickle cell disease with extensive list of references for specific topics.]

Weatherall DJ. Provan AB. Red cells I: inherited anaemias. *Lancet* 2000; 355: 1169–1175. [General, easily readable review of haemoglobinopathies and enzymopathies with useful list of references.]

Chapter 57

Haematinic deficiencies

Iron deficiency

Iron deficiency is the most common cause of anaemia and affects 20–50% of the world's population. In developing countries, about half of all cases of anaemia in women and children are the result of iron deficiency. It is usually caused by excessive loss of red cell iron from the body but may also be caused by insufficient intake. Combinations of excessive loss and reduced intake are also common. Iron deficiency is a particular problem in childhood and pregnancy when physiological requirements are high. The body has very little capacity to regulate either iron absorption or iron loss. The maximum absorptive capacity of the gut for iron is about 3.5 mg/day, and iron requirements in pregnancy are approximately 2.0 mg/day. Other factors that commonly coexist with iron deficiency and can contribute to anaemia include hookworm infestation, HIV infection, folate deficiency, infections and anaemia of chronic disease. Anaemia is one of the later manifestations of iron deficiency, and tissue function can be impaired even before there is a detectable reduction in haemoglobin level. This can lead to subtle changes in behaviour, cognition and, in children, psychomotor development.

Lecture Notes: Tropical Medicine, 6th edition.
By G.V. Gill and N.J. Beeching. Published 2009 by Blackwell Publishing, ISBN: 978-1-4051-8048-1.

Clinical features

If iron deficiency develops slowly, as in chronic hookworm infestation, physiological compensation mechanisms ensure that symptoms do not become significant until the haemoglobin has reached very low levels. Physical signs specifically associated with iron-deficiency anaemia include spoon-shaped nails (koilonychia) and angular stomatitis. Clinical examination is not a reliable method for diagnosing anaemia but is helpful to indicate some of the causes of iron deficiency. Common causes of excessive iron loss include menorrhagia, haemorrhoids, hookworm, bowel carcinoma, hiatus hernia and treatment with aspirin or non-steroidal anti-inflammatory drugs. The best dietary source of iron is red meat, so reduced iron intake is commonly associated with a vegetarian diet and can be exacerbated by phytates and tannates in cereals and tea, which inhibit iron absorption.

Investigations

In rural health facilities where specific tests to measure iron status may not be available, a reasonably firm diagnosis can be made from a well-prepared blood film. In iron deficiency, the red cells appear hypochromic (over half of the diameter of the cell is pale rather than only one-third as in normal cells) and microcytic (significantly

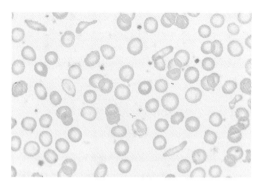

Figure 57.1 Iron-deficient red cells. The cells are paler and more irregular in shape than normal red cells. From Bain B. *Blood Cells: A Practical Guide*, 3rd edn. Oxford: Blackwell Science, 2002.

smaller than a small lymphocyte) (Figure 57.1). The red cells may also appear flattened ('pencil cells'). If an automated blood count is available, the MCV, mean corpuscular haemoglobin concentration (MCHC) and mean corpuscular haemoglobin (MCH) will all be reduced. Iron deficiency is often associated with a mildly raised platelet count which resolves as the anaemia improves.

If iron studies are available, they will demonstrate low serum iron with raised total iron-binding capacity and a low ferritin. In regions where infections and inflammatory conditions are prevalent, ferritin levels are difficult to interpret because ferritin is an acute-phase protein and can be normal or raised even in the presence of iron deficiency. In pregnancy, the haemoglobin is affected by the physiological changes in plasma volume and red cell mass, and the use of a low MCV may be misleading because of the higher proportion of larger younger red cells. The 'gold standard' investigation for iron deficiency is demonstration of a lack of iron stores in aspirated bone marrow. Tests to determine the cause of the iron deficiency should be performed and may include stool examination for hookworm ova or blood, and endoscopy or radiography of the gastrointestinal tract.

Management

Treatment of the iron deficiency itself comprises iron sulphate 200 mg three times a day; absorption can be enhanced by ascorbic acid. In true iron deficiency, early red cells should appear in the peripheral blood within 4–5 days of starting iron therapy. Early red cells are slightly larger and bluer (polychromatic) than normal red cells and can be visualized using a specific reticulocyte stain. Iron supplementation should be continued for at least 3 months after a normal haemoglobin is achieved to replenish body stores. The cause of the iron deficiency should also be rectified to prevent recurrence of the anaemia. This may involve encouraging inclusion of locally available iron-rich foods in the diet, or explaining the need for farmers to wear shoes when working in their fields to prevent hookworm infestations. Iron supplementation can reverse some developmental delays in anaemic children, even in the absence of an overall increase in haemoglobin.

Folate deficiency

Folate deficiency is usually caused by insufficient intake and less often by malabsorption. It can be exacerbated or precipitated by the excessive physiological demands for folate that occur in pregnancy and childhood, and in chronic haemolytic states. Folate is widely available in liver, yeast, spinach, green leafy vegetables and nuts, but it is easily destroyed by boiling. Bone marrow stores only last a few months. Mixed iron and folate deficiencies are not uncommon and are usually caused by poor diet. The clinical and laboratory features that result from combined deficiency are a mixture of those occurring in isolated iron and folate deficiencies.

Clinical features

In addition to general symptoms of anaemia, folate deficiency can cause anorexia, change in bowel habit, glossitis and a mild haemolytic anaemia.

Investigations

Folate deficiency results in enlarged, slightly oval red cells and hypersegmented neutrophils (six or more nuclear lobes) on the peripheral blood film

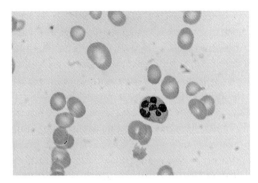

Figure 57.2 Oval macrocytes and hypersegmented neutrophils in folate deficiency. From Bain B. *Blood Cells: A Practical Guide*, 3rd edn. Oxford: Blackwell Science, 2002.

(Figure 57.2). This combination strongly suggests either folate or vitamin B_{12} deficiency, and a bone marrow examination will show typical changes of megaloblastic anaemia. On automated blood counts, an MCV over 100 fL indicates macrocytosis. Serum and red cell folate assays can provide a definitive diagnosis but are not always available in rural laboratories in poorer countries. As folate is required for DNA synthesis, severe chronic deficiency can eventually cause a reduction in white cells and platelets as well as red cells (pancytopenia).

Management

Treatment comprises folic acid 5 mg/day but, as with all anaemias, the underlying cause should be corrected. Appropriate advice should be given to maximize dietary folate intake.

Cobalamin (vitamin B_{12}) deficiency

Deficiency of cobalamin is much less common than folate deficiency, as replete body stores can last for about 2 years and absorption mechanisms are efficient. Deficiency is usually the result of impaired absorption secondary to gastrointestinal disorders, especially those that affect the small bowel and ileum (e.g. Crohn's disease, tuberculosis and tropical sprue). Cobalamin deficiency can occasionally be caused by lack of dietary B_{12}. This is particularly common in vegans and strict vegetarians.

Pernicious anaemia is a specific failure of B_{12} absorption because of a lack of intrinsic factor production by gastric parietal cells. It can be associated with antibodies to gastric parietal cells or intrinsic factor. Pernicious anaemia occurs in all races, and up to 30% of patients have relatives with the same disorder.

Clinical features

The typical neurological symptoms of cobalamin deficiency—posterolateral column degeneration, peripheral neuropathy and optic atrophy—can occur in the absence of anaemia. In severe cases, profound life-threatening anaemia may develop. As with folate deficiency, a reduction in platelets and white cells can occur. These abnormalities are generally mild, so severe infections or bleeding episodes are unusual. Features that may indicate an underlying cause of small bowel dysfunction, such as diarrhoea or abdominal pain, should be sought. Pernicious anaemia may be associated with thyroid disease, vitiligo, Addison's disease and other autoimmune disorders, and clinical evidence of these may be apparent.

Investigations

The peripheral blood film is indistinguishable from that seen in folate deficiency. Assays of vitamin B_{12} levels may be available at central laboratories and provide a definitive diagnosis. It is important to carry out investigations to determine any underlying cause.

Management

Treatment is with hydroxycobalamin injections 1 mg every 3 months after an initial loading dose (e.g. 1 mg/day for 6 days). Any underlying condition should be treated appropriately. Unless the cause of the deficiency can be eliminated, treatment will be needed for life.

Further reading

Bain B. *Blood cells: A Practical Guide*, 3rd edn. Oxford: Blackwell Science, 2002. [Atlas of haematological morphology with clear illustrations and accompanying text. Good guide to the use of the diagnostic laboratory.]

Calis JC, Phiri KS, Faragher EB *et al*. Severe anaemia in Malawian children. *New Engl J Med* 2008; 358: 888–99. [Detailed case-controlled study of the causes of severe anaemia in children under 5 years; included bone marrow studies.]

Gjorup T, Bugge PM, Hendriksen C, Jensen AM. A critical evaluation of the clinical diagnosis of anemia. *Am J Epidemiol* 1986; 124: 657–665.

Hall A. Micronutrient supplements for children after deworming. *Lancet Infect Dis* 2007; 7: 297–302. [Review of complexities surrounding haematinic supplementation and deworming programmes.]

Lewis DK, Whitty CJ, Epino H, Letsky EA, Mukiibi JM, van den Broek NR. Interpreting tests for iron deficiency among adults in a high HIV prevalence African setting: routine tests may lead to misdiagnosis. *Trans R Soc Trop Med Hyg* 2007; 101: 613–617. [Highlights difficulties of diagnosing iron deficiency in tropical setting with high HIV prevalence.]

Sazawal S, Black RE, Ramsan N *et al*. Effects of routine prophylactic supplementation with iron and folic acid on admission to hospital and mortality in preschool children in a high malaria transmission setting: community-based, randomised, placebo-controlled trial. *Lancet* 2006; 367: 133–43 and 302. [Outlines potential complications of iron therapy in malarious areas. Should be read in conjunction with related articles, as findings have been debated.]

Chapter 58

Bites and stings

Snakebite

Clinical features

There are a large number of species of venomous snakes throughout the world. These can be divided into three main categories: vipers, elapids and sea snakes. The pattern of envenoming depends upon the biting species. Only 50–70% of patients bitten by venomous snakes develop signs of envenoming.

The major clinical effects following snakebite can be divided into

1 *Local effects*—Pain, swelling or blistering of the bitten limb. Necrosis at the site of the wound can sometimes develop.

2 *Systemic effects*

- Non-specific symptoms: vomiting, headache and collapse
- Painful regional lymph node enlargement indicating absorption of venom
- Specific signs
  (a) non-clotting blood
  (b) bleeding from gums, old wounds and sores
  (c) neurotoxicity: ptosis, bulbar palsy and respiratory paralysis
  (d) rhabdomyolysis and muscle pains and black urine

(e) shock; hypotension, usually resulting from hypovolaemia.

Vipers most commonly cause local swelling, shock, bleeding and non-clotting blood. Elapids cause neurotoxicity and usually minimal signs at the bite site (with the exception of some cobras which also cause necrosis). Sea snakes cause myotoxicity and subsequent paresis. There are exceptions to this general rule; some vipers cause neurotoxicity and Australian elapids also cause non-clotting blood and haemorrhage.

First aid for snakebites

1 Reassure the patient. Many symptoms following snakebite are caused by anxiety.

2 Immobilize the limb. Moving the limb may increase systemic absorption of venom. Splinting is especially helpful in children.

3 Avoid harmful manoeuvres such as cutting, suction or tourniquets.

4 Consider a pressure bandage in regions where snakebite does not cause tissue necrosis, particularly if rapid transport to hospital is not possible. This is especially important for snakes that cause neurotoxicity. A firm crêpe bandage should be applied over the bite site and wound up the limb.

5 Transport the patient to hospital as soon as possible.

6 If the snake has been killed, take it to hospital with the patient.

Lecture Notes: Tropical Medicine, 6th edition.
By G.V. Gill and N.J. Beeching. Published 2009 by
Blackwell Publishing, ISBN: 978-1-4051-8048-1.

Diagnosis and initial assessment

Think of envenoming in unusual cases.

1 Carefully examine bitten limb for local signs.

2 Measure the pulse, respiration rate, blood pressure and urine output. The blood pressure must be watched if patients are unwell, bleeding or have significant swelling; shock is common in viper bites.

3 Look for non-clotting blood. This may be the only sign of envenoming in some viper bites. The 20-min whole blood clotting test (WBCT20; Box 58.1) is an extremely easy and useful test. This should be performed on admission and repeated 6h later.

4 Look carefully for signs of bleeding, which may be subtle (gums/old wounds/sores). Bleeding internally (most often intracranial) may cause clinical signs.

5 Look for early signs of neurotoxicity; ptosis (this may be interpreted as feeling sleepy), limb weakness, or difficulties in talking, swallowing or breathing.

6 Check for muscle tenderness and myoglobinuria in sea-snake bites.

7 Take blood for
• haemoglobin, white cell count and platelet count
• prothrombin time, activated partial thromboplastin time and fibrinogen levels if available;
• serum urea and creatinine
• creatine phosphokinase, reflecting skeletal muscle damage.

8 Take ECG if available.

Box 58.1 The 20-min whole blood clotting test.

• Place a few millilitres of freshly sampled blood in a new, clean, dry glass tube or bottle.
• Leave undisturbed for 20min at ambient temperature.
• Tip the vessel once.
• If the blood is still liquid (unclotted) and runs out, the patient has hypofibrinogenaemia (incoagulable blood) as a result of venom-induced consumption coagulopathy.

Management

General management

All patients should be observed in hospital for 12–24h, even if there are no signs of envenoming initially. They should be regularly reviewed; envenoming can develop quite rapidly. Nurse patients on their side with a slight head down tilt to prevent aspiration of blood or secretions. Avoid intramuscular injections and invasive procedures in patients with incoagulable blood. Tetanus prophylaxis should be given, but routine antibiotic prophylaxis is not required unless necrosis is present.

Antivenom

Antivenom is indicated for signs of systemic envenoming. Evidence for its efficacy in severe local envenoming is poor, but it is usually indicated if swelling extends over more than half the bitten limb. Monospecific (monovalent) antivenom can be used for a single species of snake; polyspecific (polyvalent) for a number of different species. The choice and dose of antivenom depends upon manufacturers' recommendations and local experience (see Theakston and Warrell [1991] for a list of available antivenoms; reference details in Further reading). Children require exactly the same dose as adults, as the dose is dependent upon amount of venom injected and not body weight.

• Antivenom should be diluted in 2–3 volumes of dextrose/saline and infused over an hour or so. The infusion rate should be slow initially and gradually increased.

• Adrenaline (epinephrine) should be drawn up in a syringe ready for use. Routine prophylaxis against antivenom reactions is currently unproven and should not generally be used.

• Patients should be observed closely during antivenom administration. Common early signs of an antivenom reaction are urticaria and itching, restlessness, fever, cough or feeling of constriction in the throat.

• Patients with these signs should be treated with adrenaline (0.01mg/kg) intramuscularly. An

antihistamine, for example chlorphenamine (0.2 mg/kg i.m. or i.v.), should also be given.
• Unless life-threatening anaphylaxis has occurred, antivenom can cautiously be restarted after this treatment.

The response to antivenom should be monitored. In the presence of a coagulopathy, restoration of clotting depends upon hepatic resynthesis of clotting factors. The WBCT20 should be repeated 6 h after antivenom; if blood is still non-clotting, further antivenom is indicated. After restoration of coagulation, measurement of the WBCT20 should be repeated every 6 h as a coagulopathy may recur because of late absorption of venom from the bite site.

The response of neurotoxicity to antivenom is less predictable. In species with predominantly postsynaptically acting toxins, antivenom may reverse neurotoxicity; failure to do so is an indication for further doses. However, response to antivenom is poor in species with presynaptically acting toxins.

Other therapy

• Sloughs from necrotic wounds should be excised. Skin grafting may be necessary. Severe swelling may lead to a suspicion of compartment syndromes. Fasciotomy should not be performed unless there is definite evidence of raised intra-compartmental pressure (>45 mmHg) and any coagulopathy has been corrected.
• Blood products are not necessary to treat a coagulopathy if adequate antivenom has been given.
• Endotracheal intubation should be performed to prevent aspiration if bulbar palsy develops, often obvious when difficulty in swallowing leads to pooling of secretions.
• Paralysis of intercostal muscles and diaphragm requires artificial ventilation. This can be performed by manual bagging and may need to be maintained for days, using relays of relatives if necessary.
• Anticholinesterases may reverse neurotoxicity following envenoming by some species with postsynaptic toxins.
• Careful fluid balance should be maintained to treat shock and prevent renal failure.

• Some cobras spit venom into the eyes of their victims. Rapid irrigation with water will prevent severe inflammation. 0.5% adrenaline drops may help to reduce pain and inflammation.

Epidemiology and prevention

Snakebite is mainly a rural and occupational hazard: farmers, plantation workers, herdsmen and hunter-gatherers are at greatest risk. Children also are frequently bitten as a result of their inquisitive nature. Most bites occur in the daytime and involve the foot, toe or lower leg as a result of accidentally disturbing a snake. However, some species of snake (e.g. kraits) may bite sleeping victims at night. In some areas of the world, snakebite is one of the most common causes of death, and severe morbidity can result from snakebite. Sensible footwear, discouraging handling of potentially venomous animals and keeping the grass short around dwellings can all reduce the chance of snakebite.

Scorpion stings

In some areas of the world, scorpion stings are more common than snakebites and cause significant mortality. The stinging scorpion is often not seen. A number of different species have broadly similar clinical effects. The major feature of envenoming is severe pain around the bite site, which may last for many hours or even days. Systemic envenoming is more common in children and may occur within minutes of a bite. Major clinical features are caused by activation of the autonomic nervous system (Table 58.1). Severe hypertension, myocardial failure and pulmonary oedema are particularly prominent in severe envenoming.

Table 58.1 Clinical features of scorpion stings

Tachypnoea	Muscle twitches and spasms
Excessive salivation	Hypertension
Nausea and vomiting	Pulmonary oedema
Lachrymation	Cardiac arrhythmias
Sweating	Hypotension
Abdominal pain	Respiratory failure

Management

Patients should be taken to hospital immediately; delay is a frequent cause of death. Control pain with infiltration of lidocaine around the wound or systemic opiates (with care). Scorpion antivenom is available for some species. It should be given intravenously in systemic envenoming, but intramuscular injection has been used with good effect. Prazosin is particularly effective for treating hypertension and cardiac failure. Severe pulmonary oedema requires aggressive treatment with diuretics and vasodilators.

Spider bites

Many species of spiders cause significant envenoming in the tropics. Fatal envenoming is rare.

Widow spiders

Widow spiders (*Latrodectus* spp.) are found throughout the world. Severe pain at the bite site is common. Rare cases develop systemic envenoming with abdominal and generalized pain and other features resulting from transmitter release from autonomic nerves. Hypertension is characteristic of severe envenoming. Antivenom is available in some regions and is effective for relief of pain and systemic symptoms. Opiates and diazepam are also useful for treatment of pain.

Recluse spiders

Recluse spiders (*Loxosceles* sp.) have a wide distribution and cause bites in which pain develops over a number of hours. A white ischaemic area gradually breaks down to form a black eschar over 7 days or so. Healing can be prolonged and occasionally causes severe scarring. The efficacy of antivenom and other advocated treatment (dapsone, steroids and hyperbaric oxygen) remains uncertain.

Banana (Brazilian wandering) spiders

Phoneutria spp. occur only in South America. They usually cause severe burning pain at the site of the bite, but in severe cases can cause systemic envenoming with tachycardia, hypertension, sweating and priapism. A polyspecific antivenom is available in some regions.

Funnel-web spider

Bites by funnel-web spiders in Australia may cause systemic envenoming with autonomic effects on the cardiovascular system and neurological symptoms. Antivenom is available and has helped to reduce fatalities.

Marine envenoming

Venomous fish

Many different venomous fish, for example stonefish, can sting people if they are stood on or touched. Systemic envenoming is rare. Excruciating pain at the site of the sting is the major effect. Regional nerve blocks and local infiltration of lidocaine may be effective, but most marine venoms are heat labile. Immersing the stung part into hot water is extremely effective in relieving pain. Care should be taken to avoid scalding; the envenomed limb may have abnormal sensation. Clinicians should check the water temperature with their own hand. Asking the patient to also immerse the non-bitten limb may help to avoid scalding.

Jellyfish

Venomous jellyfish have a large number of stinging capsules (nematocysts) on their tentacles that inject venom when tentacles contact skin. Pain and wheals are the usual effects but, rarely, systemic envenoming can be life-threatening. Many of the nematocysts remain undischarged on tentacles that adhere to the victim and rubbing the area of the sting causes further discharge and worsens envenoming. In box jellyfish stings, pouring vinegar over the sting prevents the discharge of nematocysts. For most other jellyfish, seawater should be poured over the stings and adherent tentacles gently removed. Ice may be useful for pain relief and hot water is effective in reducing pain for some species. Box jellyfish stings can occasionally be rapidly life-threatening. Antivenom is available and can be administered intramuscularly. The Irukandji syndrome may occur in Indo-Pacific regions when patients develop systemic envenoming shortly after a minor or sometimes unnoticed sting in deep waters. Muscle pains, spasms and hypertension with cardiac failure may occur. Treatment is supportive; intravenous magnesium has been used to reduce pain and hypertension.

Further reading

Isbister GK, Gray MR. A prospective study of 750 definite spider bites, with expert spider identification. *Q J M* 2002; 95: 723–731. [An up-to-date and extensive review of venomous spider bites from Australia.]

Meier J, White J. *Handbook of Clinical Toxicology of Animal Venoms and Poisons*. Florida: CRC Press, 1995. [A comprehensive summary of venomous animals and the effects of their bites.]

Theakston RDG, Lalloo DG. Venomous bites and stings. In: Zuckerman J, ed. *Principles and Practice of Travel Medicine*. Chichester: John Wiley and Sons, 2001: 321–341. [A practical approach to venomous bites and stings.]

Theakston RDG, Warrell DA. Antivenoms: a list of hyperimmune sera currently available for the treatment of envenoming by bites and stings. *Toxicon* 1991; 29: 1419–1470.

Warrell DA. Injuries, envenoming, poisoning and allergic reactions caused by animals. In: Warrell DA, Cox TM, Firth JD, Benz EJ, eds. *Oxford Textbook of Medicine*, 4th edn, Section 8.2. Oxford: Oxford University Press, 2003: 923–946.

Chapter 59

Non-communicable diseases

Introduction

Disease spectrum

Non-communicable diseases (NCDs) are of increasing importance all over the world, but particularly in developing countries. NCDs include all chronic disease processes, which may be treatable but are frequently not curable. By definition, they are not caused by infectious agents. Common NCDs are as f ollows:

- hypertension
- cardiovascular disease
- diabetes
- asthma
- epilepsy
- psychiatric disease
- stroke
- trauma
- cancer
- arthritis.

The pattern of NCDs encountered in tropical countries is often different from that seen in the western world. Thus, coronary artery disease is the most important form of cardiac disease in developed countries, but in many areas of the tropics the most important is rheumatic heart disease. Cardiomyopathy and hypertensive heart disease are also frequent. Similarly, although COPD is seen in the tropics, asthma is usually the most common respiratory problem encountered. Road traffic accidents (RTAs) are a particularly problematic form of trauma in developing countries, as well as the effects of war and civil unrest. Malignancy patterns vary: hepatoma, Burkitt's lymphoma, Kaposi's sarcoma, nasopharyngeal carcinoma and bladder cancer are particular tropical problems.

Mortality patterns

These are often difficult to determine in tropical countries because of diagnostic difficulties, problems of enumerating deaths outside hospital, and variable and mobile populations. In general, NCDs are globally the major cause of death, although in tropical countries infectious disease remains the major killer, as shown in Table 59.1. However, there is good evidence that the proportion of deaths caused by NCDs in developing countries is steadily increasing. Thus, in the Gambia, NCDs made up about 32% of total deaths in the 1970s but in the 1990s the proportion had risen to 49%. General projections are that, despite the HIV/AIDS epidemic, proportionate NCD mortality will overtake that caused by communicable diseases in most developing countries in the next 10–20 years.

Lecture Notes: Tropical Medicine, 6th edition.
By G.V. Gill and N.J. Beeching. Published 2009 by Blackwell Publishing, ISBN: 978-1-4051-8048-1.

Table 59.1 World patterns of proportionate mortality (communicable and non-communicable disease)

Population	Communicable disease (%)	Non-communicable disease (%)
Total world	35	65
Poorest countries	60	40
Richest countries	10	90

Box 59.1 Features of epidemiological or demographic transition.

- Urban–rural migration
- Adoption of 'western' lifestyles
- Increased food intake
- Reduced dietary quality
- Reduced exercise
- Increased alcohol intake
- Smoking
- Higher salt intake
- Pollution
- Family and social breakdown

Epidemiological transition

The reasons for the rising mortality from NCDs in tropical countries are various. Overall, mortality caused by infectious disease is falling; and even in poor countries life expectancy is slowly increasing. As many NCDs increase in prevalence with rising age (e.g. diabetes and hypertension), extended life expectancy necessarily increases the rates of such diseases. Increased vehicle use and social unrest are also leading to more traumatic deaths. A further problem is that of 'epidemiological transition'. This term refers broadly to sociocultural population changes that can have profound effects on disease patterns. Population transition is a complex process, but approximately equates to what is often referred to as 'westernization' or sometimes, more light-heartedly, as 'coca-colonization' (Box 59.1).

These processes are best seen at work in the effect on tropical populations migrating to urban environments from the country. Many studies have shown that dramatic increases in NCD prevalence occur following rural–urban migration, as shown by the figures from East Africa in Table 59.2. Obesity is a major effect of rural–urban migration, and is a major risk factor for several important NCDs (in particular, accidents, hypertension and diabetes). In Africa obesity is an especial problem in women, and in some areas up to 40% of adult urban women are significantly obese, compared with less than 5% in rural environments.

Table 59.2 Non-communicable diseases and rural–urban migration in East Africa

	Rural (%)	Urban (%)
Hypertension	13	23
Diabetes	1	6
Childhood asthma	11	26

Diabetes mellitus

Epidemiology

Diabetes is an especially important NCD in the tropics as it is common, rapidly increasing, is difficult to manage adequately, and is associated with morbidity and mortality from specific, acute and chronic complications. The latter two factors in particular make it different from and more problematic than other NCDs. Not surprisingly, its mortality is high: 20 years ago a study from Zimbabwe showed that 6 years after diagnosis, nearly 50% of diabetic patients had died—predominantly from metabolic problems (hypoglycaemia, ketoacidosis and non-ketotic hyperosmolar coma) or infections. There have been relatively few studies since, but what information there is suggests that there have been only slight improvements. However, in some communities renal failure (as a result of diabetic nephropathy) and cardiovascular disease are emerging causes of mortality. Diabetes outcome

> **Box 59.2 WHO criteria for diagnosis of diabetes.**
>
> - Fasting plasma glucose >7.0 mmol/L
> - Random plasma glucose >11.1 mmol/L
> - If no symptoms present, then abnormal tests are needed on two separate occasions

everywhere is highly dependent on local medical services, patient education and the availability of insulin and other appropriate medication.

Diagnosis

All type 1 diabetes, and much type 2 diabetes, present no diagnostic challenges, as patients present with classical symptoms (thirst, polyuria, weight loss, etc.) and obviously raised blood glucose levels. Some type 2 diabetic patients, however, have borderline values (particularly those who may be found accidentally). The WHO has recently reviewed its diagnostic criteria, as shown in Box 59.2.

A glucose tolerance test (GTT) should rarely be needed, but if so a 75 g glucose load should be used, and tests performed at 0 and 2 h only. The basal and 2 h cut-off levels are the same as for the fasting and random levels earlier. It should be remembered that although most European and North American laboratories have standardized to *plasma* glucose levels, many tropical laboratories still measure *blood* glucose. The values are not the same: a plasma glucose of 7.0 is equivalent to a blood glucose of 6.1 mmol/L; and a plasma glucose of 11.1 mmol/L is equivalent to a blood glucose of 10.0 mmol/L.

Prevalence

Fifty years ago, diabetes was thought to be rare or even non-existent in tropical countries. It was probably genuinely less common than in western countries, but high mortality prior to presentation at hospital may well have accounted for much of this 'rarity' (this remains a problem). In the last decade, type 2 diabetes in particular has

reached epidemic rates all over the world, and the rate of expansion appears to be faster in developing as compared to developed countries. The total number of people in the world with diabetes will double in the next 10–15 years, and by 2020 diabetes will (in terms of mortality) almost certainly be the most important NCD. Actual prevalence rates of type 2 diabetes vary enormously. Global prevalence was estimated as 6% in 2007, but some areas of the Caribbean have rates of 10–15%, and of the Middle East over 20%. Particularly high rates are seen in the elderly, and also in Asian migrants. In the tropics, urbanization and westernization are particular risk factors. These lead to increased body weight and reduced exercise, both of which are potent causes of insulin resistance, which is the hallmark of type 2 diabetes.

Type 1 diabetes appears to be less common in the tropics than in western countries, and contributes usually less than 10% of the total diabetic population. The incidence in Africa is about 3–5 per 100 000 per year (compared to about 15 per 100 000 per year in Europe). Enumeration difficulties, as referred to previously, may partly account for this difference. Type 1 diabetes in sub-Saharan Africa also appears to have a later age of onset than in western countries (early twenties, rather than early teens).

Causes

The causes of diabetes in tropical countries are essentially similar to elsewhere. Type 2 diabetes can be seen as a 'lifestyle' disease, rapidly increasing as a result of excessive eating and a sedentary lifestyle. The tropical townships in particular are highly 'diabetogenic'. One popular explanation for this is the 'thrifty genotype' theory. This theory suggests that genetically predisposed individuals may have reduced insulin secretory capacity or insulin resistance, which can be beneficial in a 'subsistence' or 'hunter-gatherer' situation, as ingested carbohydrate tends to be stored as fuel rather than rapidly burnt off. This 'thrifty' genotype loses its advantage when food supplies increase and exercise reduces (the urbanization situation). Here the reduced insulin reserves are overwhelmed and type 2 diabetes results. Although still theoretical, possible examples of the 'thrifty genotype' in action can be seen. Thus, in the late 1980s, a group of Africans from a famine area in northern Ethiopia were moved to Israel and within 4 years type 2 diabetes prevalence had risen from 0.1% to 8.9%.

A particular debate over the past 20 years has concerned the possible existence of a separate type of diabetes in tropical countries, distinct from type 1 and type 2 disease. This is closely associated with malnutrition—hence its usual name of malnutrition-related diabetes mellitus (MRDM). The features include the following:

- restricted to the tropics
- variable geographical occurrence
- young age
- male excess
- past or present malnutrition
- low body weight
- resistance to ketosis
- sometimes, steatorrhoea
- sometimes, pancreatic fibrosis/calcification.

There are two possible types: one in which there is definite evidence of generalized pancreatic damage (fibrocalculous pancreatic diabetes [FCPD]); and one without such features but with marked evidence of malnutrition (malnutrition-modulated diabetes mellitus [MMDM]). The exact cause of these syndromes is unknown, and even their definite status as truly separate types of diabetes is controversial.

Complications

Acute complications

These are hypoglycaemia, ketoacidosis (DKA) and hyperosmolar non-ketotic coma (HNK). They are seen more frequently in the tropics and carry a higher mortality. DKA mortality is now below 5% in Europe, but ranges from 10% to 30% or more in developing countries. Hypoglycaemia is not infrequently caused by sulphonylurea drugs; the commonly used chlorpropamide is particularly long-acting and may cause severe and prolonged hypoglycaemia.

Chronic complications

These include the classic specific complications of retinopathy, neuropathy and nephropathy, as well as the non-specific large vessel complications caused by atherosclerosis of the lower limb, coronary and cerebral arteries. Other complications include cataracts and erectile dysfunction. Diabetic complications—in particular those caused by small vessel disease—are strongly related to the degree of glycaemic control and the duration of disease. In some poorly resourced areas, the occurrence of diabetic complications may appear low; however, this may be because of inadequate surveillance or patients simply dying prematurely before complications have time to appear.

Infection

Infections are more common and more severe in diabetic patients, particularly those with poor control. Infective complications can be dramatic in the tropics—caused both by high blood glucose levels and delayed presentation. In addition to standard infections involving, for example the chest, urinary tract and foot, some particularly dramatic and specific diabetic infections can be seen in the tropics. These include severe deep sepsis of the hand and orofacial mucormycosis.

Management

Diet

Diet and exercise are the prime treatments for type 2 diabetes, particularly when associated with obesity. Unfortunately, even with good provision of expert dietetic and patient educational support, lifestyle change rarely controls diabetes adequately. Nevertheless, even in resource-poor situations, simple but firm advice should be offered.

Oral agents

Metformin should be used for obese and overweight patients inadequately controlled on diet alone, and sulphonylureas for the non-obese with similarly inadequate control. A body mass index (BMI) of 27.0 can be used for the obese/non-obese cut-off. This standard practice may be giving way to a 'metformin-for-all' policy in the future, with sulphonylureas as 'add-on' treatment.

All sulphonylurea drugs can cause hypoglycaemia, but glibenclamide and chlorpropamide are the most problematic. Oral hypoglycaemic agents should be started in low doses, and then increased as necessary. Combination treatment (metformin and sulphonylureas) can be used if control is poor on maximal doses of one drug, but beyond this insulin may be needed.

Insulin

All type 1 diabetic patients obviously require insulin for survival, but many type 2 patients ideally require insulin for control. If insulin is in short supply, it may need to be reserved for type 1 patients only. The potential benefits of insulin in type 2 diabetes also need to be weighed against potential hypoglycaemic risks (especially if patient's self blood glucose monitoring is not available). When insulin is given, as simple and safe a system as possible should be used. A twice-daily intermediate-acting insulin system (e.g. lente or isophane) may be successful. A common misconception is that patients need a refrigerator to store their insulin. Insulin is relatively stable in all but the hottest conditions, and storage in a cool and shady area of the home is sufficient.

Ketoacidosis treatment

Successful and standard protocols are widely available for the management of DKA with intravenous insulin and fluids. However, such systems often require equipment not available in developing countries. A simple system requiring no special technology is shown in Box 59.3, which assumes that only bedside reagent-strip monitoring is available. In all cases of DKA, it is also important to consider an infective precipitant such as pneumonia, urinary infection, skin sepsis (e.g. foot or hand) or malaria.

Organization of care

Although the skilled use of individual drugs and insulin is important, the real challenge of diabetes management in the tropics is of delivery of care in difficult circumstances. Particular problems are as follows:
- late presentation
- low and irregular food supply
- lack of insulin and oral agents
- absence of dietitians and podiatrists
- lack of monitoring equipment
- poor laboratory support.

Insulin shortage is a particular problem. It is an expensive drug in developing countries, and supplies are often poor and erratic. With all these problems, the aims of treatment may need to be compromised, with relief of symptoms and avoidance of hypoglycaemia the main aims. Diabetes is

---

Box 59.3 Treatment of ketoacidosis in resource-poor settings.

Fluids	Give 500 mL 0.9% saline quickly, then 500 mL hourly for 4–6 h
Potassium	Give none for the first hour, then 20 mmol KCl hourly for 3 h, then 10 mmol hourly for 2 h (diluted in the saline infusion)
Insulin	Give any soluble insulin 20 units i.m. stat, then 10 units i.m. hourly. If no soluble is available, give lente or isophane i.m. similarly
Bicarbonate	Give only if the patient is very ill and not improving. Give 50 mmol $NaHCO_3$ slowly i.v.
Monitoring	Blood glucose hourly by reagent strip
Later	When BG <15 mmol/L, convert intravenous saline to 5% dextrose. Continue i.m. insulin, and change to a subcutaneous regimen when the patient can eat

Note: BG, blood glucose.

Box 59.4 Elements of a tropical diabetes service.

- Organization and delegation
- Central hospital referral clinic
- Decentralized peripheral clinic care
- Nurse-led protocols for type 2 diabetes
- Patient and staff education system
- Medical protocols for diabetic ketoacidosis treatment
- Simple dietetic and foot care
- Sensible use of drugs and insulin
- Hypertension management
- Complication surveillance
- Gestational diabetic care

an NCD ideally suited to nurse-led and community-delivered care. The major factors in setting up a district diabetic service in a tropical country are shown in Box 59.4. Obviously, the list will need to be adapted to the geographical situation, resources available and particular clinical problems present.

Nurse-led care of type 2 diabetic patients in primary health care units is especially appropriate, and has been shown to be highly successful. Figure 59.1 shows an algorithm that has been used successfully. It assumes metformin and glibenclamide are the available drugs, but obviously must be adapted to local conditions.

Hypertension

Epidemiology

Hypertension is globally by far the most common NCD, and in the tropics it makes up approximately 40% of the total NCD burden. The major importance of hypertension is that it is a potent risk factor for stroke and, because of the frequency of raised BP, it leads to a very high population stroke risk. Effective treatment of hypertension lowers risk by at least 40%, and such treatment can involve relatively simple and inexpensive drugs. Sadly, however, much

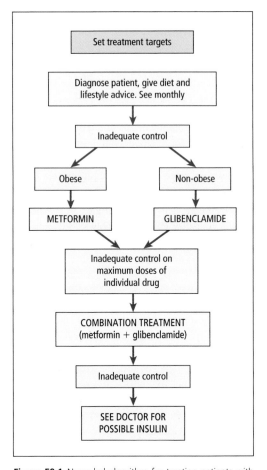

Figure 59.1 Nurse-led algorithm for treating patients with type 2 diabetes. Note: (1) The treatment target must be set locally depending on resources. Without laboratory support it should be 'absence from hyperglycaemic symptoms, and drug-induced hypoglycaemia'. Laboratory targets may be a fasting blood glucose <8.0 mmol/L, or an HbA_{1c} <8.0%. (2) Ideally, patients should see a doctor at diagnosis for complication screening. (3) Obesity can be defined as a body mass index >27.0. (4) The drugs are given in stepwise increments increasing each month as follows: metformin 500 mg/day and then 500 mg b.d., then 500 mg t.d.s., then 1 g b.d., then 1 g t.d.s. For glibenclamide, give 2.5 mg/day, then 5 mg/day, then 5 mg b.d., then t.d.s. (5) When using combination treatment, use the second drug according to the dose regimen mentioned earlier. (6) At each visit reinforce lifestyle advice, check for diabetic symptoms and possible drug side effects (hypoglycaemia with glibenclamide, and dyspepsia or diarrhoea with metformin). (7) Weigh patient and check urine at clinic visits. Always check BP and, if constantly >140/80 mmHg, treat vigorously.

hypertension remains undiagnosed, and of those cases diagnosed many are inadequately controlled.

Diagnosis

Population BP levels are continuously distributed, and there is therefore no clear dividing line between hypertensive and non-hypertensive levels. Diagnostic cut-off levels are therefore decided on the basis of risk, and these levels have been progressively decreasing. The WHO currently recommends a diagnostic cut-off of 140/90 mmHg. There is growing evidence that in certain high-risk groups (notably those with diabetes) the cut-off level should be lower—probably 130/80 mmHg.

Accurate measurement is important in diagnosing hypertension. A good quality mercury sphygmomanometer, with an adequate-sized and well-fitting cuff, remains the 'gold standard' system. However, the use of such equipment is declining, as a number of countries are restricting their use because of concerns over mercury toxicity. The alternative electronic machines are expensive and difficult to maintain. Aneroid models are a reasonable compromise, although they can read slightly lower than other systems. Overall, the major problem in accurate BP measurement is failure to use a large-sized cuff in an obese patient.

Prevalence

As may be expected, prevalence rates vary widely geographically. In some poor rural areas of the tropics, where obesity is rare, rates of well below 5% are found. Conversely, in many urban areas of sub-Saharan Africa, where obesity is very common, hypertension may be found in 40–50% of the population or more. Most tropical doctors will find themselves working in areas with hypertension prevalence rates of 10–20% at least. It should always be remembered that the prevalence of *known* hypertension (those on antihypertensive medication) always considerably underestimates the total hypertension prevalence—often by about one-half. In view of this, and the essentially asymptomatic nature of the disease,

opportunist hypertension screening should be undertaken whenever possible (e.g. at inpatient or outpatient hospital attendances, regardless of the reason for the consultation).

Causes and risk factors

About 95% of cases of hypertension is 'essential' (with no definable underlying cause). Secondary hypertension is always rare. Causes include Cushing's syndrome, Conn's syndrome, phaeochromocytoma and a variety of renal disorders. A number of aetiological factors have been suggested for essential hypertension, including genetic factors, fetal malnutrition (the 'fetal origins' hypothesis), salt retention and subtle abnormalities of the renin–aldosterone system. It is more useful to think in terms of risk factors for essential hypertension, rather than actual causes. In the tropics, the main risk factors are as follows:
- obesity (especially central)
- high salt intake
- urbanization
- excess alcohol intake
- reduced activity.

It can be seen that these make up a 'package' of adverse lifestyle factors similar to those predisposing to urban diabetes. Reduced activity and central obesity lead to insulin resistance, and this is strongly associated with hypertension, as well as diabetes. Increased salt intake is probably a major feature of tropical urbanization, and some individuals may be particularly prone to the potential hypertensive effect of increased dietary salt.

Complications

The long-term result of uncontrolled hypertension can be a variety of complications resulting from end-organ damage. These are as follows:
- stroke
- left ventricular hypertrophy
- renal failure
- coronary artery disease
- hypertensive retinopathy.

Of these, stroke is by far the most important, with hypertension leading to an excess risk of up to 10 times that in non-hypertensive subjects. Stroke in hypertensive patients can be caused by cerebral thrombosis as well as cerebral haemorrhage. Left ventricular hypertrophy is also a serious complication, which may lead to hypertensive heart failure. Hypertensive renal disease is one of the most common causes of chronic renal failure.

A rare acute complication is the 'hypertensive crisis' that occurs in severe and accelerated disease. Patients usually have a diastolic BP in excess of 140 mmHg, encephalopathy and hypertensive retinopathy (usually with papilloedema).

Management

Principles of treatment

Treatment of hypertension should follow a logical pathway, bearing in mind the following important basic principles of management below:
- *Education* is vital; patients must understand what the disease is, and how treatment will help them.
- *Non-drug treatment* includes weight reduction, reduced salt intake, reduced alcohol, avoidance of smoking and increased exercise.
- *Compliance* is a major barrier to good BP control. Try to use once daily drug systems and be sensitive to possible side effects.
- *Side effects* can be minimized by using low doses of more than one drug, rather than very high doses of a single drug.
- *Organization* of hypertension care is very important, as the number of patients involved is likely to be high.

Drug treatment

In developed countries 'cascades' of treatment, such as the 'ABCD' system are popular. The system recognizes ethnic and age-related differences in drug effectiveness. Thus angiotensin-converting enzyme (ACE) inhibitors or angiotensin receptor blockers, ARBs (A) and beta-blockers (B) work less

well in blacks and older whites, whereas calcium blockers (C) and diuretics (D) work better. Lately, beta-blockers (B) have been less favoured as antihypertensive drugs (hence the 'ACD' system), but some regard either system as too rigid, and advocate individualized treatment. Examples would be the primary use of C in those with angina and hypertension, or A in the presence of heart failure and hypertension (in both situations the antihypertensive drug is doing 'two jobs').

In developing countries, the choice will usually be dependent on cost and availability. Simple and cheap drugs such as thiazides and methyl dopa may be appropriate and effective. Side effects are rarely a problem. Thiazide doses should be low (e.g. hydrochlorothiazide 12.5 mg or bendrofluazide 2.5 mg)—at these levels adverse effects on blood glucose do not occur, and antihypertensive effect is as good as at higher doses.

Special situations

There are specific clinical situations where the standard progression of treatment (first-line, second-line, etc.) should not be followed, as specific drugs may be indicated or contraindicated. Beta-blockers should be avoided in asthma, but they are good first-line drugs in the presence of angina. Similarly, ACE inhibitors (if available) are ideally suited to patients with heart failure, or diabetes with renal complications (nephropathy or microalbuminaemia).

Hypertensive crisis

Patients should be bed-rested and observed closely, with hourly BP measurements. A simple, but often surprisingly effective treatment is simply to give methyldopa orally, 1 gm stat and then 500 mg 4-hourly. Otherwise, hydralazine 10 mg i.m. every 2–4 h is usually effective.

Organization of care

As with type 2 diabetes, routine hypertension management is ideally suited to primary health

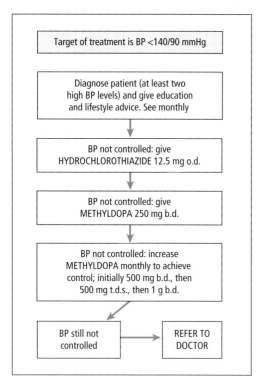

Target of treatment is BP <140/90 mmHg

Diagnose patient (at least two high BP levels) and give education and lifestyle advice. See monthly

BP not controlled: give HYDROCHLOROTHIAZIDE 12.5 mg o.d.

BP not controlled: give METHYLDOPA 250 mg b.d.

BP not controlled: increase METHYLDOPA monthly to achieve control; initially 500 mg b.d., then 500 mg t.d.s., then 1 g b.d.

BP still not controlled → REFER TO DOCTOR

Figure 59.2 Nurse-led algorithm for treating patients with hypertension. Note: (1) Any low-dose thiazide can be used. (2) Make sure BP is measured carefully and correctly. (3) At each visit, reinforce lifestyle advice and check compliance.

clinic care by suitably trained nurses. In most areas, there are large numbers of hypertensive patients, and such a system will allow medical staff to concentrate on more difficult cases. Again, as with diabetes, the protocol needs to be adapted to local needs and drug supplies. Figure 59.2 assumes that a thiazide drug and methyldopa are the main available, cheap and effective medications in use.

Initial patient education is important, and should carry two messages. First, advice should be given on non-drug aspects of treatment. Secondly, the nature and importance of hypertension should be carefully explained. In most cases hypertension is asymptomatic, and patients will not comply with long-term treatment unless they understand the benefits.

Asthma

Epidemiology

Asthma is a chronic clinical syndrome of reversible airways obstruction, characterized by wheeze and shortness of breath. Airways obstruction is caused by inflammation, resulting in bronchial oedema, mucus production and smooth muscle contraction. Asthma particularly affects younger age groups and, if poorly controlled, is likely to interfere with school or work attendance. A significant amount of asthma is undiagnosed and misdiagnosed. In the tropics, asthma is increasing and becoming a major problem in urban environments. Effective drugs are expensive and often poorly available. The death rate is unknown, but is certainly higher than in developed countries.

Diagnosis

The hallmark of asthma is reversible airways obstruction, and the key features in the history are wheeze, cough and breathlessness. Rhonchi may be present on chest auscultation, but their absence does not exclude the diagnosis, which is essentially made on the history. The wheeze is often worse at night, and may be provoked by trigger factors (e.g. allergens, cold, exercise). Sometimes, particularly in children, a dry (and often nocturnal) cough may be the only feature. In adults, breathlessness without wheeze may indicate asthma. If available, patient records of peak flow (PF) measurements are useful in making the diagnosis. PF readings will usually be variable, often low, but in particular show classical 'early morning dipping'. In doubtful cases spirometry with and without bronchodilation is useful diagnostically: classically, the forced expiratory volume in 1 second (FEV_1) is reduced (to below 80% of the predicted value), as is the FEV_1:FVC (forced vital capacity) ratio (to below 75%). Without this equipment a simple clinic PF measurement, repeated 20 min after two puffs of a salbutamol inhaler, can give similar information.

Frequently in developing countries, the diagnosis is made on history, perhaps confirmed by a trial of bronchodilator treatment. The diagnosis of asthma is summarized in Box 59.5.

Some care must be taken with the differential diagnosis. In children, simple wheezy bronchitis may be mistaken for asthma. In adults, COPD is the main alternative diagnosis. Tropical pulmonary eosinophilia should also be considered.

Prevalence

Studies of prevalence of asthma in the tropics vary widely. This is partly a result of methodological problems; for example studies of simple 'reported asthma' will clearly give lower levels than those using objective tests such as spirometry. Other factors affecting prevalence results include patient age (rates will be higher in younger age groups) and whether the environment is rural or urban. Rates are generally low in rural areas (usually below 5%), but in towns can rise to 10–15% or more. In western countries there is good evidence that asthma prevalence is increasing, and the same is probably true in the developing world.

Causes

General

There are several factors related to the causation of asthma, although the overall explanation for individual disease (and indeed increasing population trends) is often uncertain.

- *Allergens*—allergy is very important in many cases. The most important allergen is the house dust mite, but in tropical countries cockroaches and bed bugs can also be important. Other allergens include pollens and industrial fumes.

- *Genetic factors*—there is familial clustering of atopy and allergy in general, and asthma in particular.
- *'Hygiene hypothesis'*—this hypothesis is based on the observation that children who have relatively little infection or vaccination exposure early in life have a greater risk of later asthma.
- *Obesity*—the reason for this association is uncertain but asthma is certainly more common in the obese.

In addition to these, there are a number of environmental precipitants or triggers to asthma. These include some drugs (e.g. non-steroidal anti-inflammatory drugs, beta-blockers), and active or passive smoking. Nowadays atmospheric pollution in general is not thought to be a true cause of asthma. Asthma rates are steadily rising in Europe while the air gets cleaner.

Urban asthma

There are several potential causes of the marked rise in asthma prevalence seen in tropical urban, compared with rural, environments. The major reason is probably increased exposure to house dust mites, and this is supported by studies in Ethiopia. Rural dwellings tend to be spacious and well ventilated, and have rudimentary furniture. In towns, houses are smaller, and have doors and windows that reduce ventilation. There may also be curtains, carpets, easy chairs, etc. Overall, the environment is ideal for house dust mites. A further interesting factor may be the reduced childhood intestinal parasite load found in urban areas. There is evidence that increased parasite exposure in childhood reduces the risk of later asthma. Obesity increases with urbanization. Finally, the urban environment has more 'triggers' to asthma for those with a predisposition to the disease (e.g. smoking, household fires, occupational irritants).

Complications

The main complication of asthma is sudden and severe decompensation to status asthmaticus (or acute severe asthma). This is usually brought on by infection and is heralded by increasing need for reliever (bronchodilator) aerosols, reduced effect of such treatment, and severe nocturnal breathlessness. Patients at presentation usually have tachypnoea, distress and marked airways obstruction. There is often tachycardia and sometimes pulsus paradoxus. Blood gas levels are initially well preserved, but a rising pCO_2 is a dangerous sign. Cyanosis and a 'silent chest' are similarly serious signs suggesting the likely impending need for ventilatory assistance. Status asthmaticus is a serious complication of asthma with a small but significant mortality.

Management

Routine treatment

The most effective treatment is based on beta-2 agonist and steroid aerosols. Beta-2 agonists can be considered to be 'relievers'. The most commonly used is salbutamol (Ventolin) although there are several others (e.g. terbutaline). Steroid inhalers can be considered to be 'suppressors', and again there are several, although the most common is beclometasone. Reliever treatment gives rapid improvement and can be given either as needed or, if necessary, on a regular basis. Suppressor aerosols are given regularly (two puffs, twice daily), regardless of current symptoms. Asthma can be managed in a simple drug cascade system, adding in further treatment if initial management fails to control the disease or trialling reduced therapy if symptom relief is good and stable ('step up' and 'step down' treatment).

Tropical adaptations to treatment

Asthma inhalers are expensive and often difficult to obtain in developing countries. Simple identification and removal of precipitants can be very helpful. Oral bronchodilators may have to be the mainstay of treatment. These are difficult drugs to use, with a narrow therapeutic window and relatively weak bronchodilator activity. Cromoglycate (Intal) is now rarely used in modern asthma practice, but if available (and steroid inhalers are not) it is worth using as a suppressor aerosol.

Box 59.6 Treating status asthmaticus.

- High-concentration oxygen
- High-dose steroid: prednisolone 40 mg/day, *with* initially hydrocortisone 100 mg i.v. q.d.s.
- Broad-spectrum antibiotics
- Bronchodilators:
  nebulized salbutamol
  add intravenous aminophylline if necessary
- Ventilation in extreme life-threatening cases

Treatment of exacerbations

Infective exacerbations should be treated with antibiotics and a brief course of steroids (e.g. prednisone or prednisolone 40 mg/day for 5–10 days). Assuming the patient is on a beta-2 agonist inhaler (e.g. salbutamol), this should be given in a high dose (e.g. 4–8 puffs q.d.s.) via a spacer inhaler (which can, if necessary, be homemade—see later).

Status asthmaticus treatment

If asthmatic exacerbations are treated promptly and adequately, this is an avoidable complication. Nevertheless, when it does occur, it must be treated vigorously. The principles of management are shown in Box 59.6.

If nebulized salbutamol is not available, high-dose inhalers with a spacer device should be used, but intravenous aminophylline is likely to be needed. If nothing else is available, adrenaline (epinephrine) can be life-saving, used in a subcutaneous dose of 0.1 mL of 1/1000 solution per 10 kg body weight (give 0.75 mL if the patient is too ill to be weighed).

Organization of care

Patient education

Patient education is especially important if asthma treatment is to be successful, and all newly diagnosed patients should be given simple advice and training as follows:
- understanding asthma
- avoiding allergic triggers

- importance of regular treatment
- correct use of inhalers
- concept of reliever and preventer treatment
- recognizing deterioration and seeking help.

Particularly in younger asthmatic patients, attention to allergic triggers can be very successful. This includes avoiding domestic pets, good home ventilation, and regular beating and cleaning of bedclothes, mattresses and settees. Inhaler technique is vitally important—many patients find these difficult to use, and without training they will be ineffective and a waste of resources. Spacer devices are very effective, and these can be homemade. An empty plastic milk or fruit juice container is ideal—a hole is cut at or near the bottom to fit the mouthpiece of the inhaler, the required dose is delivered into the container, and then rebreathed through the top. These systems have been shown to be as effective as expensive proprietary spacers.

Doctor education

Doctor education is also important. Protocols for routine and emergency management should be widely displayed and distributed. Many patients develop acute asthma because of inadequate preceding medical treatment. In particular, steroids are widely underused—a course of prednisolone 40 mg/day for 5–7 days given on an outpatient basis frequently resolves significantly deteriorating asthma. There are few acute dangers with such short courses and, in particular, adrenal suppression does not occur. In areas where *Entamoeba histolytica* and/or *Strongyloides stercoralis* are found, asthmatic patients should be regularly screened for these infections, as steroids may cause serious deterioration of amoebic dysentery, or the hyperinfection syndrome of strongyloidiasis.

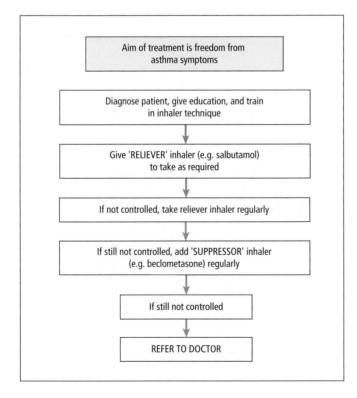

Figure 59.3 Nurse-led algorithm for treating patients with asthma. Note: (1) At each clinic visit record symptoms, measure peak flow and check inhaler technique. (2) Beyond currently taken reliever and suppressor aerosols, medical staff may have to consider oral theophylline or aminophylline preparations, or even sometimes low-dose maintenance steroids.

Nurse-led treatment protocols

As with other NCDs, basic asthma treatment is well suited to protocol-based stepwise care, delivered by nurses (Figure 59.3). Although PF measurements can be useful to detect improvement and deterioration, the basic aim of the treatment should be freedom from significant asthmatic symptoms.

Epilepsy

Epidemiology

Although epilepsy is much less common than hypertension or asthma, it is an important NCD for several reasons. Diagnosis is often difficult, and there are many with undiagnosed epilepsy. Those with known disease are frequently poorly controlled, and their continuing seizures carry a significant social stigma and life burden. The condition also carries an excess mortality of 2–5 times that of non-epileptic people. Treatment is often made difficult by a lack of modern drugs, and many doctors do not understand the basic principles of anticonvulsant therapy. There are also cultural problems affecting the person with epilepsy in the tropics. It is not always seen as a disease at all in some cultures (it may be considered a form of bewitching or possession by demons). In other societies it may be thought to be contagious.

Diagnosis

The diagnosis rests on a history of at least two typical attacks, preferably witnessed, and with the history obtained from the witness. A good description of typical grand mal (tonic–clonic) seizures should lead to a firm diagnosis, but it must be remembered that there are other less obvious types of seizure: absence attacks (or petit mal—usually in childhood); and a variety of partial seizures, with or without impairment of consciousness (e.g. focal motor epilepsy, temporal lobe epilepsy). A simple and useful modern classification of seizures is as shown in Box 59.7.

Box 59.7 Classification of epilepsy.

- Grand mal (tonic–clonic)
- Absence attacks (petit mal)
- Simple partial seizures (patient conscious), for example focal motor or temporal lobe
- Complex partial seizures (as above, but with loss of consciousness)
- Myoclonic epilepsy (rare)

Note: Partial seizures may sometimes progress to grand mal attacks.

When attacks are atypical, and especially where they are not witnessed, diagnosis may be difficult. Electroencephalography (EEG) is rarely available in tropical countries, and is anyway often unreliable. A trial of anticonvulsant therapy is sometimes a reasonable option, with the patient keeping a close record of attacks.

Prevalence

Rates of reported epilepsy in developing countries greatly underestimate the extent of the problem. Their variability also reflects diagnostic difficulties, which may alter geographically, and also local causative factors (e.g. prevalence of neurocysticercosis). Overall prevalence rates are probably around 2%. Reported studies have demonstrated prevalences of 0.5% in Ethiopia, 1.0% in Uganda, 3.0% in Tanzania and 5.0% in India.

Causes

Most epilepsy in developed countries is idiopathic, but in developing countries proportionally more cases have a definable cause. Tropical causes of epilepsy include the following:
- birth hypoxia/injury
- past head injury
- past meningitis/encephalitis (e.g. cerebral malaria, bacterial meningitis, sleeping sickness)
- HIV infection (usually caused by an associated opportunist infection or tumour such as toxoplasmosis, cryptococcosis, tuberculoma or lymphoma)
- brain tumours, cysts (e.g. hydatid)
- neurocysticercosis (*Taenia solium*)
- past stroke.

Complications

Burns and other trauma occurring during seizures are the most common complications of epilepsy. Sudden death may occur during fits. Status epilepticus is a serious complication. It normally occurs in pre-existing epilepsy and can be provoked by infection or excess alcohol. It carries significant mortality and must be treated vigorously.

Management

Drug treatment

Infections leading to epilepsy should always be treated. It has been shown that albendazole or praziquantel treatment for neurocysticercosis reduces seizure frequency, though long-term anticonvulsant treatment is generally necessary. Valproate and carbamazepine are the commonly used anticonvulsants in western countries, but these are rarely available in the tropics. Phenobarbital and phenytoin are usually available, and if used properly can be very effective. Side effects can sometimes be problematic. Phenobarbital can cause drowsiness, and sometimes behaviour change in children. Phenytoin may lead to gum hypertrophy, acne and hirsutism; as well as sedation and, in excessive doses, vertigo and incoordination. Like other anticonvulsants, phenytoin and phenobarbital are potentially difficult drugs to use as they have a narrow 'therapeutic window' of blood levels. Below this window they are ineffective, but above it they are toxic. In the absence of drug level estimations in the blood, the drugs should be started at a low dose and gradually titrated up until seizure control is obtained. Experience from India suggests that adult doses of phenobarbital should start at 30 mg/day, and be slowly titrated up to 90 mg/day (in 30 mg increments). For phenytoin the range is 100–300 mg (in 50 mg increments). Both drugs should be given once daily at night. Patients, with family members, should be seen monthly with a record of epileptic attack, and enquiries made regarding possible side effects. Effective seizure control can often be obtained using either of these drugs in this way.

Status epilepticus

If available, intravenous or rectal diazepam is ideal, but if not intravenous phenytoin can be used (this can also be given if diazepam has failed). The dose schedules are as follows:
• *Diazepam*—2 mg slow i.v. per minute (up to 20 mg).
• *Phenytoin*—18 mg/kg by slow i.v. infusion, usually 750–1500 mg over 30–60 min.

Old-fashioned paraldehyde (5 mL deep i.m. in each buttock) can still be effective (remember to use a glass syringe). In severe refractory cases, general anaesthesia with muscle relaxation and anaesthesia may be needed.

Organization of care

Education

Successful epilepsy management programmes in the tropics involve education of patients, carers and the community. As with other NCDs, patients need to understand the nature of their disease and the importance of regular treatment, particularly as most fits in established epileptic patients result from poor compliance. Other precipitants are infections, alcohol excess and some drugs which lower seizure threshold. Patients may recognize their own triggers (e.g. excessive fatigue, psychological stress and, in women, prior to menstruation). Carers should, if possible, be involved to provide support and sometimes to supervise medication. Attempts should be made at a community level to increase understanding of epilepsy, and to prevent distrust of or discrimination against the epileptic patient.

Drug treatment

Although there is less experience with nurse-led epilepsy care than with other NCDs, once the diagnosis is made and treatment initiated by medical staff, there is no reason why nursing staff cannot supervise the dose increases of phenobarbital or phenytoin mentioned earlier. Figure 59.4 illustrates a suggested protocol using phenobarbital, although an identical one could be produced with phenytoin.

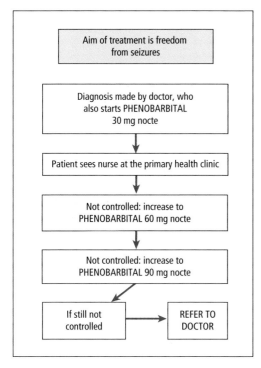

Figure 59.4 Nurse-led algorithm for treating patients with epilepsy. Note: (1) At each visit check compliance, disease understanding and any side effects of treatment. (2) Patients are asked to keep a diary of fits. PHC, primary health clinic.

Mental illness

The WHO recognizes that mental disease is an important cause of disability throughout the world but in most developing countries it has received little attention and few resources. Much mental illness presents to traditional healers, and people with serious disease such as schizophrenia may be tied up or chained for many years without effective treatment. Those with depression and anxiety are more likely to present in general medical clinics, and if the diagnosis is missed an opportunity to provide cheap and effective treatment is lost. The patient is then likely to keep on returning with his or her symptoms unresolved.

Assessment of acute mental disturbance

There are three important questions to ask when examining the acutely disturbed patient.

1 *Is this person physically ill?* Acute infections, metabolic disturbance, epilepsy or trauma may all cause confusion and sometimes frank delirium. Eliminate physical causes before assuming that the patient is mentally ill. Be careful when administering sedative drugs to patients who may be physically ill. Give only what is needed to allow safe examination and establishment of diagnosis. Benzodiazepines may be used provided the patient's conscious level is normal and there are no respiratory problems. A combination of an antipsychotic such as haloperidol with lorazepam is usually effective.

2 *Is this person under the influence of drugs or alcohol?* Use of illicit drugs and alcohol are common; ask the patient and their relative for details. Patients who appear to be simply drunk and confused may also have a head injury or metabolic disturbance: check for dehydration, hypoglycaemia and hepatic dysfunction.

3 *Is this person mentally ill?* If physical illness and drug-related problems have been eliminated, examine the patient's mental state in more detail to establish the diagnosis. Remember the patient is likely to be frightened, so needs care and kindness as well as a safe environment.

Schizophrenia

Schizophrenia is a common and serious mental disorder affecting every part of a patient's mental state. Key features are as follows:

• *Hallucinations*—the patient commonly hears people talking about him or her, often to each other and usually with an unpleasant or frightening content. There may also be disturbed perception in any other sensory modality, for example tingling or burning of limbs or body, abnormal tastes or smells.

• *Delusions*—often as a result of hallucinations, the person begins to believe things that are not true, for example that people are out to kill them or that they are being subject to mysterious forces.

- *Affective (mood) changes*—unexpected aggression, inappropriate laughter or social withdrawal may occur, again often in response to the hallucinations or delusions.
- *Disturbed behaviour*—as a result, the patient in a frightened or defensive state may hide away, run off, or express aggression to others.

Treatment

Schizophrenia in developing countries generally has a better prognosis than elsewhere. Treatment is cheap and in the setting of a primary care programme is usually very effective.

Be sure to eliminate physical causes for the psychotic symptoms (especially, illicit drugs or epilepsy). Once the diagnosis is made, the key is maintenance treatment with *antipsychotics*. If the patient has a supportive family these may be given orally, for example chlorpromazine 100 mg t.d.s. or haloperidol 5 mg t.d.s. initially. Reduce the dose once the acute phase is over, but maintain treatment to keep the patient well.

If atypical antipsychotics are available, use olanzapine for more aggressive patients. Dosage should be titrated against symptoms: check with the family as well as the patient to judge whether the psychotic symptoms are improving.

Treat side effects such as muscle stiffness and tremor with an antiparkinsonian agent, for example benzhexol 5 mg or procyclidine 5 mg two or three times a day.

If depot antipsychotics are available, these are ideal in a primary care mental health programme. Give the patient a monthly injection of fluphenazine 25 mg or flupenthixol 20–40 mg, again titrating against symptoms. Regular treatment and family and community support can transform a patient's mental health so that he can become happy and productive again.

Depression

WHO figures suggest that depressive disorder is the fourth leading cause of disease burden worldwide, and the burden of disability caused by depression comes into the same range as ischaemic heart disease, diarrhoeal disease, asthma or COPD. It is a relapsing and remitting disorder, often closely linked to events or relationships in the person's life, so a careful history is needed. In developing countries the presenting symptoms are likely to be as follows:

- low mood
- physical symptoms, for example headache, backache, general body pains and palpitations. It is helpful to learn the local language of emotional distress in order to identify the real cause of vague physical symptoms which appear to have no organic cause
- anxiety and fearfulness
- insomnia, especially with early waking
- change in appetite, usually eating less with weight loss
- poor concentration and memory
- loss of energy and motivation, withdrawal
- loss of hope and optimism

If depression is suspected, discuss the patient's life circumstances to check for an obvious cause. Often, talking over problems with a sympathetic health worker will be helpful in itself. If the patient appears becoming more severely ill, the options are as follows:

- *Antidepressants*, for example amitriptyline or imipramine in gradually increasing doses up to 150 mg at night, or fluoxetine 20–40 mg daily.
- *Cognitive behaviour therapy (CBT)*, either alone or with antidepressants. Patients with very low mood cannot concentrate well enough for psychotherapy, so will need pharmacological treatment first.
- *Electroconvulsive therapy*, a specialist treatment which may be highly effective in severe cases.

Be sure to check for suicidal ideas in any patient with depression. If the patient has clear plans and intention to harm or kill himself seek specialist help. A pathway of care for suicidal patients is shown in Figure 59.5.

Bipolar affective disorder

When the patient experiences discrete episodes of high mood as well as depression, they may have

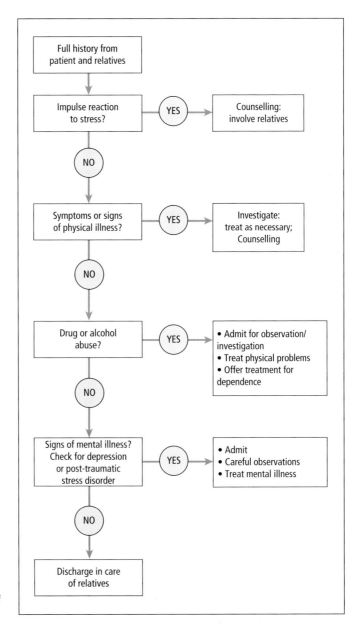

Figure 59.5 Management of suicidal patients.

bipolar disorder. This may be treated sympto-matically—antipsychotics for the high or manic mood, and antidepressants for depression.

If there is access to specialist support, better still is a mood stabilizer, for example lithium. This is excellent but needs careful monitoring includ-ing regular checks on serum levels of lithium, renal function and thyroid function. Alternative

mood stabilizers are carbamazepine and sodium valproate.

Post-traumatic stress disorder

People who have been subjected to life-threatening situations over which they have no control may develop post-traumatic stress disorder (PTSD)—a

disabling condition. Check for this in any person who has been subjected to trauma, especially in war or refugee situations. Symptoms are as follows:
- high anxiety with high vigilance
- insomnia with nightmares
- day-time 'flashbacks' (seeing images of the original trauma)
- depression and suicidal ideas.

Be alert for sexual trauma in women and girls especially. The effects are profound and long-lasting, but difficult to disclose, and the patient will need careful and sympathetic management. Treatment for PTSD is with antidepressants such as fluoxetine 20–60 mg daily, and CBT.

Organization of care

Most mental illnesses can be effectively treated in primary care.
- Include mental illness in the list of conditions managed in primary care clinics.
- Train general health workers in common signs and symptoms.
- Maintain people with schizophrenia on oral or depot antipsychotics.
- Maintain people with recurrent depression on antidepressants.
- Work with community volunteers or health workers to identify mental illness and signs of relapse in known patients.
- Work with local leaders, traditional healers and communities to reduce stigma and ensure that patients receive effective treatment.

Further reading

Gill GV, Price C, Shandu D, Dedicoat M, Wilkinson D. An effective system of nurse-led

diabetes care in rural Africa. *Diabet Med* 2008; 25: 606–611. [This article describes successful implication of a nurse-led protocol-based system of diabetes care in rural Africa.]

Mani KS, Rangan G, Srinavas HV, Srindharan VS, Subbakrishna DK. Epilepsy control with phenobarbital or phenytoin in rural south India: the Yelandur study. *Lancet* 2001; 357: 1316–1320. [An excellent report showing successful epilepsy control with appropriately delivered monotherapy.]

Parry EPO, Godfrey R, Mabey D, Gill GV, eds. *Principles of Medicine in Africa*, 3rd edn. Cambridge: Cambridge University Press, 2004. [Contains several useful chapters on NCDs—relevant to Africa and elsewhere in the tropics. These include 'Diabetes' (Mbanya J-C, Gill GV, pp. 739–767), 'Asthma' (Gordon S, Boeree M, pp. 768–778), 'Hypertension' (Walker R, Edwards R, pp. 779–797), and 'Epilepsy' (Hart Y, Prevett M, pp. 810–827).]

Patel V. *Where There Is No Psychiatrist*. London: Gaskell, 2001. [An excellent and user-friendly manual of practical psychiatry in resource-limited areas.]

Prince M, Patel V, Saxena S *et al.* Global mental health I. No health without mental health. *Lancet* 2007; 370: 859–877. [A good overview of the world impact of mental health—14% of the global burden of disease and a particular problem in the developing world.]

Chapter 60

Refugee health

Humanitarian emergencies in resource-poor countries

Most refugees/internally displaced persons (IDPs) are displaced because of complex humanitarian emergencies (CHEs) or natural disasters. CHEs are primarily internal wars in which conflicting groups compete for limited resources. CHEs are characterized by administrative, economic, political and social disruption, usually accompanied by high levels of violence. Major violations of the Geneva Conventions and Universal Declaration of Human Rights are common, and cultural, religious and ethnic groups may be at risk of extinction. CHEs frequently result in catastrophic public health emergencies as coping capacities are exceeded by need, placing vulnerable populations at greatest risk of epidemic diseases and malnutrition. CHEs may smoulder on for many years as 'chronic emergencies' with fluctuating levels of violence, displacement and disease. Natural disasters (floods, earthquakes, famine) may also become CHEs, particularly when they affect vulnerable populations in weakened or disrupted states.

Global climate change is affecting the frequency and magnitude of natural disasters, aggravating the burden of malnutrition and communicable diseases, intensifying competition for scarce resources and increasing the likelihood of conflict and population displacement.

Responding to humanitarian emergencies

Emergency phase

The initial phase of an emergency is characterized by need overwhelming available resources, resulting in increased mortality rates. Crude mortality rate (CMR) is generally used as an indicator of the severity of an emergency. Under-fives mortality (UFM) may also be used (Table 60.1).

The emergency phase of an intervention can be regarded as over when the CMR is <1 and basic needs have been met. The figures quoted in table 60.1 refer to current recommendations particularly applicable to countries in sub-Saharan Africa. Thresholds for most countries in other regions are significantly lower.

Effective action in response to a humanitarian emergency depends on individuals, governmental and NGOs working in a coordinated and complementary manner. Intersectoral collaboration is the key to success in emergency interventions. *Médecins Sans Frontières* (MSF) emphasize ten priorities in an emergency response.

Lecture Notes: Tropical Medicine, 6th edition.
By G.V. Gill and N.J. Beeching. Published 2009 by
Blackwell Publishing, ISBN: 978-1-4051-8048-1.

Table 60.1 Crude mortality rate (CMR) and under-fives mortality (UFM) used to indicate the severity of an emergency. Rates are per 10 000/day.

	CMR	UFM
Major catastrophe	>5	>10
Emergency: out of control	>2	>4
Emergency/relief programme: situation serious	>1	>2
Emergency/relief programme: under control	<1	<2
Normal rate for stable developing country	0.5	1.0

Initial assessment

The initial assessment is usually conducted in two phases.

Phase I
- Objective to enable rapid decision regarding the need for and scale of an intervention.
- Completed within 3 days.
- Focus
  (a) geopolitical context, including the background to the displacement
  (b) demographic description of the population and map of site
  (c) characteristics of the environment in which refugees have settled
  (d) availability of water, food and shelter
  (e) major health problems, epidemic diseases and mortality rates
  (f) human and material resources required
  (g) operating partners (e.g. local and national authorities, local and international organizations)

Phase II
- Conducted simultaneously with the implementation of relief actions.
- Allows more detailed programme planning and wider dissemination of information.

- Similar range of issues to Phase I, but with greater depth and emphasis.

Measles immunization

Measles can be a devastating illness in refugee populations, particularly if there is also a high level of malnutrition and vitamin A deficiency. Herd immunity is only achieved when over 90% of those susceptible have been immunized, a figure rarely achieved in any country in the world. Therefore, all children aged between 6 months and 15 years should be immunized against measles and given vitamin A.

Water and sanitation

Access to adequate supplies of water is critical in reducing the likelihood of diarrhoeal diseases. Quantity is more important than quality. A minimum of 5 L/person/day is required for essential needs such as drinking and cooking in the acute stages of an emergency. This should be increased to at least 15–20 L/person/day as soon as possible to reduce the risk of waterborne and water-washed diseases. Having sourced a sufficient quantity of water, attention can be given to assessing quality by determining the level of faecal coliforms using a field testing kit such as the Del Agua/Oxfam kit. Chlorination is the most effective way of treating water in emergencies.

During the initial stages of an emergency, it may be necessary to identify defecation areas or fields for excreta disposal. However, construction of shallow trenches or collective latrines is preferable. The target should be one latrine or trench per 50–100 people. As the situation stabilizes, the aim is for one latrine per 20 people or, ideally, one latrine per family.

Food and nutrition

Existing malnutrition in a population is exacerbated by circumstances giving rise to humanitarian emergencies. Establishing and maintaining food security (access by all people at all times to enough food for an active, healthy life) can present an enormous logistical challenge. The minimum mean population requirement is 2100 kcals/person/day. Attention must be given to ensuring that the basic food ration includes an appropriate mix of vitamins and other micronutrients. The prevalence of malnutrition among children aged less than 5 years is usually an indication of the level of malnutrition in the entire population. Therefore, the initial health assessment should include a nutritional survey of a sample of these children by measuring the weight-for-height (W/H) index and identifying children with bilateral pedal oedema.

Prevalence rates can be calculated for

Global malnutrition (percentage of children with moderate or severe malnutrition);

Severe malnutrition (children with W/H < -3 Z-Scores and/or oedema);

Moderate malnutrition (% children with W/H between -2 and -3 Z-Scores)

where 'Z-Scores' refer to the number of standard deviations above (+) or below (−) the mean in the reference population.

Mid-upper arm circumference (MUAC) is less accurate but is sometimes used for rapid screening in children aged 6–59 months if a W/H survey is impossible.

MUAC <125 mm indicates global acute malnutrition;

MUAC <110 mm indicates severe malnutrition. Bilateral pedal oedema is used as an indicator of severe malnutrition (see Chapter 61).

The results of the survey can then be used to guide the level of intervention. In addition to ensuring that general food distributions provide adequate food rations for all, there is often need for selective feeding programmes (SFPs). Blanket SFPs provide food supplements to vulnerable groups (e.g. pregnant women). Targeted SFPs provide food supplements and medical follow-up for the moderately malnourished. Therapeutic feeding programmes are used in the management of severely malnourished children and include an initial 'intensive care' phase for careful resuscitation, management of medical problems and initiation of nutritional treatment. Once complications have been brought under control and feeding has been established, the child can be transferred to a day-care unit for ongoing nutritional and medical management and follow-up.

Routine inpatient management of severe malnutrition is now being questioned. It has become evident that the traditional therapeutic feeding centre (TFC) may be suboptimal. Access to TFCs may be difficult in complex emergencies and concentration of vulnerable individuals in centres increases risk of exposure to infectious diseases, such as measles, and may also result in greater vulnerability to security threats. Carers are often dislocated from their families and communities and are unable to work or fulfil domestic responsibilities. Recently, community-based therapeutic care (CTC) has been developed as an innovative approach to management of severe malnutrition that addresses many of these issues.

The core operating principles of CTC are

• *Maximum coverage and access*—ideally, reach the entire severely malnourished population.

• *Timeliness*—begin case-finding and treatment before the prevalence of malnutrition escalates and additional medical complications occur.

• *Appropriate care*—provide simple, effective outpatient care for those who can be treated at home and clinical care for those requiring inpatient treatment.

• *Care for as long as it is needed*—by improving access to treatment, ensure that children remain in the programme until they have recovered. By building local capacity and integrating the programme within existing structures and services.

• CTC also aims to ensure that effective treatment is available for as long as acute malnutrition is present in the population.

Acutely malnourished children are identified through population screening or by community/self-referral. Three forms of treatment are provided according to the severity of malnutrition

• *Moderate acute malnutrition without medical complications*. Support in a SFP providing dry take-home rations and basic medicines.

• *Severe acute malnutrition (SAM) without medical complications*. Treat in an outpatient therapeutic programme (OTP), which provides ready-to-use therapeutic food (RUTF) and medicines for simple medical conditions. Children are managed at home with weekly OTP attendance for check-ups and supplies of RUTF.

• *Acutely malnourished with medical complications.* Treat in an inpatient stabilization centre until well enough to continue on OTP.

The CTC approach is proving effective in a wide range of contexts with outcomes equivalent to or better than those achieved in TFCs.

Shelter and site planning

Overcrowding and lack of hygiene and sanitation are major factors in the spread of communicable diseases among large populations of refugees in 'camps'. In some situations, it may be possible and preferable for refugees to be integrated among the host population.

In planning a refugee camp site, attention must be given to security, access, protection from environmental health risks and provision of essential services (reception, administration, storage, distribution, water, sanitation, cemetery, health facilities, nutrition centre(s), places for social, commercial, educational and religious activities). Careful consideration should also be given to the social, economic, health and environmental impact that refugees may have on the host population and services.

Small camps, accommodating up to about 10 000 persons, are preferable to larger camps and should be organized according to social and cultural norms, shelter and accommodation being provided on the basis of family groupings.

Health care in the emergency phase

Whenever possible, health care should be planned and implemented in consultation with national and local health authorities. Responding to the essential health care needs of refugees in camps usually requires the establishment of specific services for this population, focusing on basic curative care. Having established a central health facility, priority should be given to providing a network of peripheral health centres and health posts and developing outreach activities. There should be standardized systems for data collection and

surveillance, clear management protocols appropriate to different levels of health facility and clear guidelines for referral. Contingency plans should be developed so that appropriate action can be taken as circumstances change, for example, in response to an epidemic or in managing a sudden influx of new arrivals.

Control of communicable diseases and epidemics

Diarrhoeal diseases especially cholera and *Shigella dysenteriae* type 1, acute respiratory infections, measles, meningitis and, in many regions, malaria are among the leading infectious causes of excess mortality in refugee populations. There may also be a risk of epidemic louse-borne typhus or relapsing fever and a variety of other infections depending on the region or circumstances.

The emphasis should be on prevention, epidemic surveillance using agreed case definitions, contingency planning and epidemic response appropriate to the specific disease and circumstances of the outbreak. The number of clinical cases may overwhelm existing facilities and specific treatment centres may have to be set up and staffed.

STIs including HIV may be a serious problem in refugee populations, as a result of sexual violence or social disruption. Their long-term impact may be as devastating as any of the diseases mentioned above. Therefore, implementation of measures to prevent and treat STIs should be an early consideration following the initial emergency response.

The risk of reactivation and transmission of tuberculosis is increased in refugee populations. However, the WHO recommends that a TB control programme should not be initiated until the following criteria have been fulfilled: data indicate that TB is an important health problem; the emergency phase is over; basic needs of water, adequate food, shelter and sanitation are available; essential clinical services and basic drugs are available; security in, and stability of, the camp are envisaged for at least 6 months; sufficient funding is available for at least 12 months;

laboratory services for sputum smear microscopy are available. Similar, though even more complex, issues require consideration with regard to provision of ART for people with HIV/AIDS. Difficult ethical dilemmas face health care providers in emergency settings, who must reconcile an individual's 'right to life with dignity' with the need to adopt a public health approach for the 'greater common good'.

Public Health surveillance

Effective programme planning, implementation, monitoring and evaluation depends on a system for the collection of data on demography, morbidity, mortality, basic needs and programme activities. Simple, standardized indicators should be used. A minimum data set in the initial emergency phase should include CMR, cause-specific mortality and morbidity using simple case definitions, malnutrition rate among under-fives and indicators of access to water and sanitation facilities.

Human resources and training

Recruitment, training and management of staff are critical to the success of an intervention. It is important to determine appropriate staffing levels for a given task, prepare specific job descriptions and establish lines of management and communication. Consideration should be given to contracts, legal status and salaries. Local services can be severely disrupted when their staff are lured by superior salaries and conditions offered by refugee agencies.

Coordination

A reliable coordination mechanism and leadership should be established early in the initial phase of an emergency. Coordination requires regular meetings involving representatives from key ministries in the host government, the host community, the refugee population and the agencies involved in the response. Common objectives should be agreed and tasks determined and formally allocated. Technical guidelines and standardized policies should be introduced from the outset and procedures agreed for reporting and dissemination of data.

Post-emergency phase

The post-emergency phase commences when basic needs have been met and excess mortality has been controlled (CMR $<1/10000$/day). Continued attention is given to the 'top ten' priorities indicated in the emergency phase, whilst adapting health programmes to address additional issues that may not have been received particular attention, for example reproductive and mental health. The post-emergency phase may end with repatriation and resettlement, or, if a population faces long-term displacement, there may be a gradual process of adaptation of services according to need or integration into mainstream services for the host population.

The sphere project and humanitarian reform

The need for greater accountability and professional standards in humanitarian interventions received critical attention in the evaluation of the international response to the 1994 Rwandan genocide. Three years later a multi-agency initiative, the Sphere Project, was launched. Sphere defined minimum standards in core sectors of humanitarian assistance and advocated a universal humanitarian charter. Sphere is based on two core beliefs: first, that all possible steps should be taken to alleviate human suffering arising out of calamity and conflict and second, that those affected by disaster have a right to life with dignity and therefore a right to assistance.

Over the past decade, the frequency, magnitude, complexity and cost of humanitarian emergencies have continued to escalate. Following the Humanitarian Response Review in 2005, the international humanitarian community developed the Humanitarian Reform Agenda which aims to enhance the timeliness and effectiveness of humanitarian responses, prioritize the allocation of resources and offer more comprehensive needs-based relief and protection. The bedrock of humanitarian reform is increased capacity, predictability, accountability and partnership among humanitarian actors. This forms the foundation for the three 'pillars' of reform:

1 Improving the predictability of funding through the Central Emergency Response Fund;

2 Strengthening the Humanitarian Coordinator System;

3 The Cluster Approach coordinating effective responses through global and country cluster lead organizations addressing gaps in activities such as health, water/sanitation, logistics, nutrition, emergency shelter, camp coordination and management, emergency telecommunications, protection, education, agriculture and early recovery.

Health issues among asylum seekers in developed countries

There is a common perception in industrialized countries that asylum seekers are a threat to the health of the host population. Asylum seekers may be at risk of certain infectious diseases because of possible exposure either in their country of origin or during their migration in search of asylum; however, the risk posed by members of the host population who travel abroad on holiday or business in numbers far exceeding those of asylum seekers entering industrialized countries receives comparatively little attention. Mandatory 'screening' for infectious diseases may be perceived as threatening and stigmatizing and may deter asylum seekers from seeking health care. It is in everyone's best interest to keep a sense of proportion and encourage asylum seekers to regard access to health care as an opportunity rather than as a threat.

Health assessment of asylum seekers

In considering the health needs of asylum seekers it is important to consider the person and their predicament. Health care providers should be aware of issues related to language, communication, culture, religion, gender, family, community

and social circumstances. Social, economic, physical, psychological and emotional needs may greatly outweigh medical needs.

The 'health assessment' approach is preferable to 'screening' as the latter is often narrowly focussed and may have negative connotations from viewpoint of the asylum seeker.

The key elements in a programme for health care of asylum seekers and refugees include:
• information and encouragement
• early initial health assessment
• specialist follow-up according to need
• continuing access to specialist services
• integration into mainstream services
• communication and continuity of care
• close liaison with other services.

The history and examination should include assessment of:
• vaccination status
• nutritional status
• mental health status
• infectious diseases
• non-infectious diseases (e.g. haematological—sickle cell, thalassaemia, G6PD; cardiac—rheumatic heart disease, endomyocardial fibrosis)
• obstetric and gynaecological problems
• vision, hearing and dental problems
• presence and level of disability
• evidence of torture
• evidence of substance misuse
• risk of exposure to toxins (e.g. lead).

The choice of laboratory investigations will depend on the findings of the health assessment and whether specific 'screening' programmes are to be followed.

Assessment of children should also include: whether the child is accompanied or unaccompanied, growth and development (including language, hearing, vision) and the possibility of congenital diseases routinely screened for in neonates in the United Kingdom (e.g. hypothyroidism, phenylketonuria). Another important issue to consider in children is that of child protection, for example, certain cultural practices, notably female genital mutilation (FGM), may be traditional in the child's country of origin but illegal in the country of asylum.

Infectious diseases

Infectious diseases that are likely to be more prevalent among refugees and asylum seekers include tuberculosis, hepatitis B and C, HIV, STIs, gastrointestinal infections (bacterial/parasitic), malaria, typhoid and other tropical diseases, infestations (lice, scabies) and multidrug resistant bacterial infections. In most cases, these infections are likely to be asymptomatic. Therefore, 'screening' programmes may be recommended for specific infections, particularly those of greatest public health interest (e.g. tuberculosis, Hepatitis B/C, HIV, STIs). Issues concerning ethics, consent, confidentiality, cost-effectiveness and continuity of care deserve consideration.

Decisions regarding routine screening for intestinal helminths should be made on the basis of risk assessment. Empirical treatment with albendazole has been shown to be more cost-effective than routine screening of immigrants in the United States.

Many latent imported infections may cause clinical disease following immunosuppression, including tuberculosis, leprosy, amoebiasis, strongyloidiasis, visceral leishmaniasis, histoplasmosis, malaria, filariasis and American trypanosomiasis.

Some imported infections, if untreated, may persist for years, for example strongyloidiasis (>60 years), schistosomiasis (>30 years), melioidosis (>25 years), hydatid (>20 years) and trichinella, cysticercosis, onchocerciasis (all >15 years).

Torture and other traumatic experiences

It is estimated that 10–30% of asylum seekers will have survived torture, sexual violence or other seriously traumatizing experiences. Many will experience ongoing psychological problems including nightmares, hallucinations, flashbacks, panic attacks, sexual problems, phobias, difficulty trusting people or forming relationships, depressive illness and anxiety.

Reactions to trauma and loss may include poor concentration, memory impairment, daydreaming, intrusive thoughts and images, irritability, confusion, tiredness, lethargy, sleep difficulties and loss of motivation. Sufferers may become withdrawn and isolated and may self-harm. It is often very difficult for a person to articulate these experiences. Somatization is common and unexplained backache, headache, stomach ache or other body pains should prompt further careful enquiry. Children may, in addition, experience interrupted or uneven emotional development or failure to thrive.

The medical documentation and reporting of torture and other inhuman or degrading experiences may be a critical factor in the asylum-determination process. Guidelines and advice are available from organisations such as Physicians for Human Rights and the Medical Foundation for the Care of Victims of Torture.

Further reading

Burkle FM. Lessons learnt and future expectations of complex emergencies. *BMJ* 1999; 319: 422–426.

Coker R, Lambregts van Weezenbeek K. Mandatory screening and treatment of immigrants for latent tuberculosis in the USA: just restraint? *Lancet Infect Dis* 2001; 1: 270–276.

Collins S, Dent N, Binns P, Bahwere P, Sadler K, Hallam A. Management of severe acute malnutrition in children. *Lancet* 2006; 368: 1996–2000.

Connolly MA, Gayer M, Ryan MJ, Salama P, Spiegel P, Heymann DL. Communicable diseases in complex emergencies: impact and challenges. *Lancet* 2004; 364: 1974–1983.

Connolly MA, ed. *World Health Organization. Communicable Disease Control in Emergencies. A Field Manual. Geneva:* WHO, 2005.

Gayer M, Legros D, Formenty P, Connolly MA. Conflict and emerging infectious diseases. *Emerg Infect Dis* 2007; 13: 1625–1631. [Superb overview of recent issues in this area, public domain paper and reference source from CDC website.]

Goma Epidemiology Group. Public health impact of Rwandan refugee crisis: what happened in Goma, Zaire, in July 1994. *Lancet* 1995; 345: 339–344.

Lifson AR, Thai D, O'Fallon A, Mills WA, Hang K. Prevalence of tuberculosis, hepatitis B virus and intestinal parasitic infections among refugees to Minnesota. *Public Health Rep* 2002; 117: 69–77.

Médecins Sans Frontières. *Refugee Health: An Approach to Emergency Situations*. London: Macmillan, 1997. [This is essential reading for anyone involved in humanitarian emergencies in developing countries. Refugee Health and other key MSF books are also available on CD-ROM, and online at: http://www.msf.org/source/refbooks/E_MSFdocmenu.htm.]

Perrin P. *War and Public Health*. Geneva: ICRC, 1996. [Clear and systematic text with the added bonus of chapters on international humanitarian law and ethics. Also available online at WHO/PAHO Health Library for Disasters.]

Websites

http://www.humanitarianreform.org/. Humanitarian reform.

http://www.torturecare.org.uk/. The Medical Foundation for the Care of Victims of Torture is a registered charity that provides care and rehabilitation to survivors of torture and other forms of organized violence.

http://www.phrusa.org. Physicians for Human Rights website provides access to reports and training materials, including the 'Istanbul Protocol' (Manual on the effective investigation and documentation of torture and other cruel, inhuman or degrading treatment or punishment).

http://www.sphereproject.org/. Sphere Project: Humanitarian Charter and Minimum Standards in Disaster Response.

http://www.who.int/disasters/. WHO emergency humanitarian action website has excellent links including access to a huge range of electronic handbooks, manuals and emergency bibliography, many of which are also available on CD-ROM.

http://helid.desastres.net/. The WHO/PAHO 'Health Library for Disasters' is also outstanding.

Chapter 61

Syndromes of malnutrition

Malnutrition in children

Malnutrition in all its forms remains a major public health problem throughout the developing world and is an underlying factor in over 50% of the 10–11 million deaths in children under 5 years of age who die each year from preventable causes. Worldwide approximately 60 million children are suffering from moderate acute malnutrition and 13 million from severe acute malnutrition at any one time.

Definition

Severe acute malnutrition is defined as a weight-for-height measurement of <70% of the median or ≥3 standard deviations (SD) below the mean National Centre for Health Statistics reference values (termed wasting or marasmus), the presence of bilateral pitting oedema of nutritional origin (termed oedematous malnutrition or kwashiorkor) or a mid upper arm circumference (MUAC) of <110 mm in a child between 1 and 5 years of age. By contrast, chronic malnutrition (termed stunting) is identified using a height-for-age indicator (Table 61.1).

Aetiology

There are many factors involved in the aetiology of malnutrition, varying between geographical

regions, including famine, drought, war, poverty/social disadvantage, lack of food, infections and neglect.

The principal pattern is of a child who is underweight due to poor nutrition and recurrent infections who then develops a severe infection, for example diarrhoea or measles, which precipitates severe acute malnutrition. The varied presentations are determined by the severity, duration and complexity of interactions of specific macro- and micro-nutrient deficiencies, yet despite much research, it is not yet clear why children present with such differing clinical features.

Oedematous malnutrition is commonly seen in areas where high energy–low protein foods are the staple diet; however, the concept that protein deficiency causes this form of malnutrition has now been refuted. It is thought that oedematous malnutrition is precipitated by a variety of environmental insults, termed noxae. The child's protective mechanisms are compromised by a whole range of dietary deficiencies or depletions. Oedematous malnutrition results from an imbalance between the production of toxic radicals by the noxae and their safe disposal. The important noxae are infections, but others may be exogenous toxins such as aflatoxin and its metabolites. Oedema, aside from a low intravascular protein, is caused by the leaking membranes which have lost their integrity through oxidative stress.

Lecture Notes: Tropical Medicine, 6th edition.
By G.V. Gill and N.J. Beeching. Published 2009 by Blackwell Publishing, ISBN: 978-1-4051-8048-1.

Table 61.1 Classification of childhood malnutrition. Weight-for-height 'z-score' is defined as standard deviation (SD) below the mean for that population.

	Classification	
	Moderate malnutrition	**Severe malnutrition**
Symmetrical oedema	No	Yes (oedematous malnutrition or kwashiorkor)
Weight-for-height z-score	−3 SD to −2 SD (70–79%)	< −3 SD (<70%) (wasting or marasmus)
Height-for-age	−3 SD to −2 SD (85–89%)	< −3 SD (<85%) (stunting)

Clinical features

The principal clinical feature in children with severe wasting is wasting of muscle and fat (Figure 61.1). This can be particularly marked around the ribs, long bones and buttocks, resulting in so-called 'baggy pants'. There may be hair changes in longstanding cases. Oedematous malnutrition is characterized by:

• Oedema of a type and distribution similar to that in nephrotic syndrome, but without proteinuria (Figure 61.2). Ascites is rare.
• Progressive skin changes: hyperpigmented and dry skin is followed by flaking, peeling and hypopigmentation ('flakey paint dermatitis'—Figure 61.3).
• Enlarged fatty liver (20–40% of wet liver weight is triglyceride).
• Straightened and bleached hair which is sparse and easily pluckable (Figure 61.4).
• Mental changes ranging from irritability and apathy to semi-consciousness.
• Eye changes of vitamin A deficiency, conjunctivitis or other infections.
• Anorexia.
• Moderate anaemia which is commonly due to a mixed deficiency of iron, folic acid, riboflavin and other haematinics along with general depression of bone marrow production.

Clinical features of common infections (e.g. candidiasis, pneumonia, urinary tract infection, gastroenteritis) may complicate all types of severe acute malnutrition, although typically clinical signs may be subtle or absent.

Investigations

Malnourished children often have marked derangement of serum electrolytes. Typical changes include hypokalaemia, due to gastrointestinal (GI) losses and dietary deficiency, hypocalcaemia and hypomagnesaemia. There is an increase in total body sodium although, paradoxically, this may be accompanied by hyponatraemia.

Cell-mediated immunity is compromised; B lymphocytes and immunoglobulins are usually normal or raised, although the immune response to bacterial infections may be sub-optimal. Complement levels are reduced alongside the activity of polymorphs. Thus ensues a vicious cycle, in which infection results in malnutrition, which in turn depresses the activity of the immune system, which further leads to anorexia, weight loss and malnutrition. Serum albumin is low, as amino acids are diverted away from albumin production for synthesis of acute phase proteins and immunoglobulins.

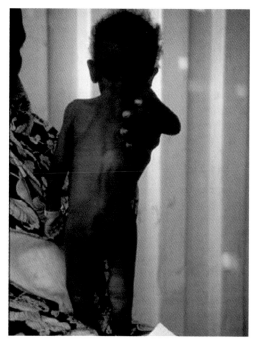

Figure 61.1 Severe visible wasting. (source IMCI teaching material).

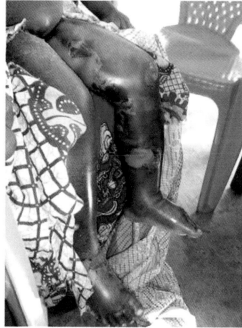

Figure 61.3 Oedematous malnutrition demonstrating hypo- and hyper-pigmented areas and flaking skin.

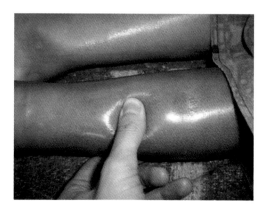

Figure 61.2 Oedematous malnutrition or kwashiorkor.

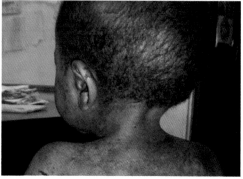

Figure 61.4 Straightened, sparse hair that is easily pluckable (in oedematous malnutrition).

Management

For all cases of severe acute malnutrition, the WHO management protocol has recommended medical and nutritional treatment regimens that are inpatient based and administered by trained healthcare professionals in ten steps in two phases, termed 'resuscitation/stabilization' (steps 1–7) and 'rehabilitation' (steps 8–10). The principal tasks during initial resuscitation/stabilization are the following:

1 *To prevent hypoglycaemia* by initiating frequent small feeds as soon as possible and continue these throughout the day and night. When hypoglycaemia is established, it should be treated

with 5 mL/kg of 10% dextrose given orally/NG/ i.v. and followed up with frequent small feeds.

2 *To treat or prevent hypothermia* by covering the child, including the head, reducing draughts and initiating kangaroo care when possible. Kangaroo care means continuous skin-to-skin nursing of the infant/child against the mother's body.

3 *To treat or prevent dehydration and shock.* Dehydration can be very difficult to recognize in a wasted child because many of the signs of dehydration will be present by virtue of the malnutrition (e.g. sunken eyes and slow skin pinch). Therefore, any child with watery diarrhoea or vomiting should be assumed to have dehydration. ReSoMal (**Re**hydration **So**lution for the **Mal**nourished—a modified oral rehydration solution (ORS)) should be commenced slowly, at an approximate rate of 5 mL/kg every 30 min for the first 2 h followed by 5–10 mL/kg every hour, until signs of improvement or a maximum of 10 h. Intravenous fluids should not be used for the treatment of dehydration in malnourished children, due to the risk of fluid overload and cardiac failure.

In malnourished children, some of the signs of shock can also be present all the time. Therefore shock is defined as:

Lethargy/unconsciousness and cold hands, plus either slow capillary refill or weak or fast pulse.

When shock is identified it should be treated with

- oxygen
- 5 mL/kg of i.v. 10% glucose or 1 mL/kg of 50% glucose
- warmth
- intravenous fluids: 15 mL/kg of fluid over 1 h. The fluid of choice is half-strength Darrow's with 5% glucose.

4 *To correct electrolyte imbalance.* Malnourished children require extra potassium (3–4 mmol/kg/ day) and extra magnesium (0.4–0.6 mmol/kg/day). If using F75 (Table 61.2), these supplements will not be necessary as the milk has a combined mineral and vitamin mix added already. Malnourished children should also receive a low-sodium diet (i.e. no salt to be added when cooking).

5 *To treat or prevent infection.* All severely malnourished children should be treated for infection,

even if there are no signs. If no complications are present, an oral antibiotic such as cotrimoxazole can be used. If complications are present (e.g. shock, hypoglycaemia, dermatosis with raw skin/fissures, pneumonia and UTI), parenteral antibiotics such as chloramphenicol and gentamicin should be used. Antibiotic choices will depend upon local microbiology knowledge and sensitivity patterns.

6 *To correct micronutrient deficiencies.* All children should receive a multivitamin supplement, folic acid 1 mg/day, zinc 2 mg/kg/day and copper 0.3 mg/kg/day. All of these are provided within F75 (Table 61.2). In addition, malnourished children will require prophylactic vitamin A and iron (3 mg/kg/day) only when the child has a good appetite and starts gaining weight. Single doses of vitamin A are: age <6 months, 50 000 IU; age 6–12 months, 100 000 IU; >12 months, 200 000 IU.

7 *To start to feed the child.* During the resuscitation phase of treatment, a low protein milk formula feed should be commenced with small volumes given every 2–3 hours. The recommended WHO feed is F75 (75 kcal/100 mL of milk; Table 61.2). Unless the child is able to take the required volume by cup, it should be given wholly or partly by nasogastric tube.

The end of the resuscitation phase is characterised by a return of appetite, along with loss of oedema.

During the rehabilitation phase of management, the principles are as follows:

8 *This is the phase of rapid catch-up growth, when the child is encouraged to eat as much as possible* (e.g.

Table 61.2 Constituents of F75 and F100 feeds

	Amount per 100 mL	
Constituent	F75	F100
Energy	75 kcal (316 kJ)	100 kcal (420 kJ)
Protein	0.9 g	2.9 g
Lactose	1.3 g	4.2 g
Potassium	3.6 mmol	5.9 mmol
Sodium	0.6 mmol	1.9 mmol
Magnesium	0.4 mmol	0.7 mmol
Zinc	2.0 mg	2.3 mg
Copper	0.25 mg	0.25 mg
Osmolarity	333 mOsmol/L	419 mOsmol/L

130–200 kcal kg/day). The WHO recommends F100 (100 kcal/100 mL of milk; Table 61.2) in addition to a normal diet and breast milk where appropriate.

9 *As the child improves, sensory stimulation and emotional support* become essential.

10 *Discharge and follow-up should be planned*. The time of discharge will vary from unit to unit; certainly, the child should have regained their appetite and have achieved a weight-for-height (W/H) measurement of 80% of the median. Recovery can take 4–6 weeks. Follow-up after recovery is essential to prevent relapse or recurrence.

Community-based therapeutic care

Despite the success of these protocols when implemented in selected units, their publication has not led to a widespread decrease in mortality in most hospitals in the developing world, which remains at 20–30% for marasmus and up to 50–60% for kwashiorkor. There are often insufficient available skilled staff and limited inpatient capacity. The centralized nature of hospitals also promotes late presentation, high opportunity costs for carers and risks of cross-infection. Therefore, an increasing number of countries have adopted a community-based model for the management of acute malnutrition called community-based therapeutic care (CTC). CTC consists of four elements:

1 Measures to mobilize the community in order to encourage early presentation and compliance.

2 Outpatient supplementary feeding protocols for those with moderate acute malnutrition and no serious medical complications.

3 Outpatient therapeutic protocols for those with severe acute malnutrition and no serious medical complications.

4 Inpatient therapeutic protocols for those with acute malnutrition also suffering from serious medical complications.

Experience over the past 5 years indicates that most cases of acute malnutrition can be successfully treated solely as outpatients, enabling intensive inpatient care to be reserved for the minority suffering from malnutrition with complications. CTC complements the existing WHO inpatient protocols using ready-to-use therapeutic foods for the majority of children. This new approach has dramatically reduced case-fatality rates. Initial data indicate that it has improved the cost-effectiveness of treating severe acute malnutrition.

Effects of HIV and tuberculosis

In sub-Saharan Africa, a high proportion of severely malnourished children admitted to nutritional rehabilitation units are now HIV positive particularly those with severe wasting. HIV and tuberculosis are increasing the workloads of units treating severe acute malnutrition through both the direct effects of infection and the indirect negative effects on livelihood and food security. HIV not only raises the prevalence of severe acute malnutrition but also increases the complication and case-fatality rates. Experience has shown that, whilst such children can achieve a full recovery using standard protocols, they recover more slowly than uninfected children.

Malnutrition in adults

Severe malnutrition in an adult population is unusual but does occur, predominantly in the context of famine or as a consequence of late stage HIV infection. The same principles apply to the classification of severe malnutrition as among children—severe wasting, represented by a significant reduction in body mass index (BMI) and oedematous malnutrition presenting as kwashiorkor. The use of the MUAC has not yet been formally validated in adults.

Managing severe malnutrition among adults should follow the same principles as those outlined in children—cautious introduction of food in the acute stage, liberal use of multivitamins and antibiotics and more aggressive rehabilitation during the 'catch-up' phase. As with children, community-based therapy may be most appropriate particularly in the context of a famine.

Specific deficiencies of one or more micronutrients may be more commonly seen in adults than in children and are occasionally a reflection of the staple elements of the diet consumed by the local population. These vary in different parts of the tropics from being predominantly rice-based in most of Asia to cassava and maize in parts of Africa. The clinical features of specific vitamin deficiencies are listed below.

Vitamin A

Vitamin A is found predominantly in green leafy vegetables. In the early stages of deficiency, there may be no clinical signs but patients may report an impairment in their night vision. The first sign of vitamin A deficiency is a dryness of the eyes, which may feel gritty, and can be clinically apparent. This is known as xerophthalmia. Bitôt's spots, grey or white plaques of damaged epithelium usually seen on the lateral aspect of the conjunctiva, were first described in the nineteenth century and are said to be a specific sign of vitamin A deficiency. As the deficiency worsens, keratomalacia may occur, in which the whole structure of the eye breaks down leading to irreversible blindness.

Vitamin B1 (thiamine)

Thiamine deficiency is classically associated with a diet consisting of polished rice—or alcohol—and ultimately results in the condition 'beriberi', a word probably derived from *beri*, the word for 'weak' in one of the Malay dialects. Two forms are described, 'wet' and 'dry'. Wet beriberi presents as a form of cardiomyopathy in which peripheral oedema is prominent. Occasionally a low output form of heart failure occurs ('Shoshun' beriberi). In either form, the response to intravenous thiamine is dramatic (100–200mg i.v. daily). Dry beriberi is characterized by a painful polyneuropathy. Thiamine deficiency is also the cause of the Wernicke–Korsakoff syndrome, or alcoholic psychosis, which is seen sporadically throughout the world. The diagnosis is usually made clinically, but in a research setting, a reduction in the red blood cell transketolase enzyme is diagnostic.

Vitamin B6 (niacin or nicotinic acid)

Niacin deficiency is primarily associated with a diet based on maize and is seen most commonly in southern Africa. Ultimately, niacin deficiency results in pellagra, a disease characterized by diarrhoea, dermatitis that predominantly affects sun-exposed skin, and dementia. A hyperpigmented rash affecting the neck and known as 'Casal's necklace' is characteristic and is not uncommon in southern Africa among marginalized adults whose diet comprises little more than maize meal porridge—*sadza* as it is known in Zimbabwe (Figure 61.5). Treatment with nicotinamide 50mg t.d.s. for 2 weeks is highly effective.

Vitamin C (ascorbic acid)

Vitamin C deficiency, or scurvy, occurs among those whose diet is deficient in any form of fruit or vegetable. Classically it produces gingivitis and ultimately bleeding—both from the gums and the skin, often around the base of the hair follicles. In practice scurvy is very rarely seen any longer. Treatment is with vitamin C 50mg t.d.s. for at least 2 weeks.

Vitamin D

Rickets is usually seen in young children but may occasionally present in young adults whose bones are still growing. Bony changes include the 'rickety rosary' caused by widening of the costophrenic junctions and a recognized association of severe protein-energy malnutrition. The radiological signs are often seen in X-rays of the wrists and forearms

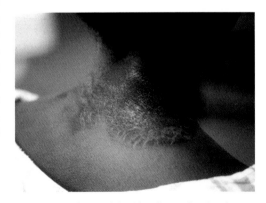

Figure 61.5 African adult with pellagra, showing the typical 'Casal's collar'.

and comprise 'cupping, splaying and fraying'. In other words, the joint spaces become wider in both longitudinal ('cupping') and transverse ('splaying') section while the joint margins become irregular ('fraying'). Involvement of the femur may result in either 'bow legs' or 'knock knees'. Although sunlight is an important cofactor in the conversion of dietary vitamin D to its active metabolite, rickets is still seen occasionally in parts of the tropics where, either for cultural or religious reasons, children are kept covered from the sun.

Other manifestations of vitamin deficiencies

Glossitis, angular stomatitis and a range of dermatoses are all features of protein-energy malnutrition in children and are occasionally seen in adults. They are a manifestation of a range of vitamin deficiencies rather than attributable to the lack of a specific vitamin. All will respond to multivitamin replacement therapy.

Further reading

Collins S, Dent N, Binns P, Bahwere P, Sadler K, Hallam A. Management of severe acute malnutrition in children. *Lancet* 2006; 368: 1992–2000. [Good up-to-date review article.]

Manary MJ, Sandige HL. Management of acute metabolic and severe childhood malnutrition. *Brit Med J* 2008; 337: 1227–30. [Useful recent review.]

WHO. *Management of Severe Malnutrition: A Manual for Physicians and Other Senior Health Workers*. Geneva: WHO, 1999. [http://whqlibdoc.who.int/hq/1999/a57361.pdf.]

Index

Note: page numbers in *italics* refer to figures and those in **bold** refer to tables and boxes

abacavir (ABC) 116
abdomen, fever 27, 187
abdominal pain 3–4, *44*
abortion, malaria 61
abscess
  amoebic 186, 187
  guinea worm 326
  melioidosis 309
  paratyphoid 286
  pyogenic 188
  spinal epidural 265
  typhoid 282
  see also liver abscess, amoebic
Acanthamoeba species 185
achlorhydria 195
aciclovir 260
acidaemia, malaria 64
Actinomycetes 330
actinomycosis 91, **314**
active immunization 269
activity, reduced 353
acute bacterial pneumonia 14
acute Chagas' disease 155
acute dermatolymphangioadenitis
  (ADLA) 142
acute disseminated
  histoplasmosis 328
Acute Filarial Lymphangitis
  (AFL) 142
acute flaccid paralysis 261
  acute inflammatory demyelinating
    polyneuropathy 262–3
  acute motor axonal
    neuropathy 263
  anterior horn cell damage
    causing 262
  clinical presentations 261–3
  definition 261
  enterovirus 71 262
  immune-mediated causes 262–3
  Japanese encephalitis virus 262
  nerve conduction studies 263
  pathophysiology 261–3
  polio 262
acute infection 323

acute inflammatory demyelinating polyneuropathy
  (AIDP) 262–3
acute motor axonal neuropathy
  (AMAN) 263
acute pneumonia 234
  differential diagnosis 235–6
  signs 234–5
  symptoms 234
acute pulmonary
  histoplasmosis 328
acute schistosomiasis 162–3, 166–7,
  168
Addison's disease 34, 340
adrenaline 343, 344, 357
adult respiratory distress syndrome
  (ARDS) 307
Aedes 142, 295, 299
Aedes aegypti 296, 299
Aedes albopictus 296
Aedes mosquitoes 245, 260, 287,
  288, 296, 299
affective (mood) changes 362
aflatoxins 223, 228
African histoplasmosis 329
African Programme for
  Onchocerciasis Control
  (APOC) 139–40
African tick typhus 305
  clinical features 305
  treatment 305
AIDS
  economic impact 107
  malabsorption 4
  mortality 98
  surveillance 104
  see also HIV infection
AIDS defining–opportunistic
  infections 109
AIDS–dementia complex 266
AIDS-related complex (ARC) 104–
  5, 109
ALA 187
  complications 188
albendazole 201, 203, 206, 327, 360

alveolar hydatid disease 232
ascariasis 209, 210
cestode infections 206
cutaneous larva migrans 318
cysticercosis 206
filariasis 144, 145
giardiasis 200
hookworm 211
hydatid cyst disease 229
loiasis 147
strongyloidiasis 324
treatment of immigrants 371
trichuriasis 212
tropical pulmonary
  eosinophilia 244–5
visceral larva migrans 213
alcohol abuse 225
  hypertension 352–4
alcoholic psychosis 378
allergens
  asthma 355–6
  avoidance 356
alpha-fetoprotein 225
alveolar hydatid disease *see*
  Echinococcus
  multilocularis
amikacin 98, 331
aminoglycoside 278, 331
aminophylline 357
aminosidine 78
amitriptyline 362
amodiaquine-artesunate 66
amoebapores 186
amoebiasis 185
  amoebic dysentery 185, 358
  amoebic liver abscess 187–8
  antigen detection and
    polymerase chain
    reaction 188–9
  clinical features 186–8
  cysts eradication 189–90
  developments 191
  endoscopy 189
  epidemiology 185
  imaging 189

380

immunosuppression, interactions
  with 190
intestinal amoebiasis 186–7
invasive amoebiasis 189
investigations 188–9
life cycle 185–6
management 189–90
microscopy 188
parasite 185–6
pathogenesis 186
practical points 190
prevention and public health
  aspects 190
serology 189
amoebic abscess 187
amoebic colitis
  differential diagnosis 187
amoebic hepatitis 187
amoebic liver abscess 27, 187–8,
  236
amoeboma 187, 190
amoxicillin 237, 251, 285
amoxicillin clavulanate 310
amphotericin B 77, 112, 190, 203,
  237, 251, 255, 329
  cryptococcal meningitis 255
  histoplasmosis 329
  liposomal 77
  visceral leishmaniasis 77
amputation
  Madura foot 331
  tropical ulcers 311, 312
anaemia 36–9
  aplastic 38
  blood transfusion 39, **39**
  breathing difficulties 12
  clinical diagnosis 36
  haemolytic in typhoid 282, 283
  history and examination **36**
  hookworm 210, 211, 212
  iron deficiency 338
  laboratory investigations 37–8
  macrocytic 37–8
  malaria 57
  management 38–9
  megaloblastic 340
  microcytic 37
  normocytic 38
  pernicious 340
  severe in *P. falciparum* malaria 60
Ancylostoma braziliense 318
Ancylostoma duodenale (hookworms)
  208, 210
angina 354

angiotensin converting enzyme
  (ACE)
  hypertension 354
angular stomatitis 376
Anopheles mosquitoes 142, 287
anterior horn cell damage 262,
  263
antibiotic resistance 239
antibiotics
  for cholera 197
  for dysentery 193
  for malaria 64
  for relapsing fever 302
  for tropical ulcer 312
  for tuberculosis 92
  for typhoid fever 284
antidepressants 362, 364
antiemetics 9, 206
antigen detection and polymerase
  chain reaction 188–9
antihistamine 344
antipsychotics 362
antipyretics 26
antiretroviral drugs
  HIV therapy 115–16
antivenom
  marine 346
  snake bites 343–4
  spider bites 345
appendicitis 3
  ascariasis 209
arboviral encephalitis 256
arboviruses 287
  chikungunya 287
  clinical syndromes 287–8
  colorado tick fever 288
  dengue virus 288
  fever–arthralgia–rash (FAR)
    arboviruses 287–8
  hosts 287
  O'nyong nyong 287–8
  ross river 288
  vectors 287
Arenavirus 291
arsenic, chronic poisoning 34
artemether 65
Artemisia annua 65
artemisinin drugs
  malaria therapy 65–6
  schistosomiasis 168
artesunate 65
arthritis 239
  guinea worm 326
  typhoid 282

arthropod-borne virus *see*
  arboviruses
Ascaris 244
Ascaris lumbricoides (ascariasis)
  191, 208, 209
  clinical features 209–10
  epidemiology 209
  investigations 210
  life cycle 209
  management 210
  parasites 209
  prevention and public health
    aspects 210
ascaris pneumonitis 209
Ascaris suum 209
ascorbic acid *see* vitamin C
aseptic meningitis 307
aspirin 338
assassin bug *see* triatomine bugs
asthma 14, 15, 235, 355–9
  beta-blocker
    contraindications 354
  care organization 357–9
  causes 356
  complications 356–7
  diagnosis 355–6, **356**
  education 357–8
  epidemiology 355
  exacerbations 357
  guinea worm 326
  intestinal parasite load in
    children 356
  management 357
  nurse-led treatment *358*, 359
  pneumonia, differential
    diagnosis of 235
  prevalence 356
  treatment use 357
  urban 356
asylum seekers 370
  health assessment 370–1
  health issues 370
atovaquone–proguanil
  malaria prophylaxis 69
  malaria therapy 68
Australian elapids 342
autoimmune disorders 340
azithromycin 193, 202, 283, 285,
  305, 307

babesiosis 31
bacillary dysentery 192
  clinical features 192–3
  epidemiology 192

bacillary dysentery (*Continued*)
 investigation 193
 management 193
 microbiology 192
 prevention and public health
  aspects 193–4
bacille Calmette–Guérin (BCG)
  vaccine
 Buruli ulcer 315
 hookworm prevalence 212
 leprosy 181
Bacillus fusiformis 311
bacitracin 203
bacterial meningitis 246
 steroids use 251–2
bacterial pneumonia 15
Balamuthia mandrillaris 185
Balantidium coli 191, 202, 203
banana spiders 345
bancroftian filariasis
 clinical effects 142, 143
 life cycle 142
barbiturate 268
BCG vaccination 96
bed nets, impregnated
 filariasis 140
 malaria 72
bedbugs 218
bedsores 260
benzhexol 362
benzimidazole 156, 227
benzyl benzoate 320
benzylpenicillin 111, 112, 237,
  251, 273
beriberi 378
beta-2 agonists 357
beta-blockers 354, 356
bilharziasis *see* schistosomiasis
biliary cirrhosis 228
biliary colic 3
 ascariasis 209
 liver fluke 227
biltricide *see* praziquantel
Biomphalaria 160
bipolar affective
  disorder 362–3
birth
 HIV transmission 105
 hypoxia/injury 359
birth weight, low in malaria 69
bites and stings
 marine envenoming 345–6
 scorpion stings 344–5

snakebite 342–4
 spider bites 345
bithionol 227
blackflies 135
blackwater fever 61
Blastocystis hominis 191, 202, 203
blindness
 leprosy 176
 onchocerciasis 136–7
blood
 cultures in respiratory
  disease 13–14
 HIV transmission 105–6
 prescribing 39
blood clotting test 343, **343**
blood pressure 353
 see also hypertension
blood transfusion 39
 HIV transmission 105
 malaria 64
body cavity myiasis 317
body lice 321
borderline lepromatous
  leprosy 176
borderline leprosy (BB) 176
borderline tuberculoid (BT) 175–6
Borrelia (relapsing fever) 301, 302
 pathology 302
Borrelia duttonii 301
Borrelia hermsii 301
Borrelia hispanica 301
Borrelia persica 301
Borrelia recurrentis 31, 301
Borrelia turicatae 301
Borrelia venezuelensis 301
bot fly 316
bowel carcinoma 338
bowel tumours 5
brain
 cysticercosis 205
 midline herniation
  syndromes 22
 Plasmodium falciparum
  malaria **59**
 tumours 359
brainstem
 damage 21
 signs 23
Brazilian wandering spider *see*
  banana spiders
breast-feeding
 HIV transmission 105
 leprosy 181

breathing
 assessment 22
 coma 19
breathlessness 11
bronchiectasis 11, 12, 91
bronchitis 356
bronchodilators, oral 357
bronchospasm 236
Brucella abortus 275, 276, 277
Brucella canis 275
Brucella melitensis 275, 276, 277
Brucella suis 275, 276
Brucellae 275
brucellosis 27, 275
 clinical features 275–6
 control 278
 diagnosis 276–7
 epidemiology 275
 follow-up 278
 pregnancy 278
 public health aspects 278–9
 treatment 278
Brugia malayi 140, 143, 244
Brugia timori 140
Bulinus 160
bullae 34
Bunyaviridae 294
Burkholderia pseudomallei 309, 310
Burkitt's lymphoma
 malaria endemic areas 63
burns
 drug eruptions 34
 epilepsy 360
buruli ulcer 311, 313
 background 313
 clinical features 313–14
 differential diagnosis **314**
 epidemiology 313
 investigations 314
 management 314–15
 microbiology 313
 prevention 315
 public health 315

Calabar swelling 146
calcium blockers 354
Campylobacter 7, 9
Campylobacter jejuni 263
Candida 107, 109, 113
candidiasis
 mouth 27, 113
 oesophageal 3, 113
Capillaria philippinensis 166

carbamazepine   360
card agglutination test for trypano-
        somes (CATT)   151
card indirect agglutination
        test for trypanosomes
        (CIATT)   151
cardiac syndrome
  leptospirosis   307
Casal's necklace   378
causal prophylactics   69
CD4 cells   107, 108
  counts   109, 115, 117
  leprosy   172
CD8 cells   173
cefixime   283, **284**
cefotaxime   250, 283
ceftazidime   310
ceftriaxone   193, 250, 278, 283,
        302, 307
cell-mediated immunity
        (CMI)   171, 217, 374
central nervous system (CNS)
  HIV infection   114
  infections   23–5
  schistosomiasis   165
  space occupying lesions   **19**
  trypanosomiasis   150, 151
cephalic tetanus   273
cephalosporins, third-generation
  Haemophilus influenzae
        meningitis   251
  meningococcal disease   250
  pneumococcal disease   250–1
cercariae   162
cercarial penetration, effects of   162
cerebrospinal fluid (CSF)
  brucellosis   276
  in CNS infections   24–5
  cryptococcosis   254
  Japanese encephalitis   257
  pyogenic meningitis   249, 250
  trypanosomiasis   151
cervical erosion   104
cervical neoplasia   108
Chagas' disease   155
  acute Chagas' disease   155
  acute stage   156
  chronic Chagas' disease   155–6
  clinical features   155–6
  control   156–7
  diagnosis   156
  epidemiology   156–7
  immunocompromise   156

indeterminate and chronic
        phase   156
  life cycle   155
  parasite   155
  parasitological techniques   156
  pathogenesis   155
  treatment   156
chagoma *see* cutaneous oedema
chancre, trypanosomal   148–9, 151
chancroid   46
  HIV infection risk   104
chemicals, ingestion of corrosive   3
chemoprophylaxis   239, 250, 251,
        252
chest pain   12
chest X-ray
  pneumonia   239
  respiratory disease   13
Cheyne–Stokes breathing   22
chiggers   316–17
chikungunya   287
child protection   370
children
  anaemia   38–9
    iron deficiency   339
  ascariasis   209
  breathlessness   14
  brucellosis   276
  Chagas' disease   155
  cholera   195
  fever   26, 28
  hepatitis B vaccination   221
  HIV infection   30, 105, 106
    prevalence   104
    transmission reduction   106
  intestinal parasite load   356
  leprosy   181
  malaria   38
    cerebral   60
  malnutrition
    aetiology   373
    classification   **374**
    clinical features   374
    community-based
      therapeutic care   377
    HIV   377
    investigations   374
    management   375–7
    tuberculosis   377
  pneumonia   233
    risk   234
  pyogenic meningitis   246
  pyrexia of unknown origin   31

refugees   370, 371
  respiratory illness   12
  Reye's syndrome   26
  schistosomiasis   162
  shigellosis   193
  snake bite   344
  swollen belly syndrome   322
  tetanus vaccination   273
Chinese paralytic syndrome *see*
        acute motor axonal
        neuropathy (AMAN)
chlamydia   46, 104
  HIV infection risk   104
chloramphenicol   111, 112, 237,
        250, 251, 283, 285, 302,
        376
  African tick typhus   305
  Haemophilus influenzae
        meningitis   251
  louse-borne typhus   304
  meningococcal disease   250
  pneumococcal disease   250–1
  resistance   305
  scrub typhus   305
chlorguanide   69
chloroquine   65, 66, 67, 190
  amoebiasis   189
  malaria prophylaxis   69, 70
  malaria therapy   65, 66, 67
chlorpromazine   344, 362
chlorpropamide   350, 351
cholangiocarcinoma, oriental liver
        fluke   228
cholangitis
  ascariasis   209
  oriental liver fluke   228
cholecystitis   3
cholera   5, 195
  antimicrobial agents   197
  control   197–8
  diagnosis   196–7
  diarrhoea   196, 197
  epidemiology   195–7
  maintenance
        hydration   197
  microbiology   195
  pandemic   196
  pathogenesis   195
  prevention   197–8
  rehydration   197
  treatment   197
  vaccine   198
cholera vibrios   9, 196

chromoblastomycosis
  diagnosis 331
  treatment 331
chronic Chagas'
      disease 155–6
chronic disseminated
      histoplasmosis 328
chronic neurological disorders 17
chronic obstructive pulmonary
      disease (COPD) 11, 14
  asthma differential
      diagnosis 356
chronic pulmonary
      histoplasmosis 328
chronic strongyloidiasis 323
chronic ulceration 312
Chrysomia bezziana (Old World
      screw fly) 317
Chrysops 146
chyluria 143, 145
cimetidine 205
cinchonism 66
ciprofloxacin 8, 112, 203
  bacillary dysentery 193
  pneumonia 237
  pyogenic meningitis 250
  relapsing fevers 302
  scrub typhus 305
  sexually transmitted
      infections 42
  typhoid carriers 285
circulation in coma 19
circumcision
  hepatitis B transmission 218
  HIV infection risk 106
classical Guillain–Barré
      syndrome *see* acute inflam-
      matory
      demyelinating
      polyneuropathy (AIDP)
classical histoplasmosis 328–9
  clinical features 328
  diagnosis 328–9
  treatment 329
clofazimine 178, 180, 181
*Clonorchis sinensis see Opisthorchis
      sinensis*
Clostridium difficile 7, 191
Clostridium tetani 272, 273
co-artem malaria therapy 66
cobalamin *see* vitamin B$_{12}$ deficiency
coca-colonization 348
codeine phosphate 110, 113

cognitive behaviour therapy
      (CBT) 362
coinfection
  hepatitis D 221
colitis
  amoebic 187, 189
colon
  pseudopolyposis 164
  strictures in amoebiasis 187
colonoscopy in amoebiasis 189
Colorado tick fever 288
coma
  cerebral malaria 59
  hyperosmolar non-ketotic 350
  P. falciparum malaria 58–9, 60
  rapid assessment 19–23
coma scale 20, **21**
commercial sex workers 102, 106
community-based therapeutic care
      (CTC) 367, 377
Community-Directed Treatment
      with Ivermectin
      (ComDT) 139–40, 146
complex humanitarian
      emergencies (CHEs) 365
condoms 47, 106, 223
Conn's syndrome 353
consciousness, altered 58–9
contractures in viral
      encephalitis 260
convulsions in malaria 64
copper 376
Cordylobia anthropophaga (Tumbu
      fly) 316
corticosteroids 3, 28, 96
cosmetic surgery 181
co-trimoxazole 237, 376
  brucellosis 278
  HIV infection and disease 98,
      111, 113, 115
  Madura foot 331
  melioidosis 310
  typhoid 283, 285
cough 11–12
  brucellosis 276
  HIV infection 111, 112
  immunosuppression 16
  relapsing fevers 302
  tuberculosis 90
Councilman bodies 300
coxsackie virus 262
Crimean–Congo haemorrhagic fever
      (CCHF) 289, 294–5

Councilman bodies 300
  management 290
crithidia *see* epimastigotes
Crohn's disease 340
cromoglycate 357
croup 12
crusted scabies 320
cryptococcal meningitis (CM) 254
  clinical features 254
  diagnosis 254–5
  organism and epidemiology 254
  treatment 255
cryptococcosis 30, 254
  HIV infection 109
Cryptococcus 266
Cryptococcus neoformans 108, 254,
      255
Cryptosporidium hominis 201
Cryptosporidium parvum 191, 200,
      201, 202
Cryptosporidium spp. 201
Culex 142, 260, 287, 288, 295
Culex pipiens 258
Culex tritaeniorhynchus 256
Culiseta mosquitoes 260
Cushing's syndrome 353
cutaneous larva migrans 318
  clinical features 318
  parasitology 318
  prevention 319
  treatment 318–19
cutaneous oedema 155
Cyclops (copepod) 326
Cyclospora 203
Cyclospora cayetanensis 191, 202
Cyclospora oocysts 202
cysticercosis 34, 205–6
  epilepsy 360
cysts, eradication of 189–90
cytomegalovirus 108

dairy products, brucellosis 275, 279
dapsone 178
  DDS syndrome 178
  pregnancy 181
DDS syndrome 178
DDT 321
  louse treatment 321
  malaria 71
  sandfly eradication 79
decorticate posturing 22–3
deep tissue invasion 312
deferiprone 335

dehydration
  in adults **6**
  cholera 195, 196
  prevention 376
  see also oral rehydration solution;
      rehydration, cholera
delayed hyperaesthesia 150
delirium, scrub typhus 305
delta hepatitis *see* hepatitis D virus
      (HDV)
delusions 361–2
demographic transition
  non-communicable diseases **348**
dengue fever (DF) 29, 296, 298
  clinical features 296–8
  dengue haemorrhagic fever
      (DHF) 298
      pathogenesis 299
  differential diagnosis **299**
  epidemiology 296
  fever in HIV infection 30
  investigations 298
  leptospirosis differential
      diagnosis 302
  management 298–9
  manifestations 299
  prevention 299
  vaccines 299
dengue haemorrhagic fever
      (DHF) 35, 296, 298, 299
dengue shock syndrome (DSS) 298
dengue virus 288
depressive disorder 362
dermacentor ticks 288
Dermatobia hominis (bot fly) 316
dermatological presentations
  bullae 34
  creeping eruptions 32–3
  papules 33
  petechial rashes 34–5
  pigmentation, changes in 34
  skin itching 32
  skin nodules 33–4
  skin ulcers 32
  urticaria 34
desferrioxamine 335
dexamethasone 28, 205–6, 243,
      251
dextrose 376
diabetes mellitus 348–52
  care organization 351–2
  causes 349–50
  complications 350

diagnosis 349
    WHO criteria **349**
  diet 350
  epidemiology 348–9
  fibrocalculous pancreatic 350
  leprosy differential
      diagnosis 177
  malnutrition-modulated 350
  malnutrition-related 350
  management 350–1
  nurse-led care 352
  pneumonia risk 234
  prevalence 349
  type 1 349
  type 2 349
diabetic ketoacidosis (DKA)
      12, 350
  pneumonia differential
      diagnosis 235
  treatment 351
      in resource-poor
          settings **351**
diamorphine 268
diarrhoea 5–9
  Campylobacter jejuni 263
  cholera 196, 197
  clinical syndromes 5–7
  dehydration **6**
  examination 5
  giardiasis 200
  history 4–5
  HIV infection 9, 113
  host factors 5
  investigations 7–9, **8**
  management 9
  pneumonia 233, 234
diazepam 260, 345, 360
Dicrocoelium dendriticum 191
didanosine (ddi) 116
diencephalon damage 21
Dientamoeba fragilis 185
diet in diabetes mellitus 350
diethylcarbamazine citrate
      (DEC) 138, 146
  provocative test 143–4
  tropical pulmonary
      eosinophilia 245
  visceral larva migrans 213
diffuse cutaneous leishmaniasis
      (DCL) 80, 81, 82
diffuse encephalopathies 20, 21
diloxanide furoate 189
diphtheria 19

tetanus and pertussis (DTP)
      immunization 273
diphyllobothriasis 206
Diphyllobothrium latum
      (diphyllobothriasis)
      206, 266
dipylidiasis 206
Dipylidium caninum
      (dipylidiasis) 206
direct agglutination test (DAT) 76
direct observation of therapy
      (DOT) 96–7
disseminated intravascular
      coagulation (DIC) 35
  malaria 61, 64
      P. falciparum 61
  splenectomy 51
disturbed behaviour 362
Dobrova virus 294
dogs
  control 271
  hydatid disease 229, 231
  leishmaniasis 78
  rabies 267
dot immunoassay tests, HIV
      testing 103
doxycycline 197, 302, 307, 310
  African tick typhus 305
  brucellosis 278
  filariasis 144
  leptospirosis 307, 308
  louse-borne typhus 304
  malaria prophylaxis 69
  onchocerciasis 139
  scrub typhus 305
dracunculiasis *see* guinea worm
      infection
Dracunculus medinensis (guinea
      worm; dracunculiasis) 326
drug users, injecting
  hepatitis B 220
  hepatitis D 221
  HIV prevalence 104
  HIV transmission 105
Duffy blood group antigen 62
dumb rabies 267
Durban's sign 187
dysentery 192
  amoebic 358
  bacillary 192–4
  trichuris 212
dysphagia 3
  HIV infection 30

dyspnoea   11
   malaria   61
   relapsing fevers   302

Eastern equine encephalitis   *259*
Ebola Cote d'Ivoire   294
Ebola fever   35, 294
Ebola Reston   294
Ebola Sudan   294
Ebola Zaire   294
Echinococcus granulosus (cystic
         hydatid disease)   229–31
   clinical features   229–30
   investigations   230
   life cycle   229
   prevention and control   231
   treatment   230–1
Echinococcus multilocularis (alveolar
         hydatid disease)   231–2
   clinical features   232
   investigations   232
   life cycle   231–2
   treatment   232
Echinococcus vogeli   229
echovirus   262
ectopic disease   241, 243
ectopic flukes   226
eczema   32
education
   asthma   358
   epilepsy   360
   HIV infection   106
   hypertension   354
efavirenz (EFV)   116
eflornithine   152, 153
elapids   342
electroconvulsive therapy   362
electrolyte imbalance   9, 376
elephantiasis, filariasis   142
ELISA testing
   brucellosis   277
   HIV testing   102
empyema   27, 236
emtricitabine (FTC)   116, 220
encephalitis   19, 256–60
   arboviral   256
   causes   256, **257**
   complications   260
   epilepsy   359
   equine encephalitis
         viruses   260
   global distribution   *259*
   Japanese encephalitis   256–8

La Crosse virus   260
   management   260
   Murray valley encephalitis
         virus   258
   St Louis encephalitis virus   258
   tick-borne encephalitis virus   258
   viral   299
   West Nile virus   258
Encephalitozoon intestinalis   203
encephalopathy   17
   metabolic   299
   reactive arsenical   152
endocarditis   239, 278
Endolimax nana   185
endoscopic retrograde cholan-
         giopancreatography
         (ERCP)   228
Entamoeba dispar (amoebiasis)
         185, 188, 189, 190
Entamoeba gingivalis   185
Entamoeba hartmanni   185
Entamoeba histolytica
         (amoebiasis)   7, 188, 190,
         191, 200, 358
   life cycle   185–6
   liver invasion   187
   virulence factor   189
Entamoeba moshkovskii   185
Entamoeba polecki   185
enteric fever   5
   see also typhoid fever
enterobacteriacae   280
Enterobius vermicularis (pinworm;
         threadworm)   191
Enterocytozoon bieneusi   191, 202,
         203
Enterotest capsule   324
enterovirus 71   262
envenoming
   marine   345–6
   scorpion stings   344–5
   snake bite   342, 343
   spider bites   345
enzyme-linked immunotransfer blot
         (EITB)   230
enzymopathies   335
   see also glucose-6-phosphate
         dehydrogenase (G6PD)
         deficiency
eosinophilia   166-7
epidemic polyarthritis   288
epidemics, control   368–9
epidemiological transition   348

features   **348**
epilepsy   359–60, *361*
   care organization   360, *361*
   causes   359
   classification   **359**
   complications   360
   cysticercosis   205
   diagnosis   359
   epidemiology   359
   management   360
   prevalence   359
epimastigotes   148, 155
epinephrine *see* adrenaline
epistaxis in brucellosis   276
Epstein–Barr virus (EBV)
   malaria endemic areas   63
equine encephalitis viruses   260
erythema nodosum   33
erythema nodosum leprosum
         (ENL) reaction   175,
         179–80
erythromycin   111, 237, 302
Escherichia coli   6, 185, 192
Escherichia coli O157:H7   193
espundia   81
ethambutol   92
extended programme on
         immunization (EPI)   221
eye disease
   leprosy   176, **177**
   onchocerciasis   136–7
eye worm *see Loa loa*
         infection
eyes
   movements   21–2
   venom spitting   344

F75 (75 kcal/100 mL of milk)   376,
         376
F100 (100 kcal/100 mL of
         milk)   376–7, **376**
fasciola excretory–secretory
         (FES)   227
Fasciola gigantica (liver fluke)   226
Fasciola hepatica (liver fluke)   191,
         226, 227
Fasciolopsis buski (intestinal
         fluke)   228
febrile illness *see* fever
feeding   376
   malnutrition   376
feeding programmes,
         selective/therapeutic   367

fever 26–31
  acute 28
  African tick typhus 305
  brucellosis 275–6
  chronic 29
  clinical problems 30–1
  examination 26–7
  history 26 26
  HIV infection 28, 30, 111, 112
  investigation 27–8
  louse-borne typhus 304
  malaria 57
  pathogenesis 26
  respiratory illness 14
  scrub typhus 305
  symptomatic treatment 26
  treatment 28–9
fever–arthralgia–rash (FAR)
        syndrome 296
  arboviruses 287–8
fibrocalculous pancreatic
        diabetes (FCPD) 350
filariasis 133
  bancroftian 142, 143
  brugian 143
  control 145–6
  diagnosis 143–4
  lymphatic 140–2, *141*
  management 144
  treatment 144–5
filariform larvae 142, 211
Filovirus 294
finger clubbing in tuberculosis 90
fish, venomous 345
fish tank granuloma 331
fish tapeworm 206, 266
fisherman's itch 162
flaviviruses 256, 262
flexible gastroduodenoscopy 324
flucloxacillin 111, 251
fluconazole 83, 113, 114
  cryptococcal meningitis 255
  histoplasmosis 329
  HIV prophylaxis 115
flucytosine 255, 331
fluoroquinolone 193, 252, 278,
        283
fluoxetine 362, 364
flupenthixol 362
fluphenazine 362
fluroquinolones 113
folate 37, 376
  deficiency 339–40

supplements in sickle cell
        disease 334
folic acid *see* folate
Fonsecaea pedrosoi
        (chromoblastomycosis)
        331
food, humanitarian
        emergencies 366–8
food contamination
  paratyphoid 280, 286
  typhoid 280
food poisoning 5
foreign bodies, ingestion 3
formol gel test (FGT) 75
fungal infections 34
  chromoblastomycosis 331
  mycetoma 330–1
  nails 111
  skin 32
  sporotrichosis 331
funnel-web spider 345
furazolidone 197, 201
furuncle 33

gastritis 3
  see also stomach
gastrointestinal infections in refu-
        gees/asylum seekers 371
gastrointestinal presentations
  abdominal pain 3–4
  diarrhoea 4–9
  dysphagia 3
  haematemesis 3
  malabsorption 4
  see also named regions
generalized tetanus 272
Geneva Convention 365
genital herpes simplex 104
genital mutilation, female 370
genital ulcer disease 40, **41**, *45*, 46
gentamicin 112, 251, 278, 376
Giardia 199, 200, 201
Giardia duodenalis 199
Giardia intestinalis 199
Giardia lamblia 4, 199, 200
giardiasis 199
  clinical features 199–200
  differential diagnosis 200
  epidemiology 199
  investigations 200
  life cycle 199
  management 200–1
  parasite 199

prevention 201
public health 201
gibbus 265
GlaxoSmithKline (GSK) 146
glibenclamide 351, 352
Global Alliance for the Elimination
        of Lymphatic Filariasis
        (GAELF) 145–6
Global Buruli Ulcer Initiative 315
Glossina fuscipes 153
glossitis 379
glucose, blood levels
  malaria 64
glucose-6-phosphate dehydrogenase
        (G6PD) deficiency 61, 62,
        68, 178, 335, 336
  clinical features 335–6
  diagnosis 336
  epidemiology 335
  management 336
glucose–electrolyte solutions 197
glucose tolerance test (GTT) 349
gonorrhoea 46
  HIV infection risk 104
ground itch 211
growth retardation, whipworm 212
Guillain–Barré syndrome 19, *261*,
        262, 263
guinea worm infection
  clinical features 326
  control 327
  diagnosis 326
  distribution *327*
  life cycle 326
  treatment 327

haematemesis 3
haematinic deficiencies
  cobalamin deficiency
        clinical features 340
        investigations 340
        management 340
  folate deficiency
        clinical features 339
        investigations 339–40
        management 340
  iron deficiency
        clinical features 338
        investigations 338–9
        management 339
haemoglobin
  genotype 63
  measurement 38

haemoglobin (*Continued*)
  sickle 333
haemoglobinopathies 333
  β thalassaemia 335
  clinical features 334
  diagnosis 334
  epidemiology 334
  management 334–5
  protection against malaria 334
  sickle cell anaemia 333
haemoglobinuria, malaria 61
haemolytic anaemia 178, 282
haemolytic uraemic syndrome 193
Haemophilus ducreyi 104
Haemophilus influenzae 14, 111,
  237
Haemophilus influenzae type b
  (Hib) 239, 246
  epidemiology 248
  management 251
  vaccines 248
haemoptysis 12
haemorrhage 187
haemorrhagic fever with renal
  syndrome (HFRS) 290,
  294
haemorrhoids 338
hairy string test 324
hallucinations 361
halofantrine 68
haloperidol 361, 362
Hansen's disease 171
  see also leprosy
Hantaan fever **290**, 294
Hantaan virus 294
hantavirus pulmonary
  syndrome 294
HBeAg 217, *218*
HbF 37, 333
HbS 333, 334
HBsAg 216, 217
  endemicity *219*
head injury 359
head lice 321
headache 19
Heaf test 86
health care, in humanitarian
  emergencies 368
health care workers
  HIV prophylaxis 115, 117, 118
  HIV transmission 105–6
heart failure, hypertensive 354
Helicobacter pylori 3, 191, 199

helminths, soil-transmitted *see*
  soil-transmitted helminths
hemiparesis 22
hemispheric signs 23
HemoCue Hb 301 system 37
Henoch–Schönlein purpura 35
hepatitis
  amoebic liver abscess differential
    diagnosis 188
  dengue 299
  fever 27
  viral 215
hepatitis A virus (HAV) 216, 223
hepatitis B virus (HBV)
    216–20, *217, 218*
  asylum seekers 371
  immunization 220–1
hepatitis C virus (HCV) 222–3
  asylum seekers 371
hepatitis D virus (HDV) 221–2
hepatitis E virus (HEV) 223, *224*
hepatocellular carcinoma
    (HCC) 216, 223, 225
hepatoma *see* hepatocellular
    carcinoma
hepatomegaly 27
  fever 27
  leishmaniasis 74
  liver fluke 226
  oriental liver fluke 228
  relapsing fevers 302
hepatosplenomegaly, scrub
    typhus 305
herpes simplex 104
herpes viruses 266
herpes zoster 110–11
hiatus hernia 338
highly active antiretroviral therapy
    (HAART) 17, 31, 75
Histoplasma capsulatum var
    capsulatum 328, 329
Histoplasma capsulatum var
    duboisii (African
    histoplasmosis) 328
histoplasmosis 328
  African histoplasmosis 328–9
  classical histoplasmosis 328–9
  disseminated 328
  HIV infection 329
  pulmonary 328
HIV-1 101–2
HIV-2 101–2
HIV infection 101–20

antiretroviral therapy 115–16
asylum seekers 371
clinical problems 110–14
control strategies 106–7
cough and fever 111–12
cutaneous leishmaniasis 82
disease mechanisms 107–8
early disease 109
economic impact 107
epidemiology 103–4
epilepsy 359
fever 30
HIV-1 101–2
HIV-2 101–2
late disease 110
latent phase 109
leishmaniasis coinfection 75
malaria 62
natural history 109–10
pathogenesis 107
prophylaxis 114–20
public health 40
refugees 368
respiratory illness 15–16
seroconversion 109
seroprevalence 104
skin problems 110
staging 108–9
surveillance 103–4
and TB 89, 90–1, 98–9, 377
testing 47, 102–3, **103**
toxoplasmosis 114
transmission 104–6
  infected blood 105–6
  risk 104–5
  sexual 104
  vertical 105
viruses 101
see also AIDS
HIV myelopathy 266
hookworm
  clinical features 211
  epidemiology 210
  investigations 211–12
  iron deficiency 338
  life cycle 211
  management 212
  parasites 211
  prevention and public health
    aspects 212
hookworm folliculitis 318
house dust mites 356
human herpes virus 8 113

human resources/training,
humanitarian
emergencies 369
human T lymphotrophic
virus type 1 (HTLV-1) 266
humanitarian emergencies 365–9
communicable diseases
control 368–9
coordination 369
emergency phase 365, **366**
epidemics control 368
food 366–8
health care 368
human resources and training 369
initial assessment 366
measles immunization 366
mid-upper arm circumference 367
nutrition 366–8
post-emergency phase 369
public health surveillance 369
in resource-poor countries 365
shelter and site planning 368
water and sanitation 366
Hyalomma 294
hydatid cyst disease *see Echinococcus*
granulosus
hydatid disease 229
Echinococcus granulosus 229–31
Echinococcus multilocularis 231–2
hydralazine 354
hydrocele, filariasis 142
hydrocephalus 205
hydrophobia 267
hydroxycobalamin injections 340
hygiene
amoebiasis prevention 190
ascariasis 209
asthma 356
giardiasis 201
helminth infections 208
shigellosis 193–4
hymenolepiasis 206
Hymenolepis diminuta 206
Hymenolepis nana 191, 204, 206
hyperosmolar non-ketotic coma
(HNK) 350
hyper-reactive malarial
splenomegaly 50–1
hypertension 352–5
care organization 354–5
causes 353
complications 353–4
diagnosis 353

epidemiology 352–3
management 354
prevalence 353
risk factors 353
hypertensive crisis 354
hypertrophic lichen planus 34
hyperventilation 22
hypnozoite 55
hypochlorhydria 5
hypoglycaemia
diabetes mellitus 350
malaria 64
P. falciparum 61
malnutrition
prevention 375–6
hypothermia prevention 376

imipramine 362
immunosuppression
amoebiasis 190
cough 16
HIV 108–9
malaria 63
impetigo, bullous 34
indirect fluorescent antibody test
(IFAT) 63
infants
exposure to sandfly bites 83
hepatitis B virus 218
vaccination 221
low birth weight in malaria 69
infections
asylum seekers 370
asylum seekers 371
diabetes mellitus 350
log–normal distribution 161
malnutrition 376
multidrug-resistant 371
refugees 371
see also fungal infections
infectious mononucleosis
fever 27
infectious neurological diseases 17
inflammatory diarrhoea
clinical features **6**
pathogens in **7**
insect bites 32
see also bites and stings
insecticide-treated nets (ITNs) 72
insulin 351
Integrated Management of Childhood
Illness (IMCI) strategy 14
interferon-γ (IFN-γ) 172

interleukin 1 26
interleukin 2 172
interleukin 6 26
intermittent presumptive
therapy (IPT) 69
internally displaced persons
(IDPs) 365
international normalized ratio
(INR) 215
intestinal amoebiasis 186–7
intestinal cestode infections
cysticercosis 205–6
diphyllobothriasis 206
hymenolepiasis and
dipylidiasis 206
life cycle 204–5
management 206
parasites 204–5
prevention 206
intestinal flukes 228
intestinal obstruction 3
ascariasis 209
intestinal parasite load 356
intestinal protozoal infections 201
Balantidium coli 202
Blastocystis hominis 202
clinical features 201
Cryptosporidium parvum 201
Cyclospora cayetanensis 202
investigations 202
Isospora belli 201–2
life cycle 201
management 202–3
microsporidia 202
parasite 201
intestinal TB 4
intracranial pressure, raised
cerebral malaria 60
cryptococcal meningitis 255
lung fluke 243
viral encephalitis 260
intravenous magnesium 273, 346
invasive amoebiasis 189
iodoquinol 190
iron chelation 335
iron deficiency
clinical features 338
investigations 338–9
management 339
iron-deficient red cells 38
isoniazid 92, 115
tuberculosis 92
preventive therapy 96

Isospora 113, 202, 203
Isospora belli 190, 201–2
Isospora oocysts 202
itching, skin 32
itraconazole 83, 329, 331
ivermectin 213, 319, 320, 324–5
 loiasis 146
 microfilariae 144, 145
 onchocerciasis 138–9, 140
Ixodes ticks 258

Japanese encephalitis 262
 clinical features 257
 epidemiology 256–7
 future developments 258
 investigations 257
 management 257
 prevention and public
  health 257–8
 transmission cycle *258*
Jarisch–Herxheimer reaction 302
jaundice 188, 335
 causes *216*
 malaria 57
jellyfish, venomous 345–6
jiggers *see* chiggers

K39 test 76
Kaposi's sarcoma 34, 82, 101,
  113–14
 nodules 34
 pulmonary 111
Katayama fever 26, 162, 165
 oriental liver fluke (similar
  syndrome) 227
Kérandel's sign 150
keratomalacia 378
Kernig's sign 17, 21
ketoacidosis *see* diabetic ketoacidosis
ketoconazole 83, 331
kissing bugs *see* triatomine bugs
Koplick's spots 27
kraits 344
kwashiorkor 373, 377
 pneumonia risk 234

La Brea 222
La Crosse encephalitis *259*, 260
labetolol 273
lactase deficiency 4
lagophthalmos 176, 180
lamivudine (3TC) 116, 220
Lantana camora 153
large bowel, diarrhoea 5, 7
larva currens 33, 318

clinical features 323
 rash 324
larva migrans 32
 cutaneous 318–19
 hookworm 211
 ocular 213
 prevention 318–19
 visceral 213
laryngotracheobronchitis 12
Lassa fever 35, 290, 291
 management 293
latrines, refugee camps 366
Latrodectus (widow spiders) 345
left ventricular hypertrophy 354
*Leishmania*80
 lifecycle 73–4
Leishmania chagasi 73, 80
Leishmania donovani 73, 76, 80
Leishmania infantum 73, 75, 80
Leishmania tropica 73, 75, 80
leishmaniasis, cutaneous 80–4
 clinical features 80–2
 diffuse 81
 investigations 82
 management 82–3
 nodules 34
 prevention 83–4
 sporotrichosis differential
  diagnosis 331
 treatment 83
leishmaniasis, lupoid 81
leishmaniasis, mucocutaneous
  80, 82
leishmaniasis, mucosal 80
leishmaniasis, post-kala-azar dermal 34, 78
leishmaniasis, visceral 73–9
 circumstantial evidence 75
 clinical features 74
 epidemiology 73
 fever 27
 hepatomegaly 74
 HIV coinfection 73, 75
 host elimination 78
 investigations 75–6
 life cycle 73–4
 lymphadenopathy 74
 management 77–8
 massive tropical
  splenomegaly 49–50
 parasite 73–4
 parasitological evidence 76
 post-kala-azar dermal
  leishmaniasis 78

prevention 78–9
 serological evidence 75–6
 splenic aspirate 76
 splenomegaly 74
 vector elimination/
  avoidance 79
 viscerotropic 75
leishmaniasis recidivans (LR) 80, 82
leishmanin test 82
Lemierre's syndrome 29
lepromatous leprosy (LL) 82, *173*,
  176
leprosy 19, 27, 171–81
 anaesthesia 173, 175
 BCG vaccine 181
 borderline 176
 borderline lepromatous 176
 borderline states 173
 borderline tuberculoid 175–6
 cell-mediated immunity
  171, 173
 chemotherapy 177
 children 181
 classification 175–6
 clinical features 173–5
 clofazimine 178
 control 181
 dapsone 178
 delayed hypersensitivity
  reaction 179
 diagnosis 176–7
 differential diagnosis 177
 disability prevention 180–1
 elimination 181
 epidemiology 171
 eye 176
 foot care *180*
 forms 176
 granuloma formation 172
 hand care *180*
 immune response 172–3
 immunological features *172*
 incidence 171
 lepromatous 176
 leprosy provision, in general
  health services 181
 management 177–80
 microbiology 171–2
 multibacillary disease 175,
  178–9
  children 181
 multidrug therapy 178–9
 nerve damage 173–5
 neuritis 179, 180

nodules 33
paucibacillary 175, 177
    children 181
pigmentation change 34
polar 175
pregnancy 181
prevention 181
    of disability 180–1
reactions and nerve
        damage 179–82
reconstructive surgery 180–1
rifampicin 177–8
skin lesions 173
slit skin smears 177
tuberculoid 171, 172–3
tuberculoid leprosy 175
type 1 reactions 179
vaccines 181
women 181
see also erythema nodosum
        leprosum (ENL)
        reactions
Leptospira 306, 307
Leptospira bireflexa 306
Leptospira interrogans 306
leptospirosis 306
    aseptic meningitis
    cardiac syndrome
    clinical features 306–607
    diagnosis 307
    epidemiology 306
    microbiology 306
    pathogenesis 306
    prevention 308
    pulmonary syndrome
    treatment 307–8
    Weil's disease
leucopenia 298
leukaemia38
    chronic myeloid 49
levamisole 210, 212
Lhermitte's sign 266
lice 321
lichen planus 34
liposomal amphotericin B
        (AmBisome) 77
Liv-52 215
live attenuated oral vaccine
        (Ty21a) 285
liver 67, 74, 150
    schistosomal fibrosis 164–5
liver abscess
    amoebic 27, 112, 187, 236
        aspiration 190

complications 188
differential diagnosis 188
drainage 190
pneumonia differential
        diagnosis 236
treatment 189, 190
ascariasis 209
liver cancer,
        cholangiocarcinoma 228
    see also hepatocellular carcinoma
liver failure, dengue 299
liver flukes 226
    clinical features 226
    epidemiology 226
    investigations 227
    management 227
    oriental 227–8
    parasites and life cycles 226
    prevention and public health
        aspects 227
Loa loa infection 133, 139, 140,
        145, 146
localized tetanus 273
Löffler's syndrome 209
log–normal distribution 161–2
loiasis 133
    diagnosis 146
    treatment 146–7
lopinavir/ritonavir 116
louse 301
    body 301, 304, 321
    head 301, 321
    infestation in refugees/asylum
        seekers 321
    pubic 321
louse-borne relapsing fever
        (LBRF) 31
    clinical features 302
    diagnosis 302
    epidemiology 301–2
    fatality rate 302
    pathology 302
    prevention 303
    treatment 302–3
louse-borne typhus 304, 321
    clinical features 304
    treatment 304
lower respiratory tract infection
        (LRTI) 14, 233
Loxosceles (recluse spider) 345
lumbar puncture (LP) 23–5, 27, 28
    pyogenic meningitis 249
lung fluke 241
    clinical features 241

diagnosis 243
distribution *242*
ectopic disease 241, 242
life cycle 241
lung disease 241
treatment 243
lung function testing 14, 244
lungs/lung disease 89
    histoplasmosis 238
    hookworm larval migration 211
    hydatid cyst disease 230
    leptospirosis pulmonary
        syndrome 307
    lung fluke 241
    pathology 188
    pneumonia risk 234
    schistosomiasis 164
    trans-thoracic aspirate 236
lupus vulgaris 82
lymphadenitis, tuberculosis 89, 90
lymphadenopathy
    African tick typhus 305
    brucellosis 276
    fever 27
    filariasis 140
    leishmaniasis 74
    scrub typhus 305
lymphatic filariasis (LF) 140–2
    distribution *141*
    individual and community
        chemotherapy **140**
lymphoedema
    management 145
lymphoma 266
    fever 27
    massive tropical
        splenomegaly 49
    primary CNS 108

macrocytic anaemia 37–8, 266
macrolide 42, 237
macrophages 74, 107, 281
Madura foot *see* mycetoma
Madurella mycetomatis
        (mycetoma) 330, 331
magnesium 273, 346
magnetic resonance imaging
        (MRI) 189
malabsorption 4
    diarrhoea 7
malaria 55–72
    anaemia 59
    asylum seekers 371
    cerebral 59–60

malaria (*Continued*)
    protective effect of
        ascariasis 208
    chemoprophylaxis 69–70
    children 38, 39
    clinical features 57
    complicated 58, 59
    congenital 62
    control 71–2
    diagnosis 63–4
    diarrhoea 5
    drug resistance 68
    epidemiology 70–1
    fever27, 28, 30, 57
        classical stages 57–8
    G6PD protection 335
    global eradication 71–2
    HIV infection 30, 62
    hyper-reactive malarial
        splenomegaly 50–1
    immune disorders 62–3
    immunity 62–3, 71
    immunosuppression 63
    importance and distribution 55
    individual precautions 72
    intermittent presumptive
        therapy 69
    jaundice 57
    leptospirosis differential
        diagnosis 307
    life cycle 55–7, *56*
    massive tropical
        splenomegaly 49–50
    measuring in community 70–1
    morbidity 70
    mortality 70
    peculiarities 58–61
    placental 69
    precautions 72
    pregnancy 61–2
        intermittent presumptive
        therapy 69
    protective factors 62
    quartan 57
    refugees 371
    relapse 69
    severe 58, 61, 65
    splenomegaly 57
    stable 71
    subtertian 57
    tertian 57
    treatment 64–8
        chemotherapy 64–8
        combination therapy 68

    supportive 64
    unstable 71
    untreated 58
Malarone 68
malathion 321
malnutrition
    in adults 377–9
        vitamin A 378
        vitamin B1 (thiamine) 378
        vitamin B6 (niacin or nico-
            tinic acid) 378
        vitamin C (ascorbic
            acid) 378
        vitamin D 378–9
        vitamin deficiencies
            manifestations 379
    in children 373–7
        aetiology 373
        classification **374**
        clinical features 374
        community-based
            therapeutic care 377
        HIV 377
        investigations 374
        management 375–7
        tuberculosis 377
    definition 373
    humanitarian emergencies 365
    humanitarian emergencies 366–7
    oedematous 373
    tuberculosis 89
    viral encephalitis 260
malnutrition-modulated diabetes
        mellitus (MMDM) 350
malnutrition-related diabetes
        mellitus (MRDM) 350
Malta fever *see* brucellosis
Mansonia 142, 143
Mantoux test 86
marasmus, pneumonia risk 234
marburg haemorrhagic
        fevers 294
marine envenoming
    jellyfish 345–6
    venomous fish 345
mass chemotherapy 169–70
massive splenomegaly 49–50
mature flukes 161, 226
Mazzotti reaction 138, 144, 146
mean corpuscular haemoglobin
        (MCH) 339
mean corpuscular haemoglobin
        concentration
        (MCHC) 339

measles 27, 28
    immunization 366
    pneumonia risk 234
mebendazole 209, 210, 212, 213,
        232
    alveolar hydatid disease 232
    ascariasis 210
    hookworm 212
    trichuriasis 212
    visceral larva migrans 213
mefloquine
    malaria prophylaxis 70
    malaria therapy 67–8
mega-oesophagus 3
meglumine antimonate
        (Glucantime) 77
melarsoprol 152, 153
melioidosis
    clinical features 309
    diagnosis 309
    epidemiology 309
    pathogenesis 309
    prognosis 310
    treatment 310
meningism 17, 20
    coma 23
    pneumonia 234
meningitis 19
    aseptic in leptospirosis 307
    cryptococcal17, 28, 246, 248
        HIV infection 255
        pyogenic meningitis
            differential diagnosis
            248
        raised intracranial
            pressure 255
    epilepsy 359
    meningococcal 250, 252
        control of epidemics 252
    pneumonia 234
    pyogenic 246
        clinical features 248
        complications 251–2
        diagnosis 249–52
        differential diagnosis **248**
        empirical therapy 251
        epidemic control 252
        epidemiology 246–8
        management 249–52
        vaccination 247
    tuberculosis 265
    typhoid 282
    vaccination 248
meningitis belt 246, *247*

meningococcal disease
  in Africa 247
  empirical therapy 251
  epidemic control **252**
  epidemiology 246–7
  management 250
  vaccines 248
meningococcus 252
meningoencephalitis 262, 302
  brucellosis 276
  louse-borne typhus 304
menorrhagia 211, 338
mental illness 361–4
  assessment 361
  bipolar affective disorder 362–3
  care organization 364
  depression 362
  post-traumatic stress
        disorder 363–4
  schizophrenia 361–2
    treatment 362
mercaptoethanol 276
Merck & Co. Inc 146
meropenem 251
merozoites 55–6, 57
mesenteric adenitis 3
metabolic acidosis 12
  cholera 197
  P. falciparum malaria 58
metacercariae 227, 228
metformin 250, 351, 352
methyldopa 354, 355
metriphonate 168
metronidazole 189, 190, 200, 203,
        273, 327
microbicides, vaginal 107
microhaematocrit (MHCT) 151
micronutrient deficiencies 376
microscopic agglutination
        (MAT) 277
Microsporidia 202
mid-upper arm circumference
        (MUAC) 367
migrants
  louse-borne typhus 304
  urbanization **348**
milk, brucellosis 275
miltefosine 77–8, 83
minianion exchange column
        technique (MAEC) 151
minocycline 179
mite typhus 305
mites, scabies 320
mononeuritis multiplex 19

Montenegro test 80
mosquitoes
  anopheline55, *56*
  arboviral encephalitis 256, 258,
        260
  arboviruses 287
  control 145–6
  dengue fever 296, 298
  filariasis vector 142
  Japanese encephalitis 256
  yellow fever 287
motor axonal neuropathy, acute
        (AMAN) 261, 263
motor neurones, spastic
        paralysis 264
mouth
  fever 27
  Kaposi's sarcoma 113–14
  see also candidiasis
moxifloxacin 99
mucosal leishmaniasis (ML) 81,
        82, 83
multidrug therapy 178–9, 181
mumps 249, 276
Murray valley encephalitis
        virus 258, *259*
mycetoma
  clinical features 330
  diagnosis 330–1
  epidemiology 330
  treatment 331
mycobacteria
  atypical infection 331
  faecal 113
  other than tuberculosis
        (MOTT) 85–6
Mycobacterium avium
        complex 30
Mycobacterium leprae (leprosy) 171,
        172, 173, 175, 177, 178,
        179, 181
  cell-mediated immunity 171
  delayed hypersensitivity
        reaction 179
  detection 177
  microbiology 171–2
Mycobacterium marinum (fish tank
        granuloma) 331
Mycobacterium tuberculosis
        (tuberculosis) 85, 93, 108,
        112, 119, 233,
        236, 249
Mycobacterium tuberculosis MTB
        complex 85

  culture 91
  delayed-type hypersensitivity
        reaction 86
  microbiology 85
  purified protein derivatives
        (PPD) 86, 92
Mycobacterium ulcerans (Buruli
        ulcer) 313
Mycobacterium vaccae 315
mycoplasma pneumoniae 265–6
myelitis 19
myelodysplastic syndrome 38
myelofibrosis 49
myiasis 316
  body cavity myiasis 317
  bot fly 316
  chiggers 316–17
  furuncular 33
  nasal 317
  Tumbu fly 316
Médecins Sans Frontières
        (MSF) 365

Naegleria fowleri 185
nails, fungal infections 111
nasal myiasis 317
natural disasters 365
Necator americanus (hook-
        worms) 208, 210
neck flexion 266
neck stiffness 21
needlestick injuries
  HIV prophylaxis 115
  HIV transmission 105–6
Neisseria gonorrhoea 41
Neisseria meningitidis 246
  see also meningococcus
neonatal anaemia 335
neonatal tetanus 272–3
nephropathy, diabetic 350
nephrosis, malarial 62
nephrotic syndrome 234
nerve damage 173–5
nerve tissue vaccines 270
neuritis, leprosy 179, 180
neurocysticercosis 205, 359, 360
neurological disorders 17–25, 27
  assessment 19–23
  causes **18, 19**
  chronic 17
  examination 20–2
  lumbar puncture,
        indications and contraindi-
        cations for 23–5

neurological disorders (*Continued*)
  pathology 19
  space occupying lesions 19
  syndromes 17, 19
neurological injury 12
neurological signs, focal 19, 248,
    256, 257
  coma 23
neuropathy 19
  diabetic 350
neuropsychiatric disorder,
    brucellosis 276
neuroschistosomiasis 165, 167, 169
neurotoxicity, snake bites 342, 344
nevirapine (NVP) 106, 116
niacin *see* vitamin B6
niclosamide 169, 206
nicotinic acid *see* vitamin B6
nifurtimox 153, 156
nitazoxanide 191, 202, 209
  ascariasis 210
  cestode infections 206
  giardiasis 201
  liver fluke 227
  trichuriasis 213
nitrofuran 336
nitrosamines, dietary 228
Nocardia brasiliensis
    (mycetoma) 330
nocardiosis 331
nocturnal dyspnoea 11
nodules, subcutaneous in
    onchocerciasis 136
non-communicable diseases
    (NCDs) 347–64
  asthma 355–9
  diabetes mellitus 348–52
  epidemiological transition 348
  epilepsy 359–60, *361*
  hypertension 352–5
  mental illness 361–4
  mortality patterns 347, **348**
  spectrum 347
non-governmental organizations
    (NGOs) 365
non-Hodgkin's lymphoma 108
non-infectious neurological
    disorders 17
non-inflammatory diarrhoea
  clinical features **6**
  pathogens in **7**
non-nucleoside reverse
    transcriptase inhibitors
    (NNRTI) 116

non-steroidal anti-
    inflammatory drugs
    (NSAIDs) 3, 338
  asthma trigger 356
non-typhi *Salmonella* (NTS) 108,
    112
normochromic anaemia 152
norovirus 191
norwegian scabies 110, 320
nose, mucosal leishmaniasis 81
nucleoside (or nucleotide) reverse
    transcriptase inhibitors
    (NRTI) 116
nutrition, humanitarian
    emergencies 366–7

obesity 348
  asthma incidence 356
  hypertension 353
occupation, respiratory illness 12
ocular larva migrans (OLM) 213
oculocephalic (doll's eye) reflex
    21
oculovestibular reflex 21–2
oedematous malnutrition 373,
    374, *375*
oesophageal carcinoma 3
oesophageal varices 3
oesophagitis 3
ofloxacin 179
Old World screw fly 317
older people
  pneumonia risk 234
Onchocerca volvulus 137, 139
  life cycle 133, 135
onchocerciasis 32, 34, 133
  clinical features 135–6
  control 139–40
  diagnosis 137–8
  distribution 133, *134*
  epidemiology 135
  finding microfilariae 137–8
  individual and community
    chemotherapy **140**
  life cycle 133, 135
  nodules 33
  pigmentation change 34
  subcutaneous nodules 136–7
  treatment 138–9
Onchocerciasis Control Programme
    (OCP) 139
Onchocerciasis Elimination
    Programme for the
    Americas (OEPA) 140

Oncomelania 160
Opiates 345
Opisthorchis felineus 227
Opisthorchis sinensis (liver
    fluke) 227
Opisthorchis viverrini (liver
    fluke) 227, 228
oral chloroquine 189
oral hypoglycaemic agents 350–1
oral rehydration solution 7
  cholera 197, 198
  refugee camps 9
oral rehydration therapy 6
orbital oedema 155
orchitis, brucellosis 276
oriental liver flukes
  clinical features 227–8
  epidemiology 227
  investigations 228
  life cycles 227
  management 228
  parasites 227
  prevention and public health
    aspects 228
Orientia tsutsugamushi (scrub
    typhus) 305
Ornithodoros 301
Orthopnoea 11
osteomyelitis 239
oxamniquine 168
oxygen supplementation 237
O'nyong nyong 287–8

pain response 22–3
PAIR (Puncture, Aspiration,
    Injection,
    Re-aspiration) 231
paludrine 69
pancreatitis
  ascariasis 209
  oriental liver fluke 228
papule 33, 80, 320
paracetamol 26, 64, 298
Paragonimus westermani 241
paraldehyde 360
paralysis 17
  acute flaccid 261–3
    anterior horn cell
      damage 262, 263
    immune-mediated
      causes 261, 262
  rabies 263, 268
  spastic 264–6
    causes 264–6

paralytic poliomyelitis 262
paratyphoid 280
    mode of infection 286
paravertebral plexus,
        schistosomiasis 165
parenteral penicillins 237
parkinsonian syndrome 257
paromomycin 83, 189, 201, 202,
        203
parotitis 193
particle agglutination tests, HIV
        testing 103
pathogens
    opportunistic 108
    stool 113
Pediculus capitis (head louse) 301,
        321
Pediculus humanus 301, 305, 321
pellagra 34, 378
pelvic inflammatory disease 27
pemphigus 34
penicillin 41, 145, 302,
        307
    meningococcal disease 250
    pneumococcal disease 250, 251
    pneumonia 237, 239
    resistance 239
    sickle cell disease 334
    tropical ulcer 312
penicillinase-resistant
        penicillin 111
Penicillium marneffiei 30
pentamidine
    trypanosomiasis 151, 152, 153
    visceral leishmaniasis 77
pentavalent antimonials 77
peptic strictures 3
peptic ulceration 3
perforated peptic ulcers 3
peripheral nervous system,
        leprosy 173
peritonitis 187
    amoebiasis 187
    fever 27
    granulomatous in ascariasis 210
permethrin 72, 305, 320, 321
pernicious anaemia 266, 340
pets 199
phaeochromacytoma 353
pharyngitis 27, 29
phenobarbital 360
phenothiazine 268
phenytoin 360
Phoneutria (banana spider) 345

Phthirus pubis (pubic louse) 301,
        321
phytates 338
pigmentation changes in skin 34
piles 79, 193
piperazine 210
pityriasis versicolor 32, 34
pivmecillinam 193
plaques 173, 176, 313, 314
Plasmodium falciparum 55, 56, 57,
        61, 63, 65, 66, 68, 69, 70, 208
    complicated malaria 58, 59
    diagnosis 63
    hyperpyrexia 58
    immunity 62
    infection peculiarities
        58–61, **59**
    protective factors 62
    untreated attack 58
Plasmodium knowlesi 55
Plasmodium malariae 55, 56, 57, 62
    untreated attack 58
Plasmodium ovale 55, 56, 57
    relapse 68
    untreated attack 58
Plasmodium vivax 55, 56, 57
    protective factors 62
    relapse 68
    untreated attack 58
pleural aspiration 236
pleural effusions 15, 90, 91, 146,
        236
pleural fluid 14, 15
pleurisy, tuberculosis 86, 89, 91
pneumococcal disease 115
    epidemiology 247–8
    management 250–1
    vaccines 248
    see also pneumococcal
        pneumonia; *Streptococcus
        pneumoniae*
pneumococcal pneumonia 15,
        236, 239
pneumococcal vaccines 240
Pneumocystis carinii pneumonia
        (PCP) 91, 237, 239
Pneumocystis jirovecii
        pneumonia 30, 31, 108,
        111, 115
Pneumocystis pneumonia 111, 115,
        236
pneumonia 5, 112, 254
    active vaccination 239
    antibiotic resistance 239

bacterial 11
chemoprophylaxis 239
children 233, 234, *235*, 237
clinical features 234–6
complications 237–9
diarrhea 5
differential diagnosis 235
epidemiology 233–4
fatality rate 234
fever 27
future developments 239–40
HIV infection 111, 112–13
inpatient therapy 237
investigations 236–7
louse-borne typhus 304
management 237–9
microbiological tests 236–7
microbiology 233
outpatient therapy 237
pleural aspiration 236
pneumococcal vaccines 109,
        240
prevention 239
radiology 236
risk factors for 234
sputum gram stain 236
sputum Ziehl–Neelsen stain 236
trans-thoracic lung aspirate 236
typhoid lobar 282
vaccination 239
viral encephalitis 260
pneumonitis
    ascaris 209
    hookworm 210
poisoning
    food poisoning 5
    pneumonia differential
        diagnosis 236
polar leprosy **175**
polio 262
poliomyelitis 261
polymerase chain reaction
        (PCR) 64, 67, 76, 138, 144,
        290, 302, 314
    and antigen detection 188–9
polymyositis 282
polyradiculopathy 19
porphyria 34
portal hypertension 27, 49, 74, 76,
        164, 167
post-dysenteric ulcerative
        colitis 187
posterior cervical
        lymphadenopathy 151

post-kala-azar dermal
    leishmaniasis (PKDL) 34,
    74, 78
post-traumatic stress disorder
    (PTSD) 363–4
Pott's disease 264
poverty and tuberculosis 97
praziquantel 168, 205, 206, 226,
    228, 231, 243, 360
  cestode infections 205
  cysticercosis 205
  lung fluke 243
  oriental liver fluke 228
prazosin 345
prednisolone 147, 179, 180, 181,
    357, 358
pregnancy
  brucellosis 278
  HIV testing 102
  HIV transmission 105, 106
  hypoglycaemia in
    P. falciparum malaria 60
  iron deficiency anaemia 338
  leprosy 181
  malaria 61–2
    intermittent presumptive
      therapy 69
  pigmentation 34
  and pneumonia 234
  tetanus vaccination 273–4
prevention of mother to child trans-
    mission (PMTCT) 106
primaquine 68, 336
proctitis, granular 193
procyclidine 362
proglottids 204, 229
proguanil 51, 67, 69
protein-losing enteropathy 193
pruritus, HIV infection 110
pseudopapillomas 164, 167
psychosis, typhoid fever 27
pubic and head lice 321
public health
  ascariasis 210
  brucellosis 278–9
  Buruli ulcer 315
  catastrophic emergencies 365
  giardiasis 201
  hookworm 212
  humanitarian emergencies 369
  Japanese encephalitis 257–8
  schistosomiasis 169–70
  sexually transmitted
    infections 40

shigellosis 193–4
toxocariasis 214
pulmonary eosinophilia
  pneumonia differential
    diagnosis 236
  see also tropical pulmonary
    eosinophilia
pulmonary Kaposi's
    sarcoma 16, 111
pulmonary syndrome
  of leptospirosis 307
punch biopsy 138
punctate keratitis 137
pupils, light reaction 21
purified protein derivatives (PPD)
    skin test 86, 92
Putzi fly 316
Puumula virus 294
pyogenic meningitis 246
  clinical features 248
  diagnosis 249–52
  differential diagnosis **248**
  epidemic control 252
  epidemiology 246–8
  management 249–52
pyrantel pamoate
  ascariasis 210
  hookworm 212
pyrazinamide 92
pyrexia of unknown origin
    (PUO) 31
pyrimethamine 203

quantitative buffy coat (QBC)
    technique 64, 151
Queensland tick typhus 305
quinacrine 201
quinfamide 190
quinine 61, 65, 66–7
quinolone 112

rabies 19, 267
  active immunization 269
  clinical features, in
    humans 267–8
  diagnosis 268
  in dog 267
  dumb 267
  first aid treatment 269
  flexibility, need for 270
  furious 267
  immediate treatment 269
  nerve tissue vaccines 270
  in animals 267

paralytic 263, 268
passive immunization 269
postexposure treatment 268–9
postexposure vaccine
    regimens 269–71
postmortem diagnosis 268
precautions with patients 268
pre-exposure immunization
    271
prevention 271
treatment 268
WHO recommended
    schedules 270
rabies immune globulin 269
rapid assessment procedures
    for loiasis (RAPLOA) 147
rapid dignostic test (RDT) 63
rash
  HIV infection
    children 115
    seroconversion 109
  larva currens 318
  meningococcal 25, 27
  onchocerciasis 135
  schistosomiasis 162
  typhus
    African tick 305
    louse-borne 304
    scrub 305
reactive arsenical encephalopathy
    see encephalopathy
recluse spiders 345
rectal prolapse 7, 193, 212
rectal strictures, amoebiasis 187
recurrent ulceration 312
red cells
  sickle haemoglobin 333
red flies 146
redcurrant jelly 193
reduviid 155
refugees 365–71
  asylum seekers 370–1
  children 370
  cholera 196
  diarrhoea 5, 9
  HIV infection 368
  humanitarian emergencies
    365–9
    communicable diseases
      control 368–9
    coordination 369
    emergency phase 365
    food and nutrition 366–8
    health care 368

human resources and
training 369
initial assessment 366
measles immunization 366
public health
surveillance 369
shelter and site
planning 368
water and sanitation 366
infectious diseases 371
louse-borne typhus 304
post-emergency phase 369
sexually transmitted
infections 368
shigellosis 194
sphere project
and humanitarian
reform 369–70
torture 371
trauma 371
tuberculosis 369
rehabilitation 376
malnutrition 376–7
rehydration 64
cholera 197
see also oral rehydration
solution
Reiter's syndrome,
post-dysenteric 193
relapsing fevers 301–3
renal disease
hypertension 353, 354
typhoid 282
ReSoMal (Rehydration Solution for
the Malnourished) 376
respiratory infections, acute
HIV infection 106
respiratory tract disorders 11–16
assessment 11–13
in HIV-infected adults 15–16,
15
investigation 13–14
presentations 14–15
respiratory tract infection,
lower 14
resuscitation, pneumonia 237
resuscitation/stabilization 376
malnutrition 375–6
retinoblastoma 213
retinopathy
cerebral malaria 59, *60*
diabetic 350
Reye-like syndrome 299
Reye's syndrome 26

rhabditiform larvae 211, 322
rheumatic heart disease 27
ribavirin 222
treatment 295
viral haemorrhagic fevers
290, 293, 294, 295
rickets 378
Rickettsiae 304
fever 29
tick-borne 27
Rickettsia africae 305
Rickettsia conorii 305
Rickettsia orientalis 305
Rickettsia prowazekii 304
Rickettsia tsutsugamushi 305
Rickettsial infections
African tick typhus 305
louse-borne typhus 304
scrub typhus 305
rifampicin 177–8, 181, 250, 305,
314
brucellosis 278
leprosy 177–8
pregnancy 181
tuberculosis 92, 94, 97, 98
Rift Valley fever (RVF) 290, 295,
300
Ringer's lactate solution 193, 197
river blindness *see* onchocerciasis
riverine tsetse flies 153
road traffic accidents (RTAs) 347
Rock fever *see* brucellosis
Rocky Mountain spotted
fever 305
Romaña's sign *see* orbital oedema
Ross River virus 288
rotavirus 191
roundworms, intestinal 34
rubella 27

salbutamol 357
Salmonella
diarrhoea 5
non-typhi 108, 112
septicaemia 30, 285
Salmonella enterica 280
Salmonella enterica ser Paratyphi
C 280
Salmonella paratyphi
(paratyphoid) 280
Salmonella typhi (typhoid) 280
salt intake, increased 353
sandflies 73, 74, 79, 83
sanitation

amoebiasis prevention 185, 190
giardiasis 199, 201
helminth infections 209, 210,
212, 213
humanitarian emergencies 366
oriental liver fluke 228
shigellosis 193–4
'Santa Marta' fever 222
Sarcoptes scabiei (scabies) 320
scabies 32, 320–1
onchocerciasis differential
diagnosis 137
refugees/asylum seekers 371
scarification 218
Schistosoma haematobium 162, 165,
167, 285
clinical features
bladder calcification 164
bladder pathology 163–4
genital schistosomiasis 164
obstructive uropathy 164
squamous cell
carcinoma 163–4
diagnosis 165
eggs 163
life cycle 158, 160–1
urine filtration 166
urine sedimentation 165–6
Schistosoma intercalatum 158
Schistosoma japonicum 162, 165,
167
clinical features 165
diagnosis 166
eggs 163
life cycle 158, 160–1
Schistosoma mansoni 7, 158,
161, 162, 164–5, 166,
167, 285
clinical features 164
diagnosis 166
eggs 163
life cycle *160*
schistosomiasis 26, 158
acute 162–3, 166–7
Ag–Ab complex formation 162
asymptomatic infection 168–9
biopsy techniques 166
bladder calcification 164
bladder pathology 163–4
cercarial penetration 162
clinicopathological
features 162–5
contact reduction 169
cor pulmonale 164

schistosomiasis (*Continued*)
  direct diagnosis 165
  distribution 158, *159*
  drug treatment 168–9
  epidemiology 161–2
  exposure 161
  fever 26, 27
  future developments 170
  genital 164
  granuloma 164
  hepatic fibrosis 3, 216
  immunity 161
  immunodiagnostic tests 166
  indirect diagnosis 166
  infection in children 162
  investigation 165–7
  Katayama syndrome 34, 162, 165
  life cycle 158–61
  log–normal distribution 161–2
  magnitude of problem 161
  management 168–9
  mass chemotherapy 169–70
  massive tropical
      splenomegaly 49
  neuroschistosomiasis 165, 167
  obstructive uropathy 164
  parasitology 158–61
  pathology 165
  prevention and public health
      aspects 169–70
  progression to disease 162
  pseudopolyposis of colon 164
  pulmonary complications 15, 16
  reservoir hosts 161
  Schistosoma haematobium
      165, 167
    clinical features 163–4
    and lung 164
  Schistosoma japonicum 165, 166,
      167
  Schistosoma mansoni 166, 167
    clinical features 164
    and liver 164–5
  snail clearance 169
  squamous cell carcinoma 163–4
  tissue reaction to retained
      eggs 163
  transmission, requirements
      for 161
  treatment monitoring 169
  urine filtration 166
  urine sedimentation 165–6
  urticaria 34

water contamination
    reduction 169
schizogony 55, 56, 57
schizonticides 65, 69
schizophrenia 361–2
scorpion stings 344–5
  clinical features **344**
  management 345
scrub typhus
  clinical features 305
  leptospirosis differential
      diagnosis 307
  treatment 305
sea snakes 342
seizures
  P. falciparum malaria 59
  viral encephalitis 260
  see also epilepsy
selective feeding programmes
    (SFPs) 367
Seoul virus 294
septicaemia
  fever 28
  melioidosis 309
  meningococcal 24, 34, 250
  paratyphoid 286
  Salmonella 30
  splenectomy 51
serodiagnosis 63, 282–3
sex education 106
sexually transmitted infections
    (STIs) 40–7
  asylum seekers 371
  flow charts usage 44–6
  hepatitis B 218
  HIV risk 104
  HIV testing 47
  HTLV-1 266
  local adaptations 41–2, *42, 43,*
      44
  partner notification/
      treatment 47
  public health 40, 47
  refugees 368, 371
  syndromes 40, 41
  syndromic management 40,
      46–7
  treatment 106
  treatment-seeking behaviour *47*
  WHO flow charts 42, *42, 43, 44,*
      44–6, 45
shelter, humanitarian
    emergencies 368

shiga toxin 193
Shigella 192
  multidrug resistance 193
Shigella boydii 192
Shigella dysenteriae 192, 193
Shigella flexneri 192
Shigella sonnei 192, 193
Shigellosis 5, 192
  clinical features 192–3
  epidemic 194
  investigation 193
  management 193
  prevention 193–4
  public health 193–4
shingles 110
shock
  hypovolaemic 197, 290
  in malnourished children 376
Shortness of breath 11, **12**
Siberian tick typhus 305
sickle cell anaemia *see* sickle cell
    disease
sickle cell crisis 334
sickle cell disease 333–5
  clinical features 334
  diagnosis 334
  management 334–5
  pneumonia prevention 239
  pneumonia risk 234
sickle cell trait 62
sickle haemoglobin (HbS) 333, 334
sickle–haemoglobin C (SC)
    disease 247
Simulium (blackflies) 135
Simulium damnosum 135, 140
Simulium metallicum 135
Simulium naevei 135
Simulium ochraceum 135
Sin Nombre 294
sinusitis
  pneumococcal 109
skin
  bullae 34
  creeping eruptions 32–3
  diseases 32–5
  fever 27
  infections in HIV 111
  lesions 173, *174*, 177
  nodules 33–4
  onchocerciasis 135–6
    diagnosis 137–8
  papules 33
  pigmentation, changes in 34

ulcers   32, 80, 187
  see also larva currens; larva
      migrans; rash
skin-snip microscopy   138
sleeping sickness *see*
      trypanosomiasis, African
'slim disease'   113
slit lamp   138
small bowel
  biopsy   200
  malabsorption   7
  secretory diarrhoea   6
smoking
  asthma trigger   356
snakebite
  clinical features   342
  diagnosis   343
  epidemiology   344
  first aid   342
  management   343–4
  prevention   344
sodium stibogluconate   77
soil-transmitted helminths   208
  ascariasis   209–10
  hookworm   210–12
  toxocariasis   213–14
  trichuriasis   212–13
South American haemorrhagic
      fevers   293
'Sowda'   136
space-occupying lesions   19
spacer devices   358
spastic paralysis   264
  anatomy   264
  assessment of patient with   264
  causes   264
  tropical causes
      HIV myelopathy   266
      spinal epidural abscess   265
      subacute combined
          degeneration, of spinal
          cord   266
      transverse myelitis   265–6
      tropical spastic
          paraparesis   266
      tuberculosis   264–5
spider bites
  banana spiders   345
  funnel-web spider   345
  recluse spiders   345
  widow spiders   345
spinal cord
  compression   264

subacute combined
      degeneration   266
spinal epidural abscess   265
spine, radiology of   **277**
splenectomy   51
splenic aspirate   76
splenic dysfunction   247
splenomegaly   27, 49–51, 74
  differential diagnosis   74
  hyper-reactive malarial   63
  malaria   49, 50–1, 57
  massive tropical   49–50
  relapsing fevers   302
spontaneous eye movements   21
Sporothrix schenckii
      (sporotrichosis)   331
sporotrichosis
  clinical features   331
  diagnosis   331
  treatment   331–2
sputum culture   28
sputum examination   13
sputum gram stain   236
sputum Ziehl–Neelsen stain   236
squamous cell carcinoma   163–4,
      312
St Louis encephalitis virus   258, *259*
standard agglutination test
      (SAT)   276
staphylococcal infection, skin
      sepsis   27
staphylococci   246
Staphylococcus aureus
  pyogenic meningitis   246
  spinal epidural abscess   265
status asthmaticus   356
  treatment   **357**
status epilepticus   360
stavudine (d4T)   116
Stercoralis stercoralis   322
steroids   206
  inhaled   357
  meningococcal disease   250
  pyogenic meningitis   251–2
  tuberculosis   89
      adjunctive   96
  typhoid   285
stings and bites *see* bites and stings
stomach
  gastric carcinoma   3
  gastric ulcers   3
  Giardia lamblia colonization
      4, 199

Stop TB strategy   99
streptococcal infection, skin
      sepsis   27
Streptococcus pneumoniae   14, 233
  chloramphenicol activity   237
  HIV association   108
  penicillin resistance   239
  pneumonia   233
  pyogenic meningitis   246
  symptoms   234–5
Streptococcus suis   246
Streptomyces somaliensis
      (mycetoma)   330
streptomycin   278
  buruli ulcer   314
  Madura foot   331
  tuberculosis   92, 93
stricture   187
  amoebiasis   189
stridor   12, 15
string test   200, 324
stroke   352, 353–4
Strongyloides fülleborni (swollen belly
      syndrome)   322
Strongyloidiasis (*Strongyloides
      stercoralis*) 4, 33, 34, 113,
          166, 191, 208,
          318, 322, 358
  acute infection   323
  autoinfection cycle   322–3
  chronic strongyloidiasis   323
  clinical features   323
  control   325
  diagnosis   324
  epidemiology   325
  hookworm differential
      diagnosis   211
  hyperinfection   323–4
      prevention   291
      steroids   324
  hyperinfection syndrome   323–4
  larva currens   33, 318
      rash   324
  life cycle   322
  treatment   324–5
  tropical pulmonary
      eosinophilia differential
      diagnosis   244
suckling mouse brain (SMB)
      vaccine   270
suicidal patients, management
      of   *363*
sulfadiazine   250

sulfadoxine–pyrimethamine
(Fansidar) 67
sulfamethoxazole 203, 310, 331
sulphonamides 67, 203, 336
sulphonylureas 350, 351
sulphur ointment 320
sunburn 34
superficial fungal infection 32
superinfection 221
supratentorial focal damage 20
suramin 151, 152, 153
swimmer's itch 162
swollen belly syndrome 322
symmers pipestem fibrosis 164
syndromic management
sexually transmitted
infections 40, 46–7
syphilis 40, 46
fever 27
gumma 188
HIV infection risk 104
systemic lupus erythematosus
27, 31

T-helper cells 107
tachypnoea 12–13
Taenia asiatica 205
Taenia saginata (tapeworm) 191,
204, 205
Taenia solium (tapeworm) 204, 205
taeniasis 205
clinical features 205
Tannates 338
tapeworms 204–7
tattooing 81, 218
tendon transfers 181
tenofovir (TDF) 116, 220
terbinafine 331
Ternidens diminutus 211
tetanolysin 272
tetanospasmin 272
tetanus 272
bacteriology 272
breathing difficulties 12
cephalic 273
clinical manifestations 272–3
diagnosis 273
epidemiology 273–4
generalized 272
localized 273
neonatal 272–3
pathogenesis 272
prevention 273–4

treatment 273
tropical ulcer 312
vaccination 273–4
tetanus immunoglobulin 273
tetanus toxoid 273–4
tetmosol 321
tetracycline 4, 29, 190, 197, 302
African tick typhus 305
brucellosis 278
louse-borne typhus 304
pneumonia 237
resistance 305
scrub typhus 305
thalassaemia 37
β thalassaemia
clinical features 335
diagnosis 335
epidemiology 335
management 335
thiazides 354
thiosulphate citrate bile salt sucrose
(TCBS) agar 196
third-generation
cephalosporins 250, 283,
285
thrifty genotype theory 349
thrombocytopenia 29, 58, 66, 298
thyroid disease
breathing difficulties 12
vitamin B$_{12}$ deficiency 340
tiabendazole
chromoblastomycosis 331
cutaneous larva migrans 319
hyperinfection syndrome
strongyloidiasis 325
visceral larva migrans 213
tick-borne encephalitis 258, 259
tick-borne relapsing fever
(TBRF) 301
clinical features 302
diagnosis 302
epidemiology 301–2
fatality rate 302
pathology 302
prevention 303
treatment 302–3
tick paralysis 263
tick typhus 305
Tifomycin 250, 251
tine test 86
tinea corporis 111
tinidazole 189, 190, 201
tobacco smoke 11

torture 371
toxaemia in typhoid 282
toxic megacolon 190
Toxocara canis (toxocariasis) 213
toxocariasis
clinical features 213
epidemiology 213
investigations 213
life cycle 213
management 213
ocular larva migrans 213
parasites 213
prevention 214
visceral larva migrans 213
Toxoplasma gondii 108, 115
toxoplasmosis
fever 27, 30
HIV association 109, 114
ToxR 195
trans-thoracic lung aspirate 236
transverse myelitis 265–6
trauma
epilepsy 360
refugees 371
travellers
hepatitis A 216
hepatitis E 223
rabies immunization 271
trematodes 226, 241
trench fever 321
triatomine bugs 155
tribendimidine 209
Trichomonas vaginalis
(trichomoniasis) 46, 191
HIV infection risk 104
Trichostrongylus 212
trichuriasis
clinical features 212
epidemiology 212
investigations 212
life cycle 212
management 213–14
parasites 212
prevention 214
Trichuris suis 212
Trichuris trichiura (whipworms)
7, 166, 187, 191,
208, 212
triclabendazole 226, 227,
243, 331
trimethoprim–sulfamethoxazole
see co-trimoxazole
Triplopen 250

trophozoite   9, 56, 185, 186, 187, 199, 200
tropical pulmonary
        eosinophilia   14, 142, 244–5
    asthma differential diagnosis 356
    clinical features   244
    diagnosis   244–5
    epidemiology   244
    investigations   244
    prevention   245
    treatment   245
tropical spastic paraparesis   266
tropical sprue   4, 340
Tropical ulcer
    clinical features   311
    complications   312
    epidemiology   311–12
    microbiology   311
    prevention   312
    treatment   312
Trypanosoma brucei   148
Trypanosoma brucei gambiense   148, 150
    control   153–4
    diagnosis   151–2
    epidemiology   153
    surveillance   153–4
    treatment   152–3
Trypanosoma brucei rhodesiense   148, 149, 150
    control   153–4
    diagnosis   151–2
    epidemiology   153
    surveillance   153–4
    treatment   152–3
Trypanosoma cruzi   155
    see also Chagas' disease
trypanosomiasis, African   148
    clinical picture   150
    diagnosis   151–2
    disease   148–9
    distribution   149
    epidemiology   153
    fever   27
    life cycle   148
    parasites   148
    skin itching   32
    surveillance   153
    treatment   152–3
    vector   153
        control   154

trypanosomiasis, South American
    see Chagas' disease
tsetse fly   148, 153
Tsutsugamushi fever (scrub typhus)   305
tubercle bacilli   85, 91
tuberculoid leprosy   174, 175
tuberculoma   248, 265
tuberculosis   235, 264–5, 85–99
    amoebic liver abscess
        differential diagnosis   188
    amoeboma differential diagnosis   187
    annual risk of infection (ARI)   97
    asylum seekers   370
    BCG vaccination   96
    brucellosis differential diagnosis   277
    case-finding   97, 98
    chemotherapy   92–6
    clinical features   89–91
    clinical manifestations   86
    corticosteroid therapy   89
        adjunctive   96
    cough   11–12, 16
    cutaneous   82
    diagnosis   91
    differential diagnosis   91
    disseminated   27, 110, 112
    DOTS strategy   97
    epidemiology   86–9, 87
        HIV effect   89
    extrapulmonary disease   89, 90
        clinical features   89
    fever   27
    future developments   99
    HIV infection   13, 15, 29, 30, 89, 90–1
        association   102
        clinical presentation   90
        coinfection   111
        early disease   109
        TB chemoprophylaxis   115
    hospital admission   95–6
    immunity   86
    incidence   86, 87
    infection   86
    intestinal   3
    investigations   91–2
    isolation   95–6
    malnutrition   89
    management   92–6
    meningitis   248, 249

    microbiology   85–6
    mortality   96
    multidrug-resistant   97
    pneumonia differential diagnosis   235
    pneumonic illness   233
    postprimary lesions   88
    poverty   97–8
    prevention   96–9
    progression to disease   86, 88
    public health aspects   96–9
    pulmonary disease   90
        differential diagnosis   91
        signs/symptoms   90
    pyogenic meningitis
        differential diagnosis   248
    refugees   370, 371
    risk factors   88–9
    spastic paralysis   265–6
    sporotrichosis differential diagnosis   331
    systemic symptoms   89–90
    transmission   86
    treatment
        monitoring   95
        outcomes   **95**
        regimens   93, 94
    vitamin B$_{12}$ deficiency   340
Tumbu fly   316
tumour necrosis factor α (TNF-α)   172
Tunga penetrans (chiggers)   316
20-min whole blood clotting test (WBCT20)   **343**, 344
type 1 (reversal) reactions   179
typhoid fever   280
    amoxicillin   285
    asylum seekers   371
    azithromycin   285
    carrier state   285
    chemotherapy   283–5
    chloramphenicol   285
    clinical signs   281
    complications   281–2
    co-trimoxazole   285
    diagnosis   282–3
    leptospirosis differential diagnosis   307
    mode of infection   280
    organisms   280
    paratyphoid A and B   286
    paratyphoid C   286
    psychosis   27

typhoid fever (*Continued*)
  refugees   371
  steroids   285
  treatment   283–5
  vaccine   285–6
typhoid nodules   281
typhus
  African tick   305
  louse-borne   304
  scrub   305
    leptospirosis differential
      diagnosis   307

ulcerative colitis,
      post-dysenteric   187
ulcers
  Buruli   313–15
  chronic   312
  genital   131
  guinea worm   326–7
  recurrent   312
  skin   32, **33**, 80
    amoebiasis   189
  tropical   311–12
Universal Declaration of Human
      Rights   365
urbanization   311, 349, 353
ureters, schistosomiasis   164
urethral discharge   41, *42*
urinary bladder calcification   167
uropathy, obstructive   164, 167
urticaria   34
  guinea worm   326

vaccines/vaccination
  cholera   198
  dengue   299
  hepatitis B   220–1
  HIV   107
  leprosy   181
  measles   366
  pneumococcal   240
  pneumonia   239
  pyogenic meningitis   247, 248
  rabies postexposure   269–70
  tetanus   273–4
  typhoid fever   285–6
  yellow fever   300
vaginal discharge   *43*
vaginal flora   104
valproate   360
vancomycin   251

var *gattii*   254
var *grubii*   254
var *neoformans*   254
varicella-zoster virus   108
Venezuelan equine
      encephalitis   *259*, 260
venomous fish   345
verapamil   273
Vibrio cholerae (cholera)   198
  classification   *196*
  El Tor biotype   195
  serotype 0139   195
vipers   342
viral haemorrhagic fevers
      (VHFs)   289
  Crimean–Congo
      haemorrhagic fever   294–5
  dengue and yellow fever   295
  diagnosis   290
  differential diagnosis   290
  ebola   294
  epidemiology   289
  identification   289–90
  lassa fever   291, 293
  management   289, 290–1
  marburg   294
  nosocomial spread   291
  overview   **290**
  pathogenesis   289
  rift valley fever (RVF)   295
  South American   293
  transmission   *291*
  with renal syndrome   294
viral hepatitis   215
  general clinicoepidemiological
      features   215–16
  hepatitis A   216
  hepatitis B   216–20
    immunization   220–1
  hepatitis C   222–3
  hepatitis D   221–2
  hepatitis E   223, *224*
  hepatocellular carcinoma
      223, 225
viral load testing   103
viral meningitis   246
visceral larva migrans (VLM)   213
visceral leishmaniasis (VL) *see* leish-
      maniasis, visceral
vitamin A supplements   28–9, 193,
      366, 378
vitamin B1 (thiamine)   378

vitamin B6   378
vitamin B$_{12}$ deficiency   37, 266, 340
vitamin C   378
vitamin D   378–9
vitamin deficiencies   19, 379
vitiligo   34, 340
voluntary counselling and
      testing (VCT)   47, 102, 106

Wakana syndrome   211
wasting in HIV infection   113
water supply
  amoebiasis prevention   190
  chlorination   169
  filtration   201, 327
  giardiasis   199
  guinea worm   327
  humanitarian emergencies   366
  refugee camps   9
WBCT20   **343**, 344
WC-B vaccine   198
weight-for-height (W/H) index   367
weight loss, HIV infection   30
Weil–Felix test   304, 305
Weil's disease   306, 307
Wernicke–Korsakoff syndrome   378
West Nile virus   258, *259*
Western blots   103
westernization   348, 349
wheeze   15, 355
  asthma   355
whipworm   208, 212
whooping cough   12
Widal test   282–3
widow spiders   345
Wolbachia   133, 135, 137, 142
women, leprosy   181
Wuchereria bancrofti (filariasis)
      140, 142, 244

xerophthalmia   378

yaws   34
yellow fever
  clinical features   299–300
  control   300
  epidemiology   299

Zenker's degeneration   282
Zidovudine (AZT)   106, 116